HIV Scale-Up and the Politics of Global Health

The global expansion of HIV programming and the growth of global health in the past decade have reshaped politics, power, civic relations, and citizen subjectivities in countries across the globe. The race to treat and prevent HIV in resource-poor contexts catalyzed a global 'scale-up' of programs, policies, and strategies that set the stage for many subsequent global health initiatives. This volume contemplates 'scale-up' (and, subsequently, 'scale-down') as an object of analysis and a culture of practice in the politics of response to global crisis. The transnational shifts and expansions brought about by scale-up necessitate further critical evaluations across social science and public health disciplines. This book draws on interdisciplinary research from numerous sites in the Global South to examine the political dimensions of the expansion of HIV and global health programming. Collectively, the authors paint a complex global portrait of a unique period in the social history of HIV, as the pandemic enters its fourth decade and the global response reaches its peak. By collecting diverse perspectives on the political legacies of HIV and global health, this book provides a unique history of the present, cataloguing emerging global health practices and policies that will have long-term social impacts.

This book was originally published as a special issue of *Global Public Health*.

Nora J. Kenworthy is an interdisciplinary researcher in public health, political science, and anthropology. Her work focuses on the political impacts of global health endeavours. She is currently assistant professor in the School of Nursing and Health Studies at the University of Washington Bothell, USA.

Richard Parker is a pioneer scholar of structural and political-economic factors shaping HIV/AIDS globally and the politics of HIV and global health policy. He is currently professor of sociomedical sciences and anthropology and director of the Center for the Study of Culture, Politics and Health at Columbia University, USA.

HIV Scale-Up and the Politics of Global Health

Edited by
**Nora J. Kenworthy and
Richard Parker**

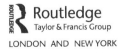

LONDON AND NEW YORK

First published 2015
by Routledge
2 Park Square, Milton Park, Abingdon, Oxon, OX14 4RN, UK

and by Routledge
711 Third Avenue, New York, NY 10017, USA

Routledge is an imprint of the Taylor & Francis Group, an informa business

© 2015 Taylor & Francis
Chapter 14 © The Author(s). Published by Taylor & Francis

British Library Cataloguing in Publication Data
A catalogue record for this book is available from the British Library

ISBN 13: 978-1-138-84318-9

Typeset in Times New Roman
by RefineCatch Limited, Bungay, Suffolk

Publisher's Note
The publisher accepts responsibility for any inconsistencies that may have
arisen during the conversion of this book from journal articles to book chapters,
namely the possible inclusion of journal terminology.

Disclaimer
Every effort has been made to contact copyright holders for their permission to
reprint material in this book. The publishers would be grateful to hear from any
copyright holder who is not here acknowledged and will undertake to rectify
any errors or omissions in future editions of this book.

Contents

CONTENTS

Citation Information

The chapters in this book were originally published in *Global Public Health*, volume 9, nos. 1–2 (January–February 2014). When citing this material, please use the original page numbering for each article, as follows:

Chapter 15
AIDS policy responsiveness in Africa: Evidence from opinion surveys
Ashley M. Fox
Global Public Health, volume 9, nos. 1–2 (January–February 2014) pp. 224–248

Please direct any queries you may have about the citations to
clsuk.permissions@cengage.com

INTRODUCTION

HIV scale-up and the politics of global health

Nora J. Kenworthy[a] and Richard Parker[b]

[a]Nursing and Health Studies Program, University of Washington Bothell, Bothell, WA, USA; [b]Department of Sociomedical Sciences, Mailman School of Public Health, Columbia University, New York, NY, USA

HIV has a political and social history that is unlike any other disease in modern times. As we move forward into the fourth decade of responses to AIDS, it is impossible not to view the pandemic in terms of its sociopolitical, as well as epidemiological, evolution. The AIDS activist movements that began in the late 1980s indelibly shaped our collective understanding of HIV and the public responses it mandated (Parker, 2000, 2011; Smith & Siplon, 2006). Activist and civil society movements bravely appropriated and challenged scientific process (Epstein, 1996), built dynamic and flexible transnational movements for treatment access (Petchesky, 2003) and forcefully demanded that governments address HIV by breaking through the most trenchant social prejudices and mitigating the inequalities driving infections (Berkman, Garcia, Munoz Laboy, Paiva, & Parker, 2005; Parker, 2009, 2011). Elsewhere, especially in the Global South, quieter forms of solidarity were also forged, as AIDS service organisations (ASOs) developed community-based care models that broke through stigma and assuaged suffering (Altman, 1994; Daniel & Parker, 1993; Rau, 2006).

Now, however, we find ourselves in an undeniably different political landscape. From activist movements, to 'activist states' (Biehl, 2007), to the global governance of HIV intervention, the vast mobilisation of resources, commitment and expertise involved in the expansion of global treatment access dramatically changed the nature of the politics of HIV. Activists have increasingly been 'domesticated' (Parker, 2011, p. 34): drawn into service provision, given expert positions of their own and incorporated into institutional networks of non-governmental organisations (NGOs) and governments. Paradoxically, just as the global institutional architecture responding to HIV expanded rapidly and began to acknowledge the demands of activist movements for universal access to treatment, the HIV agenda was distilled into a focus on 'administering the epidemic' – a predominantly technocratic shuttling of drugs into bodies (Parker, 2000; Smith & Siplon, 2006). The very response many had so long fought for not only brought hope, and extended lifespans, but also arrived with its own 'anti-politics' (Ferguson, 1994; Taylor & Harper, 2013), in which therapeutic regimes outpaced attention to the broader social conditions of HIV infection and the survival of those already infected (see, for example, Biehl, 2007;

Kalofonos, 2010; Marsland, 2012). With HIV treatment 'scale-up', the defining characteristics of the politics of response shifted from transnational activism to global governance and donor-driven agendas.

Thus, we embark on this special issue at a particular disjuncture in the history of the epidemic. Just over 10 years ago, the President's Emergency Plan for AIDS Relief (PEPFAR) was launched, shortly after the introduction of the Global Fund to Fight AIDS, Tuberculosis and Malaria (GFATM). What followed was a race to treat and prevent HIV in resource-poor contexts – a global 'scale-up' that set the stage for many subsequent global health initiatives. For many, scale-up represented a primarily technocratic and infrastructural challenge: a focus on how donors, agencies, NGOs and community-based organisations (CBOs) could develop the kinds of health system capacities necessary for the large-scale implementation of treatment regimens. Now, however, we appear to be at the twilight of this acute period of scale-up: many perceive the long-awaited expansion of treatment as unfinished, cut short by the global financial crisis (Medecins Sans Frontieres, 2011; UNAIDS & The World Bank, 2009). Many now speak of 'scale-down' as an inevitability, rather than the potential consequence of shifting funding priorities [see the articles by Naukushu & Kapilashrami and Amaya, Caceres & Balabanova in this issue; see, also, Ford, 2010; Kaiser Family Foundation (KFF) & UNAIDS, 2010]. Other global health concerns seem well-poised to eclipse the once exceptional focus on HIV/AIDS.

In the past decade, scale-up has become a social force of its own. Though it involves pharmacological flows and therapeutic processes, it represents more than a simple expansion of services, strategies and treatments. 'Scale-up' is an assemblage of vast resources, manpower, expertise, strategies and technologies, all of which are presumed essential for the implementation of complicated, multifaceted global health interventions throughout and among recipient nations. Similar to Strathern's (2000) 'audit cultures', scale-up has also become a culture of practice in which new ideological frameworks become dominant and normalised. These include but are not limited to: guiding philosophies such as community participation, empowerment, political commitment, national ownership, accountability and sustainability; powerful institutional hierarchies that shape policy-making and priority-setting practices; donor, foundation and expert-led agendas of 'best-practices' for achieving desired outcomes; and tenets regarding the boundaries for appropriate spaces, objects and populations of intervention.

In the past decade, scholars across a number of disciplines have engaged in critical conversations concerning the content, direction and approaches of what we now call global health initiatives (Biehl & Petryna, 2013; Pfeiffer & Nichter, 2008). This collective endeavour has simultaneously attempted to call into question the taken-for-granted norms of emerging cultures of practice in global health and to maintain a scholarly focus on the central importance of alleviating and addressing the biological and social suffering of populations with acute health needs (Biehl & Petryna, 2013; Farmer, 2004; Feierman, Kleinman, Stewart, Farmer, & Das, 2010; Fullwiley, 2004; Nichter, 2008; Pfeiffer, 2004; Swidler, 2009; Whiteford & Manderson, 2000). Politics has emerged as a powerful theoretical focal point in these conversations, providing a bridge between structures, economies and inequalities, and their socio-physiological manifestations in bodies and everyday lives (see, for example, Altman & Buse, 2012; Feierman et al., 2010; Labonte, Schrecker, & Sen, 2005; Nguyen, 2010; Redfield, 2005; Whyte, 2009).

Historically, the engagement of political science with questions of HIV has been limited, with a few notable exceptions primarily exploring the conditions under which countries craft effective responses to the epidemic (Lieberman, 2009; Parkhurst, 2001; Patterson, 2005; Poku & Whiteside, 2004). Although such research was remarkably limited during the first three decades of the epidemic, in recent years, some crucial headway has been made in addressing this disciplinary gap, encouraging a deeper engagement with HIV in political science (Altman & Buse, 2012). The broader political concerns with global health, however, arise not only from within a positivist science of politics. They also emerge from the acknowledgement that the global responses to HIV and other diseases are themselves political forces, impacting how governments, citizens, civil society and transnational institutions function in the world, relate to one another and alter collective norms (Biehl, 2007; Birdsall et al., 2007; Kapilashrami & O'Brien, 2012; Lewis, 2007; Parker, 2011; Sparke, in press; Swidler, 2009). Recent work recognises that the global AIDS response created new measures of valuable and appropriate politics – eliciting demonstrations of political 'commitment', 'ownership' and 'accountability' from recipient countries in exchange for funding and support [see the articles by Esser, Fox and Gore, Fox, Goldberg & Barnighausen in this issue; see, also, Nattrass, 2008; Organization for Economic Cooperation and Development (OECD), 2008; Swidler, 2009]. Finally, the expanded emphasis on politics includes a number of thoughtful explorations into lived experiences of the political dimensions of global health and the broad social ramifications of the hierarchies and powerful inequities that persist in such endeavours (Biehl & Petryna, 2013; Fort, Mercer, & Gish, 2004; Good, Hyde, Pinto, & Good, 2008; Maternowska, 2006; Nguyen, 2010; Whiteford & Manderson, 2000). This focus has allowed many scholars to offer important critiques of the objectives and practices of many initiatives carried out under the guise of global health and HIV projects, while retaining a concern for, and solidarity with, those most often deemed 'recipients' of such programmes.

The articles in this issue draw on anthropology, sociology and political science to understand contemporary changes brought about by global health. They approach politics, variously, as a bureaucratic functioning and the deployment of policy (see the articles by Amaya et al., Gore et al., Naukushu & Kapilashrami, and Qureshi in this issue); as an unfolding set of microcosmic and transnational social changes (see Colvin, Kenworthy, Kalofonos, and Reynolds in this issue); as the everyday experience of the sculpting conditions of life chances (see David and Winchester in this issue) and as the institutionalisation of powerful hierarchies (see Esser, Fan, Fox, Høg, and Kapilashrami in this issue). In doing so, the work in this issue represents a broad, transdisciplinary approach to grappling with 'the political' in our changing world.

In addition, the authors in this issue appear to share some common concerns about, and aspirations for, future global health endeavours. They reflect a growing recognition that pharmaceutical or biomedical treatment does not make a person whole, and that vertical, technical health interventions cannot substitute for glaring absences in the social contract and social safety nets in many recipient countries. In a related vein, many seem to retain biopower as a theoretical touchstone, and biological or therapeutic citizenship as an increasingly important theoretical development in this field (see David, Reynolds and Winchester in this issue). In particular, there are concerns with the strange logics of programmatic politics: the 'therapeutic sovereignty' of HIV policies and practices to decide who belongs in treatment and under what conditions; the lived experience of exceptionality in various HIV programmes; and the sheer normative and disciplinary force of global HIV policy and practice (Nguyen, 2010; see David, Esser, Høg and Winchester in this issue). As global health evolves, the earlier lessons of development and globalisation studies hold increasing truth, though global health reveals new political patterns, structures and possibilities (see Esser and Kenworthy in this issue). And there is an abiding concern with the implicit normative frameworks that shape priorities, policy-making and implementation at multiple levels (see Colvin, Esser, Fan, Fox, Gore et al., Høg, Kalofonos, Kenworthy, and Reynolds in this issue). Finally, as we look over the precipice at the potential scale-down of HIV funding and commitments, there are significant questions about the pragmatic realities of such a process, as well as the lasting lessons scale-up may leave in its wake (see Amaya et al., Naukushu & Kapilashrami, and Qureshi in this issue).

Writing during what appears to be the twilight hours of one of the most vast and resource-intensive health initiatives in world history, we take this issue as an opportunity to reflect on the politics of a passing era, while at the same time recognising that HIV scale-up has institutionalised political dynamics that will long outlive its period of prominence. In many ways, the transnational activism of, and consequent global response to, HIV created a lasting mould for subsequent initiatives that now make up what we collectively recognise as global health. In light of this, we trust that the articles included in this special double issue of *Global Public Health* do not simply provide a reflection on the scale-up of the response to HIV and AIDS over the past decades. They offer important insights into the transnational trends and politics of an unfolding global health paradigm – a still emergent history of the present whose lessons will hold relevance far beyond HIV and well into future decades of global public health.

References

Altman, D. (1994). *Power and community: Organizational and cultural responses to AIDS*. London: Taylor & Francis.

Altman, D., & Buse, K. (2012). Thinking politically about HIV: Political analysis and action in response to AIDS. *Contemporary Politics*, *18*, 127–140. doi:10.1080/13569775.2012.674334

Berkman, A., Garcia, J., Munoz Laboy, M., Paiva, V., & Parker, R. (2005). A critical analysis of the Brazilian response to HIV/AIDS: Lessons learned for controlling and mitigating the epidemic in developing countries. *American Journal of Public Health*, *95*, 1162–1172. doi:10.2105/AJPH. 2004.054593

Biehl, J. (2007). *Will to live: AIDS therapies and the politics of survival*. Princeton, NJ: Princeton University Press.

Biehl, J., & Petryna, A. (Eds.). (2013). *When people come first: Critical studies in global health*. Princeton, NJ: Princeton University Press.

Birdsall, K., Kelly, K., Moteetee, M., Kadzandira, J., Munthali, A., Costa, D., ... Nyirenda, C. (2007). *Pioneers, partners, providers: The dynamics of civil society and AIDS funding in Southern Africa*. Johannesburg: CADRE/OSISA.

Daniel, H., & Parker, R. G. (1993). *Sexuality, politics and AIDS in Brazil*. London: Taylor & Francis.

Epstein, S. (1996). *Impure science: AIDS, activism, and the politics of knowledge*. Berkeley: University of California Press.

Farmer, P. (2004). An anthropology of structural violence. *Current Anthropology*, *45*, 305–325. doi:10.1086/382250

Feierman, S., Kleinman, A., Stewart, K., Farmer, P., & Das, V. (2010). Anthropology, knowledge-flows and global health. *Global Public Health*, *5*, 122–128. doi:10.1080/17441690903401338

Ferguson, J. (1994). *The anti-politics machine: "Development," depoliticization, and bureaucratic power in Lesotho*. Minneapolis, MN: University of Minnesota Press.

Ford, N. (2010, July 17). Not the time to scale down funds for HIV treatment. *Financial Times*, p. 5. London (UK).

Fort, M. P., Mercer, M. A., & Gish, O. (Eds.). (2004). *Sickness and wealth: The corporate assault on Global Health*. Cambridge, MA: South End Press.

Fullwiley, D. (2004). Discriminate biopower and everyday biopolitics: Views on sickle cell testing in Dakar. *Medical Anthropology*, *23*, 157–194. doi:10.1080/01459740490448939

Good, M.-J. D., Hyde, S. T., Pinto, S., & Good, B. (2008). *Postcolonial disorders*. Berkeley: University of California Press.

Kaiser Family Foundation & UNAIDS. (2010). KFF/UNAIDS report finds donor nation support for AIDS relief was flat in 2009 during world economic crisis, with US$7.6 billion provided during the year [Press Release]. Retrieved from http://www.unaids.org/en/media/unaids/contentassets/dataimport/pub/pressrelease/2010/20100718_pr_funding_en.pdf

Kalofonos, I. A. (2010). "All I eat is ARVs": The paradox of AIDS treatment interventions in Central Mozambique. *Medical Anthropology Quarterly, 24*, 363–380. doi:10.1111/j.1548-1387.2010.01109.x

Kapilashrami, A., & O'Brien, O. (2012). The Global Fund and the re-configuration and re-emergence of "civil society": Widening or closing the democratic deficit? *Global Public Health, 7*, 437–451. doi:10.1080/17441692.2011.649043

Labonte, R., Schrecker, T., & Sen Gupta, A. (2005). *Health for some: Death, disease and disparity in a globalizing world*. Toronto: Centre for Social Justice.

Lewis, B. (2007). New global health movement: Rx for the world? *New Literary History, 38*, 459–477. doi:10.1353/nlh.2007.0045

Lieberman, E. (2009). *Boundaries of contagion: How ethnic politics have shaped government responses to AIDS*. Princeton, NJ: Princeton University Press.

Marsland, R. (2012). (Bio)sociality and HIV in Tanzania: Finding a living to support a life. *Medical Anthropology Quarterly, 26*, 470–485. doi:10.1111/maq.12002

Maternowska, C. (2006). *Reproducing inequities: Poverty and the politics of population in Haiti*. New Brunswick, NJ: Rutgers University Press.

Medecins Sans Frontieres (MSF). (2011). *Reversing HIV/AIDS? How advances are being held back by funding shortages*. Paris: Author.

Nattrass, N. (2008). Are country reputations for good and bad leadership on AIDS deserved? An exploratory quantitative analysis. *Journal of Public Health, 30*, 398–406. doi:10.1093/pubmed/fdn075

Nguyen, V.-K. (2010). *The republic of therapy: Triage and sovereignty in West Africa's time of AIDS*. Durham, NC: Duke University Press.

Nichter, M. (2008). *Global health: Why cultural perceptions, social representations, and biopolitics matter*. Tuscon: University of Arizona Press.

Organization for Economic Cooperation and Development (OECD). (2008). *The Paris declaration on aid effectiveness and the Accra agenda for action*. Paris: Author.

Parker, R. G. (2000). Administering the epidemic: HIV/AIDS policy, models of development, and international health. In L. Whiteford & L. Manderson (Eds.), *Global health policy, local realities: The fallacy of the level playing field* (pp. 39–56). Boulder, CO: Lynne Rienner.

Parker, R. G. (2009). Civil society, political mobilization, and the impact of HIV scale-up on health systems in Brazil. *Journal of Acquired Immune Deficiency Syndrome, 52*, 49–51. doi:10.1097/QAI.0b013e3181bbcb56

Parker, R. G. (2011). Grassroots activism, civil society mobilization, and the politics of the global HIV/AIDS epidemic. *Brown Journal of World Affairs, 17*, 21–37.

Parkhurst, J. O. (2001). The crisis of AIDS and the politics of response: The case of Uganda. *International Relations, 15*, 69–87. doi:10.1177/004711701015006006

Patterson, A. (2005). *The African state and the AIDS crisis*. Burlington, VT: Ashgate.

Petchesky, R. (2003). *Global prescriptions: Gendering health and human rights*. New York, NY: Zed Books.

Pfeiffer, J. (2004). Condom social marketing, pentecostalism, and structural adjustment in Mozambique: A clash of AIDS prevention messages. *Medical Anthropology Quarterly, 18*, 77–103. doi:10.1525/maq.2004.18.1.77

Pfeiffer, J., & Nichter, M. (2008). What can critical medical anthropology contribute to global health? *Medical Anthropology Quarterly, 22*, 410–415. doi:10.1111/j.1548-1387.2008.00041.x

Poku, N., & Whiteside, A. (2004). *The political economy of AIDS in Africa*. Cape Town: Ashgate.

Rau, B. (2006). The politics of civil society in confronting HIV/AIDS. *International Affairs, 82*, 285–295. doi:10.1111/j.1468-2346.2006.00531.x

Redfield, P. (2005). Doctors, borders, and life in crisis. *Cultural Anthropology, 20*, 328–361. doi:10.1525/can.2005.20.3.328

Smith, R. A., & Siplon, P. D. (2006). *Drugs into bodies: Global AIDS treatment activism*. Westport, CT: Praeger.

Sparke, M. (in press). Health. In R. Lee, N. Castree, R. Kitchin, V. Lawson, A. Paasi, S. Radcliffe, & C. Withers (Eds.), *The SAGE handbook of progress in human geography*. London: Sage.

Strathern, M. (Ed.). (2000). *Audit cultures: Anthropological studies in accountability, ethics and the academy*. New York, NY: Routledge.

Swidler, A. (2009). Responding to AIDS in sub-Saharan Africa: Culture, institutions, and health. In P. A. Hall & M. Lamont (Eds.), *Successful societies: How institutions and culture affect health* (pp. 128–150). Cambridge: Cambridge University Press.

Taylor, E. M., & Harper, I. (2013). The politics and anti-politics of the Global Fund experiment: Understanding partnership and bureaucratic expansion in Uganda. *Medical Anthropology*. Advance online publication. doi:10.1080/01459740.2013.796941

UNAIDS & The World Bank. (2009). *The global economic crisis and HIV prevention and treatment programmes: Vulnerabilities and impact*. Geneva and Washington, DC: UNAIDS and The World Bank.

Whiteford, L., & Manderson, L. (Eds.). (2000). *Global health policy, local realities: The fallacy of the level playing field*. Boulder, CO: Lynne Rienner.

Whyte, S. R. (2009). Health identities and subjectivities: The ethnographic challenge. *Medical Anthropology Quarterly*, *23*(1), 6–15. doi:10.1111/j.1548-1387.2009.01034.x

'All they do is pray': Community labour and the narrowing of 'care' during Mozambique's HIV scale-up

Ippolytos Kalofonos

Department of Psychiatry and Behavioral Sciences, University of Washington Medical Center, Seattle, WA, USA

This paper tracks the intertwined biographies of a community home-based care (CHBC) volunteer, Arminda, the community-based organisation she worked for, Mufudzi, and the HIV scale-up in Mozambique. The focus is on Arminda – the experiences, aspirations, skills, and values she brought to her work as a volunteer, and the ways her own life converged with the rise and fall of the organisation that pioneered CHBC in this region. CHBC began in Mozambique in the mid-1990s as a community-level response to the AIDS epidemic at a time when there were few such organised efforts. The rapid pace and technical orientation of the scale-up as well as the influx of funding altered the practice of CHBC by expanding the scope of the work to become more technically comprehensive, but at the same time more narrowly defining 'care' as clinically-oriented work. Over the course of the scale-up, Arminda and her colleagues felt exploited and ultimately abandoned, despite their work having served as the vanguard and national model for CHBC. This paper considers how this happened and raises questions about the communities constituted by global health interventions and about the role of and the voice of community health workers in large-scale interventions such as the HIV scale-up.

Introduction

When I first arrived, Beatriz would do that thing, go to the clinic one day, then follow other programmes. Go to a traditional healer for treatments, go to the clinic, round and round. I proposed another mechanism [to her husband]: 'will you accept, starting today, your wife accompanies us, begins new consultations?' I spoke about this with her father, who then spoke with his son-in-law. I took them to the testing center. They were all positive. Now they are all following their treatment, I keep visiting them, checking on them, but they are well! (Arminda, Community Home-Based Care volunteer, Chimoio, October 2005)

A single mother of three in her sixth decade of life, Arminda[1] was a community home-based care (CHBC) volunteer in the central Mozambican city of Chimoio. This passage from an explanation of how the availability of AIDS treatment changed her work with her patient, Beatriz, provides a glimpse into the arduous nature of her work as she counseled ill individuals and their families, recruited them for HIV testing, monitored and accompanied them through treatment, and offered assistance with daily activities as well as spiritual and emotional support. According to UNAIDS, volunteers such as Arminda constitute one of the 'key pillars' of AIDS treatment programmes (UNAIDS, 2010).

The intersection of the AIDS epidemic with structural adjustment policies gutting public health and social welfare systems contributed to the epidemic's catastrophic toll in Mozambique and sub-Saharan Africa (Pfeiffer & Chapman, 2010). This lack of infrastructure has been a defining challenge to the expansion of HIV programming and services (or HIV scale-up) in sub-Saharan Africa. CHBC is an example of an intervention, following the neoliberal principles guiding structural adjustment, where 'civil society' and 'the community' are called upon to perform voluntary basic health care services to compensate for an absent safety net (Comaroff & Comaroff, 1999; Ferguson, 2006).

This paper tracks the intertwined biographies of CHBC, Arminda, and the community-based organisation (CBO) she worked for, Mufudzi.[2] The intertwined biographies framework positions Mufudzi as a 'crossover point between biography and history,' a site that makes visible the intersection of Arminda's individual experience with the historical temporalities of the HIV epidemic and the scale-up (Hansen, 1997, p. 9). My focus is on Arminda, the experiences, aspirations, skills and values she brought to her work as a volunteer, and the ways her own life converged with the rise and fall of the organisation that pioneered CHBC in this region and with the scale-up. CHBC began in Mozambique in the mid-1990s as a community-level response to the AIDS epidemic at a time when there were few such organised efforts. Rapid HIV testing and antiretroviral treatment (ART) were not broadly available until the early to mid-2000s. Mufudzi, a Christian organisation, adapted a CHBC approach modeled on pastoral visits of local churches, involving visiting all chronically ill individuals in a neighbourhood to educate them and their families about HIV, offering comfort-oriented basic care as well as emotional and spiritual support, and referral to appropriate health and social services. CHBC was 'scaled-up' in the early 2000s when a national ministry of health (MISAU) working group incorporated significant aspects of Mufudzi's manual and approach into what became the national CHBC model. As the only CHBC organisation operated and run by laypersons in Mozambique, Mufudzi was the exemplar for the scale-up. At the same time, a concern that volunteers were 'just praying' led the working group to focus on establishing 'minimum quality standards' for clinically-oriented care, such as adherence to medications, tuberculosis screening, and management of opportunistic infection prophylaxis. As a consequence of the scale-up, CHBC returned to Mufudzi through standardised protocols and increased donor funding that catalysed changes. The rapid pace and the technical orientation of the scale-up altered the practice of CHBC by expanding the scope of the work to become more technically comprehensive, but at the same time more narrowly defining 'care' as clinically-oriented work. The context within which CHBC was practiced also changed, altering the volunteers' own relationship to the work and the organisation. Over the course of the scale-up, Arminda and her colleagues felt exploited and ultimately abandoned, despite their work having served as the vanguard and national model for CHBC. This paper considers how this happened and in doing so raises questions about the communities constituted by global health interventions and about the role of and the voice of community health workers (CHWs) in large-scale interventions such as the HIV scale-up.

Arminda and her colleagues were pulled between competing conceptions of what care entailed. Alex Nading discusses the ambivalence of CHWs in Nicaragua that resulted from 'a split understanding of community health work' that demanded both 'technical rigidity,' and 'compassionate flexibility' (2013, p. 85). A similar tension is inherent in the two basic constituents of the term 'care': emotional and technical/practical (Kleinman &

Van Der Geest, 2009). Mufudzi recruited 'motherly' women who were considered wise, capable of mantaining confidentiality and of confronting suffering and death gracefully and compassionately. For the volunteers, prayer and spirituality played a principle role in this work. While the community embeddedness and dedication of the volunteers was seen as a strength by MISAU, the use of prayer marked the work as suspect and potentially opposed to the clinical priorities the working group identified. This was represented by the phrase I often heard repeated by nongovernmental organisation (NGO) and MISAU officials as well as health professionals in reference to Mufudzi's volunteers: 'all they do is pray.' As the scale-up progressed, technical aspects were increasingly emphasised and the volunteers were found to be lacking. At the same time, even as more resources became available for HIV programmes, Mufudzi insisted the work be done voluntarily lest it be tainted by selfish motives.

A gendered division of labour anchored this positioning – indeed the official name of the volunteer position included the title '*Mãe*,' Portuguese for 'Mother.' Care, particularly the nontechnical aspects conducted within households, is marked as a woman's activity and marginalised within a global political economy organised around technology as the driver of improved health (Kleinman & Hanna, 2008). It is a taken for granted and naturalised form of labour that is frequently reinforced as relating to local gender norms (Akintola, 2008; Du Preez & Niehof, 2008). Locally marked in this way, the volunteers had a tenuous connection to the global space of the scale-up, demarcated by actors, resources, expertise and discourse of transnational biomedical technology (Ferguson, 2006; Prince, 2014; Sullivan, 2011; Wendland, 2012). Caught between profesionalisation and preservation of the 'volunteer spirit' (Maes, 2012) and the technical and emotional dimensions of care, the volunteers were trapped in a marginal position.

Methods

I conducted ethnographic research in Mozambique for a total of eighteen months between 2003 and 2010 on a project exploring the narratives and networks of care emerging around HIV/AIDS interventions.[3] Data for this paper draws on participant-observation and semi-structured interviews with CHBC volunteers and programme administrators in local organisations and in the national capital. The majority of fieldwork was conducted in Chimoio, capital of Manica province, though I also visited CHBC programmes in other regions of Manica, Sofala, and Gaza provinces that allowed me to make comparisons across locations. I accompanied volunteers in Chimoio from the two principle organisations performing CHBC on their regular visits to patients' homes and conducted semi-structured interviews with a convenience sample of 25 volunteers. This paper focuses on a volunteer from one of these organisations. I also interviewed officials and administrators from government and NGOs. Interviews ranged from 30-minute single encounters, to many hours spread over the years of my involvement. This longitudinal engagement allowed me to build relationships with volunteers, people living with HIV/AIDS (PLWHA), and administrators and to witness changes over time. Interviews and fieldnotes were recorded in real-time as well as at the end of each day of fieldwork and were analysed using thematic and narrative analyses. The majority of the interviews were conducted in Portuguese by the author and when necessary, in Chiteve, with the aid of an interpreter. Conclusions were reviewed with key informants to ensure accuracy and the combination of participant-observation across a range of settings and the contents of conversations, interviews and fieldnotes provided detailed triangulation.

Contexts: CHBC, central Mozambique, and Arminda

CHBC is an internationally circulating model defined by the WHO as: 'any form of care given to sick people in their homes' (2002). Its emergence in 'resource-limited settings' is appropriate because:

> [it] draws on two strengths that exist throughout the world: families and communities. Families are the central focus of care and form the basis of the CBHC team. Communities are places where people live and a source of support and care for individuals and families in need. (WHO, 2002, p. 8)

UNAIDS called CHBC 'one of the outstanding features of the epidemic and a key coping mechanism for mitigating impact' (2002, p. 3). As the scale-up has progressed UNAIDS continues to reaffirm CHBC as a key component of HIV treatment (2010). The WHO's (2002) framing relies on taken-for-granted ideas of 'family' and 'community' as pre-existing resources to be tapped by development initiatives to stand-in for underfunded public health systems (Maes, 2012). This turn to civil society was a part of structural adjustment programmes implemented in Africa during the 1980s, diverting foreign aid toward the private sector, and devolving responsibility for care onto citizens themselves (Foley, 2010). One of the earliest African models of CHBC was The AIDS Support Organisation of Uganda (TASO), whose activists trained and supported family members caring for PLWHA at home in the late 1980s (Iliffe, 2006). CHBC volunteers are an incarnation of CHWs, global health actors often seen as a 'homogenous and unchanging "resource" in the provision of health care' (Swartz, 2013, p. 140). In the Alma Ata Declaration of 1978, the WHO identified CHWs was one of the cornerstones of comprehensive primary health care and as community advocates for social change (Lehmann & Sanders, 2007). Following this model, newly independent Mozambique's comprehensive national health system was fronted by a cadre of CHWs called *Agentes Polivalentes Elementares* (APEs) and made impressive population health improvements in a brief period (Walt, 1983). An externally funded civil conflict and structural adjustment-imposed austerity measures decimated much of this infrastructure. Though APEs survived in some regions and have been revitalised in recent years (Simon et al., 2009), the role of post-structural adjustment CHWs has shifted from 'change agent' to 'extension worker,' oriented towards technical and community management functions (Lehmann & Sanders, 2007, p. 6). Structural adjustment measures introduced in 1987 initiated privatisation of public services and industries, cuts in education and health, removal of price subsidies for food and fuel and reduction of other social services and safety nets (Hanlon, 1996; Pitcher, 2002). Health and social programmes were outsourced to foreign nongovernmental organisations (Hanlon, 1991), effectively hollowing out and fragmenting the public health sector (Pfeiffer, 2003). The number of health centres remains below prewar levels (Hanlon & Smart, 2008). The same period has seen a 'Pentecostal fervour' spread throughout central and southern Mozambique as over half of the peri-urban poor belong to healing churches that have become venues for seeking support and care (Pfeiffer, 2011).

Arminda was part of Mufudzi's first volunteer cohort and remained a volunteer throughout this fieldwork. Like many of her generation, her life story was defined by the region's violent political transitions. She grew up in a colonial village liberated by Frelimo[4] during the war of independence against Portugal in the 1960s. As Frelimo ascended and supported African nationalist movements in neighbouring Rhodesia and

South Africa, Rhodesian forces fought back, first directly, then by fostering a proxy war through Renamo,[5] a Mozambican insurgency. She recalled:

> We suffered the war out there in the bush, the war of our neighbour, Ian Smith [Rhodesian prime minister]. He came with airplanes, dropping bombs. We ran carrying bundles in our hands, whatever we could fit on our heads. I was a girl at the time but my mother was pregnant so I had to carry my baby brother.

As Zimbabwean independence ended 'Smith's War,' Mozambique's conflict escalated thanks to continued support for Renamo from South Africa and the USA. Arminda's family fled to Zimbabwe, then moved to Beira in 1990 before settling in Chimoio. As much as 40% of the Mozambican population was estimated to have been displaced during this period. Rural inhabitants moved to neighbouring countries or urban centres along the international highway (Hanlon, 1996). Arminda and her daughters lived behind the market stall she operated in one of Chimoio's cane city neighbourhoods.

Chimoio grew from a colonial railway stop into a city around a Portuguese textile factory built in 1944 (Artur, 1999). Nationalised in 1975 and privatised in the late 1980s, TextÁfrica employed between 2500 and 5000 residents when it closed in 2000 (AIM, 2002; Guerreiro, 2003; Magalhães, personal e-mail communication, February 20, 2006; Pitcher, 2002). Chimoio's population grew from 50,000 at independence in 1975 to 250,000 (INE, 2008). Most residents live in the 'cane city,' shanty towns which ring the former colonial 'cement city.' This zone dramatically grew during the post-independence civil war and has continued to expand. Households in the cane city combine wages or income from the informal market with production on subsistence plots outside the city. The dominant languages are Portuguese and *Chiteve*, a variant of Shona.

Origins: Mufudzi and the emergence of CHBC

Mufudzi was founded in 1995 through a partnership between *Muchengeti* (The Care Giver), a Zimbabwean faith-based NGO seeking a Mozambican partner to support refugee repatriation and a European faith-based NGO working in Zimbabwe. Muchengeti identified HIV/AIDS as a concern in refugee communities, and the initial goal was to mobilise Mozambican churches with ties to congregations across the border. These partners found eight Mozambican churches (four Pentecostal, three Evangelical, and one Catholic) willing to work with them. Mufudzi became a single organisation that operated through its member churches and individual volunteers who did not have to belong to member churches or be Christian. The first ten members were nine Mozambican representatives of these churches and a European volunteer from the faith-based NGO.

Muchengeti's Shona-language training materials were employed. Mufudzi's European member recalled:

> People were just coming out of the war and were eager to learn anything. I think they came to the trainings partly to get a free meal, but as they learned about HIV, people became really interested. They said: 'we have these problems here'.

A Mozambican founding member emphasised the early challenges:

> The initial reception was difficult because the pastors didn't accept this word, HIV/AIDS, in church. They thought those with AIDS were people with immoral lives and not people in the church. It wasn't relevant to them. We kept working on sensitising them, until we

encountered the story of a pastor who got sick and died of HIV/AIDS. That alerted the pastors that HIV/AIDS doesn't distinguish amongst churches or morality.

Even as this stigma seemed to lessen over the course of scale-up, the themes of poverty, hunger and interventions representing opportunity for education as well as material support would persist in narratives around HIV treatment interventions. CHBC was one of Mufudzi's early initiatives.[6] According to a founder, the first group of 28 volunteers were women in their 40s or 50s, 'good in caring, not afraid of cleaning or of intimacy with those who were sick and dying, who really were motherly.' Half were literate. They had been identified by their churches as 'wise, able to maintain confidentiality, strong in faith, and wanting to do the work without pay. It was more of a calling, a biblical mandate.' This was a defining aspect of CHBC that Mufudzi leadership maintained throughout the intervention: volunteers needed to be motivated by altruism rather than personal gain, and therefore the work needed to be freely given rather than remunerated.[7] This stance would become a source of tension between Mufudzi, funders, MISAU, and volunteers as the landscape of HIV care was transformed by the scale-up, but nobody felt it was an issue at this early stage, when there was little money available for CHBC.

CHBC was explicitly based on the model of pastoral visits that many local churches engaged in: visiting ailing parishioners and offering support, including prayer, help with household work, and material assistance. The difference was that Mufudzi visited people irrespective of church affiliation and was oriented towards caring for people with AIDS and other chronic diseases.[8] Volunteers attended a two-week workshop on CHBC focused on HIV transmission, the signs of AIDS, and how to care for an HIV-positive person at home, often bed bound. This included assessing for dehydration, malnutrition, fever, open wounds and bedsores, bathing and washing bedclothes, and doing basic physical therapy. Alongside this bodily care were techniques for counselling and educating about HIV, as well as spiritual support. Volunteers were officially assigned up to five or six patients to follow but in practice they might follow many more than that. They could routinely spend 2–3 days a week on their visits. When the project began in the mid-1990s, the task of the volunteers was to provide palliative care and support to people who were facing imminent death, if not actively dying. An HIV/AIDS clinic opened on the grounds of the provincial hospital, but it only offered treatment for opportunistic infections, not HIV itself. Volunteers and health care providers recalled overwhelmed hospital staff sending people home to die, telling their family members there was nothing more to be done. Volunteers spoke of the need to bring compassion and dignity to people who felt abandoned.

In keeping with studies of CHBC in other African settings, Mufudzi's volunteers had multiple motivations.[9] Arminda first learned about Mufudzi from a colleague in the market and was recruited by a fellow church member active in the organisation. Arminda converted to the Universal Church of the Kingdom of God, an international Pentecostal church, soon after she moved to Chimoio in the mid-1990s, after she saw her daughter's persistent illness successfully healed by prayer in this church. She recalled hearing about 'this association where many people come together from different countries, from Zimbabwe, Zambia, Malawi, they get together and exchange opinions…about civilisation, how to live with others religiously. I said, I think I could benefit from that.' It reminded her of an association she had been a part of as a refugee in Zimbabwe:

We had a partnership there, we made a contribution and then there was help for all in times of illness or death. We also studied ideas together…[Mufudzi] could help me like that association from Zimbabwe did. So I liked it and entered that first training. It was about how to do business, to help orphans, the sick, how to help people…that was my motivation, religious union, about life, studying about these positive diseases.

Arminda's recollection of her motivations to become a volunteer speaks to her sense of multiple potential benefits, including opportunities to enact prosocial, altruistic, and spiritual values of service alongside desires for education, self-improvement, and a proximity to a cosmopolitanism that the Zimbabwean association and her own church represented, and that this CBO, which was supported by Zimbabwean and European colleagues, based on regionally circulating CHBC models, and part of the emerging global fight against AIDS, seemed to promise. By joining Mufudzi, Arminda was placing herself on a 'forward moving trajectory' (Prince, 2014). Arminda proudly displayed the certificates she had earned as tangible evidence of this progress.

In Arminda's telling, her own biography led her into the work. She had experience caring for a daughter and a brother with AIDS. Her father was a *curandeiro*, a traditional healer. She recalled what she inherited and learned from him:

> I have a personal spirit for this. My father was a *curandeiro*…sick people always came [to our house]. So this work was nothing new. My patients also, those who can walk, they come here and tell me their stories. Sometimes they feel isolated at home, there are things they can speak to me about that maybe they are too proud to share with their families. Its not difficult for me, because in my father's house, we always ate together [patients and family], we were all one family.

Arminda's spiritual calling prevented her from tiring and provided protection and guidance:

> There could be a demon in that house that wants to kill. First I get the Lord's blessing that he may help me, bring me strength, intelligence. Its not luck, its not knowledge…without the Lord in my heart I would get upset, leave. But with the power of the Lord, I win those people over and take them to the hospital.

These syncretic notions of spirits acting in the world are characteristic of contemporary African Pentecostal churchs (Honwana, 2002; Meyer, 2004) and are widely shared in Chimoio's cane city, where the majority of residents are Christian and consider spiritual alongside natural causes when discussing etiologies of affliction (Chapman, 2010; Pfeiffer 2005).

Arminda took pride in the trust that her neighbours granted her by opening up to her about their HIV status and their personal challenges. The ill and their family members sought her out: 'they say "*Mamá*, I can tell you my secret".' In other cases, Arminda would gradually approach families, taking her time to familiarise herself with the situation and to gain their trust. Visits nearly always began with a prayer. The patient and all family members present were invited to join hands and participate. When asked about the role of prayer in their work, volunteers gave a variety of answers. One common saying amongst both volunteers and patients was 'prayer is medicine.' In keeping with local Pentecostal church practices, volunteers prayed for God or the Holy Spirit to directly intercede and heal. The work was seen to be therapeutic on not only an individual level, but on a communal level as well. This was reflected in another phrase volunteers used: 'God sends misfortune so that people may be united.' Christian notions of forgiveness were also mobilised to address guilt and blame within individuals and families. Volunteers saw their response to the HIV epidemic as a way to enact both individual and communal healing.

Faith in the power of prayer was accompanied by a concern for basic needs. Volunteers consistently pointed to poverty and hunger as the principle challenges their patients faced. When long-time volunteers recounted the history of the CHBC programme, they recalled that women were initially ashamed of visiting sick people empty-handed. Initially, volunteers began bringing their patients small amounts of food from their own homes, until Mufudzi began growing food for their patients. This notably improved the success volunteers had in recruiting patients. As one of the early coordinators recalled: 'Families hid their sick at first...but they opened their doors for food.'

Much like prayer, food was conceived as a family and communal intervention as much as for an individual's health. Chronic illness frequently drained the resources and energy of families. In the case of AIDS, an illness with no cure, families were faced with the choice of where to allocate scarce resources, a form of 'life boat ethics' where the 'pragmatics of saving the savable' is evoked over more egalitarian principles (Scheper-Hughes, 1992, p. 405). Some families withdrew material support from sick family members who were felt to be on the brink of death in order to benefit the more productive members. It was this phenomenon with political-economic dimensions as well as notions of kinship obligation and multiple coexisting etiologies of illness causation that was frequently labeled 'stigma' by HIV/AIDS interventions and addressed via educational interventions that assumed a lack of knowledge. In this context, food had more than nutritional value. One volunteer explained that if a sick person can 'bring benefits' to the entire family, they would be more likely to unite and mobilise the family around them. During the early years of CHBC, volunteers focused on palliative and comfort-oriented care, education and improving basic health and social relationships through a diverse set of techniques and approaches, including bodily care, prayer, food, help with domestic chores, compassion and counselling.

Scaling-up

Mozambique's scale-up grew exponentially with significant aid packages from the World Bank and the Global Fund in 2001, the Clinton Foundation in 2003, and PEPFAR in 2004, which altogether would rival MISAU's entire budget (Matsinhe, 2006; Oomman, Bernstein, & Rosenzweig, 2007). Rapid testing became broadly available in the public sector in 2002–2003 with ART following in 2004–2005. This would impact CHBC volunteers in three ways. First, the work of CHBC shifted from palliative care of the bed-ridden, chronically ill to recruiting individuals for testing and supporting ART initiation and maintenance. Second, the incorporation of CHBC into the National Strategic Plan to Combat HIV/AIDs introduced an increasingly technical definition of care. Finally, dissent around the issue of payment led to fracture within Mufudzi. These changes would ultimately marginalise a significant number of volunteers and contribute to the demise of Mufudzi's CHBC programme.

Technicisation of care

Mufudzi was well-positioned to benefit when the scale-up increased momentum. CHBC was a UNAIDS Best Practice already implemented in much of Southern and Eastern Africa. MISAU convened a working group on CHBC in 2000 to develop a national plan that included members of government, and national and international NGOs. Mufudzi was officially a part of the working group, but their participation was limited to email contact as there was no funding to transport anyone from Chimoio, a flight or full day's drive from Maputo. The two CHBC programmes operating in the country were Mufudzi in Chimoio and a nurse-run intervention in Maputo. Mufudzi became the unofficial model for the national programme because it was a community-operated programme designed for lay volunteers. At the same time, however, a working group member shared with me the group's concern that volunteers 'were just praying, and a lot more could be done, even without ART, to prolong life and make people more comfortable and less stigmatised.' The national CHBC manual was based on Mufudzi's, but Mufudzi members were upset that spiritual components of care, prominent in their version, were nearly absent in the national manual. Nonetheless, MISAU encouraged organisations interested in starting CHBC programmes to visit Mufudzi and learn from their approach. Volunteers became accustomed to frequent visits from MISAU officials and AIDS organisations from around the country.

CHBC was given a central role in the initial model for HIV/AIDS treatment services scaled-up in Mozambique, termed the Integrated Health Network. According to MISAU's national HIV/AIDS strategy manual: 'the link between the HIV/AIDS clinic and home-based care is the cornerstone for the monitoring and treatment of PLWHA' (MISAU, 2004, p. 43). In its definition of CHBC, however, the MISAU distinguished between 'home-based care' and 'home visits':

> 'Care' is defined as the attention provided at home to PLWHA and their families, which includes: health, education, HIV/AIDS prevention and counselling, evaluation and care of symptoms, adherence to drugs and a referral system between the National Health Services and the community and other social sectors, with a view to the reduction of HIV transmission and the integrated care of PLWHA, while home 'visits' generally have social, emotional and spiritual support as their objective. (MISAU, 2004, p. 43)

Care was defined as an activity with a technical orientation that mostly related to a biomedical conception of health and disease and that involved referral and connection to biomedical services.[10] Visits that were not technically oriented were simply home visits, and did not qualify as home-based care. The working group concern that volunteers were 'just praying' can be read into these definitions, as social, emotional and spiritual support did not constitute 'care'. Though Mufudzi's community orientation made it the favoured initial model, national certification courses were taught by nurses trained in CHBC and in order to accommodate increasing amounts of technical information, the official CHBC training manual doubled in size between 2002 and 2006, from 83 to 160 pages.

Volunteers had always collected data for Mufudzi and funders. The national data collection form, which had both words and pictures for the many illiterate volunteers, required a new level of detail. The data were pooled at the organisation level and 'uploaded' to the MISAU and donors. The 2006 version included number of visits, death, loss to follow-up, enrollment in antiretroviral or tuberculosis treatment, and a set of appropriate referrals, to the HIV clinic, supplemental food support, education for children, legal issues, number of orphans and income. By 2010, the form was more streamlined, including pictures for enrollment in antiretroviral and tuberculosis treatment, use of antibiotic prophylaxis, pregnancy, enrolled in the clinic, loss to follow-up and death. Notably absent were the majority of 'social' categories, including supplemental food support and income problems.[11] Altogether, the changes indicate an increasing focus on biomedical issues and away from issues defined as social such as nutrition and employment.

The needs of CHBC patients changed during the scale-up. As availability of testing and treatment increased, there was less need for palliative care of bed-bound individuals and support for domestic chores and more need for counselling, monitoring, documentation, and an ability to master increasingly complex domains of knowledge that the expanding training module encompassed. These changes shifted the desired qualifications for volunteers to a minimum criteria of 6 years of schooling and ability to read and write. In effect, this shifted the profile from the older, 'motherly,' individual Mufudzi sought, to a more educated, and therefore, likely younger profile that MISAU preferred.

Scale-up incorporated CHBC into the Integrated Health Network and made more resources available for the intervention. Though the national programme was modelled on Mufudzi's, changes introduced at a national level pushed CHBC in a more technical direction, which would have ambivalent impacts on Mufudzi's volunteers as they were increasingly told their skill-set was obsolete by officials from MISAU and partner organisations. In tandem with this technicisation, the rapid and massive infusion of resources would also have an impact on Mufudzi and CHBC volunteers.

Professionalisation of a CBO

Mufudzi increased and expanded in step with the scale-up. A formal organisation structure with a constitution and a governing assembly was established at the founding. The first salaried positions were created in 1999, for the director, chief administrator, and the heads of the CHBC, pastor education and youth programmes. The professional staff would grow to as many as 56, only four of whom had been founding members. An initial budget of just over US$600, spent on trainings and renting a shared office space would mushroom in the 2000s to US$10,000 and then US$700,000. While initial funding was from European, religiously-oriented donors, later and larger quantities of funding came from US sources, including PEPFAR, through a partnership with a locally-operating American NGO. Over 80 churches became members and the scale of activities similarly expanded. There were as many as 130 CHBC volunteers in Chimoio, and a total of 240 for the five districts of province as programmes were initiated in urban centres throughout the region. Mufudzi moved from a borrowed back room to rent its own office space in the early 2000s, to finally build its own office in 2008. Mufudzi expanded its activities to include a support group of PLWHA with over 700 registered members and programmes for Orphans and Vulnerable Children (OVC).[12]

With the rapid treatment scale-up leading to a growing number of CHBC organisations, MISAU recommended an incentive rate of 60% of the minimum wage (amounting to about US$24/month) for volunteers, with maximum allowable payment not to exceed the minimum wage (MISAU, 2006, p. 10). According to a working group participant, the consensus within the group was that poor women caring for others deserved to be paid something. The recommendation was also meant to prevent one particularly well-resourced NGO from paying volunteers higher salaries than nurses and attracting their labour from the public sector.

Payment was a controversial issue for Mufudzi. In the mid-1990s, nobody was paid for working with people with HIV, and most Mufudzi members indeed said they started the work without the expectation of payment. As the scale-up progressed and the amount of money available nationally for HIV/AIDS exponentially increased and was channelled into Mufudzi, the assumption the volunteers would not be paid remained, even as the organisation professionalised. Volunteers, however began requesting their share of the funding, particularly when a second NGO in Chimoio began providing CHBC modelled on Mufudzi's practice and provided its volunteers the incentive. At one meeting, a programme coordinator scolded the volunteers raising this issue:

> This work should come from the heart. It should not be done for payment, but to help our neighbours, our brothers and sisters. It is our work that we do. If we get paid, it is not a bad thing, but we do not do this work in order to be paid, and we do the work even when we are not being paid.

Mufudzi's administrators feared that payments would distort the work and attract opportunists who would be less effective than those motivated by altruism and a religious calling. Most of those who objected to paying CHBC volunteers had salaried positions themselves, however.

WHO and MISAU guidelines encouraged nonmonetary incentives: refresher trainings and exchanges with other groups, during which volunteers were provided with snacks and lunches, certificates, organisation t-shirts and wraps, and annual bonuses of rice, corn, oil or soap. Mufudzi attempted to meet the recommended incentive by providing group rather than individual incentives and experimented with a micro-credit project and a community garden for volunteers, but nothing was sustained. Finally in 2008, under pressure from Mufudzi's CHBC funder to provide volunteers their incentives and in response to increasing frustration from the volunteers, it was agreed that volunteers would be paid the recommended amount, but the number of CHBC volunteers was reduced by 40% as the available funding would only cover a limited number. According to a Mufudzi administrator, the funder would or could not support group payment schemes, such as funding a group microcredit project, and insisted on monetary incentives for individual volunteers as stipulated in the grant. Those removed – older and less educated volunteers – were invited to work with OVC, which did not provide monetary incentives.[13] Most of these volunteers held out hope they might be reinstated to CHBC.

The volunteers had mixed responses to the changes the scale-up brought. They welcomed the changes that they could see resulted in improvements for their patients, despite the increased workload. They desired trainings and education and so did not protest the technical shift. They continued with the same approach, but worked to incorporate the increased clinical aspects and demands for referral and documentation. Those who could not read and write did struggle with documentation, but worked around it by recruiting literate colleagues and family members to help them. Neighbourhood CHBC teams tended to have at least one literate member who organised documentation. Volunteers appreciated the closer connection with the health services and the increase in treatments their patients accessed. They did complain, however, about not always being respected or treated well by clinical staff when they accompanied patients to clinic. Another welcome change that the scale-up brought was a contract with the World Food Programme (WFP) which provided monthly food baskets to patients. This became divisive, however, when volunteers were told not to share the available food amongst all their patients, as had been their practice, but rather to target those receiving ART and TB treatment. This produced resentment and jealousy amongst their patients. As the numbers on treatment increased, the amount of food aid did not keep pace, generating intense competition around the acquisition of the WFP ration cards (Kalofonos, 2010). When volunteers finally were awarded monetary incentives, after several years of acrimony, the fact that nearly half of the volunteers were removed was demoralising.

Volunteers felt they were able to continue to provide appropriate and quality care through the changes. As the scale-up proceeded, however, the assessments of those around them changed. In 2003, one administrator of an NGO that worked with Mufudzi told me: 'I think its horrible to pay church women to visit their neighbours when they are sick. Shouldn't they just do so because it's the right thing to do?' The comment 'all they do is pray' was a frequent characterisation of Mufudzi's CHBC programme in the mid to late 2000s and indicated that Mufudzi's CHBC no longer resembled 'care' despite the fact that their practices were embedded in the national manual. A young official in the provincial health department with whom I discussed CHBC in 2010, even denied that Mufudzi had ever served as the model for CHBC, asking how illiterate and uneducated women could be expected to provide effective home-based care. These informal comments point to not only an overwhelmingly technical and clinical conception of care, but also to the ways community labour are naturalised and gendered. While Mozambican CHBC began in Chimoio as a holistic intervention run by church-based volunteers, it became technicised through the scale-up to the extent that the practices of the vanguard of CHBC were no longer recognisable to those implementing the scale-up. While the volunteers continued to be dedicated to their work, the landscape around them shifted considerably.

Chica: 'yes, I am better. But my stomach hurts!'

In 2010, Mufudzi was having multiple organisational challenges and CHBC was no longer a top priority of the funding partner. Mufudzi would lose the majority of its CHBC funding that year and the organised CHBC programme would come to an end by 2012. I was in Chimoio in 2010 and accompanied Arminda on her visit to Chica, a woman whom she had recruited for testing and treatment. Arminda was concerned about Chica's difficulties in adhering to her medications. We arrived at Chica's house around lunchtime. A young woman was cooking peas in front of the family hut, while an elderly woman and two children ate porridge with the characteristic beige colour of USAID corn-soy blend. On the far side of the yard, another young woman and man sat selling *nipa*, a fermented sugarcane brew. We entered the hut. Arminda initiated the visit with a prayer and proudly introduced Chica, saying: 'Here is my patient. I can tell you she is much better!' Chica added: 'Yes, I am better. But my stomach hurts!'

In the months since Arminda had first seen her, Chica's health and appearance had improved significantly, despite spotty adherence and clinic attendance. Antiretrovirals were commonly said to cause hunger in central Mozambique (Kalofonos, 2010) and indeed Chica endorsed this:

> This medicine, it bites. Its not like a normal hunger. If I don't eat when I take it, I tremble and shake. It is said this medicine will kill you if you don't eat with it. If I take my pills at night, my stomach wakes me up, and I have to eat. In the morning when I awake, I have to eat again.

She had been awarded a WFP ration card, entitling her to receive 10 kilograms of corn-soy blend and 1 kilogram of legumes per month,[14] an amount that, when shared amongst her 3 children, 2 grandchildren, and her elderly mother, lasted 4 days. She also sold *nipa* and sought odd jobs. When she did not have food to eat, Chica skipped her ART. Arminda listened and discussed possible avenues of support. Chica disclosed that she engaged in serial short-lived sexual relationships with men who could provide her with material support and did not always use condoms. Her current stomach pain was accompanied by a foul-smelling vaginal discharge that she was ashamed to reveal to a clinician lest she be rebuked for having unprotected sex. She occasionally treated it with antibiotics, when she could afford to seek treatment. Arminda arranged to accompany Chica to the clinic later that week to be assessed and also encouraged her to stay adherent to her antiretrovirals. Arminda would visit daily for the rest of the week, bringing food from her own home for Chica to take with her antiretroviral medications. With a wrinkled brow, Arminda expressed mixed feelings following the visit:

> That's the difficulty of this work. When a patient doesn't have food, doesn't have soap to wash her clothes, no way of getting to the hospital when she is ill, with children who depend on her…I bring her things from my own home, because I can't let a patient die of hunger. You have to take a bit of whatever you have. Sometimes she'll come herself to my house, '*Mamá*, I'm hungry!' But what can I do? I'm a person too.

Arminda and her fellow volunteers were acutely aware of their limitations, and they were often overwhelmed by the needs of their patients. While they experienced considerable satisfaction when their patients recovered, they were distressed by their inability to address their patients' basic needs, especially food. They also endured losses, as more of Arminda's patients had died than were alive: 'we are used to seeing them greet us, having conversations, looking for a way forward together. That makes us proud of work done well. But when a patient dies, we feel it.' Volunteers often took setbacks personally and suffered through feelings of guilt and sleepless nights. One of Arminda's colleagues told me: 'I get this nervousness, a kind of stress, and loneliness, because there is often nothing more I can do.' Arminda's comment above, 'I'm a person too,' is a reminder that the volunteers were in similar situations of chronic uncertainty as their patients, and were often HIV-positive themselves or caring for family members with AIDS.

We can't find this spirit of help

Arminda had hoped her certifications and experience would translate into steady employment: 'when we were trained, we were told we would be needed one day [as salaried workers]. Well, that day has not come.' The recommended monthly incentive was usually half the amount Arminda made through her market stall, a significant sum despite being set below minimum wage, yet it was inconsistently provided for a relatively brief period. Arminda expressed her frustration:

> We are expected to carry the burden of labour but not the benefits? Our organisation has built a nice office. Those people who work in the office, they go to work in cars. But those of us who do the work in the neighbourhoods? This is not our office, and that hurts. We built that office, we built the organisation. We arrive at the homes of the sick, and they say, '*Mufudzi* is here.' We are *Mufudzi*. But we [volunteers] are the last to receive and the first to lose. Perhaps we should discuss selling the office.

'Work in the neighborhoods' involved relating to and accompanying patients and their families. Arminda maintained it was unfair that the organisation's administration materially benefited from her work, while her aspirations for greater security went unfulfilled. It was not simply insufficient remuneration that bothered Arminda, however, as much as the sense that she and her colleagues had been used and abandoned in the scale-up.

Arminda recalled her initial vision for the project, of a collective effort for self and communal improvement, with disappointment. She herself could be counted a success story: as a volunteer she enrolled in night school and became literate enough to compile the data and the monthly summary report for the group of volunteers she managed. But she noted her story was exceptional when she told me the majority of the volunteers she had initially trained with had died. We had just visited another volunteer that had suffered a stroke resulting in partial paralysis. Arminda reflected on the irony that this long-time volunteer was now worse off than their patients, as her affliction was not amenable to ART, and therefore, did not qualify for the services for which they recruited. She was left with few protections despite her many years of service: '*Mamá* is sick, her arm is paralyzed, she can't work, what will she eat? A person who was working. Today she has stopped and what benefits does she have?' She reflected on the prosocial spirit of the volunteers and lamented the absence of this spirit in other quarters:

> There are many volunteers, and since they started they've been given what? Soap, tshirts, finally we were given something from the cashbox, money that came from other countries, but now, the well is empty. What are we to do, wait five more years to refill this empty well? We know how to help one another, and we have our patients who rely on us…but who wants to work for nothing? Those of us with this spirit, we still visit the sick. You can't just call this work…this isn't an enterprise or a business, its more like a church…but this spirit doesn't appear for everyone. We've got this situation amongst the volunteers. We are dying and being buried in disgrace. We lack transportation, we lack coffins, nothing to cover even ourselves. Where is Mufudzi? They have fallen on hard times. They depended on foreign countries, why don't we have our own funds for our volunteers? I think of that association in Zimbabwe, we started it alone, made our own contributions. We would all go sew seeds in someone's *machamba* today, tomorrow in someone else's. We built our houses together as well. We made the bricks, got the wood, men cut, women collected. It wasn't easy, but there was this spirit of help, support. Here in the city, we can't find this spirit of help.

While CHBC began as a grassroots effort based on solidarity, service and sacrifice, the influx of resources and shifts in values introduced by the scale-up contributed to the fracturing of the organisation and the collective identity of the volunteers. This loss of solidarity that Arminda experienced on a personal level with Mufudzi resonates with the larger transformations in the politics of governance and aid contributing to growing inequality in Mozambique (Hanlon & Smart, 2008; Pfeiffer, 2003). Despite her frustration, Arminda maintained that she and her fellow volunteers would continue following their patients. But she noted a double standard, that while they selflessly served their patients, they could not expect the same from their organisation. This may reflect the difficult reality of CBOs whose fortunes are tied to 2- and 5-year grant cycles. Neither the burden of labour nor the chronic uncertainties that the volunteers faced were equally shared, however.

On the uses of CHBC volunteers

This paper uses the framework of intertwined biographies to foreground Arminda as an individual who brought her own life course, aspirations and expertise to her work as a volunteer with Mufudizi and to the scale-up of CHBC. This emphasis on Arminda's singular experience highlights the importance of going beyond the notion of the CHW as a resource, an undifferentiated labour pool to be exploited in the name of cost-effectiveness and sustainability and who can be counted on to implement global health directives without bringing individual thought and biography to bear.

CHBC began as disparate and desperate local action in the face of overwhelming need. It had a pragmatic, palliative and spiritual orientation towards relieving suffering and addressing material deprivation, that emphasised individual and collective well-being and the importance of relationships in care. As the scale-up gained momentum and life-saving technologies of HIV testing and ART became available, CHBC also became more technically defined. The original model of CHBC became a stand-in and a stop-gap for what was constructed as truly effective care that was clinically-oriented, a crisis plan rendered obsolete by the arrival of appropriate techology. This move devalued both the non-technical skills of CHBC and the people who were seen to embody and represent them: older, poorly educated women.

Following Ferguson's metaphor, derived from extractive mineral industries, of contemporary modes of governance dividing Africa into a patchwork of secured, cared-for, usable 'enclaves' and unusable, abandoned terrain, the scale-up extracted volunteer labour from a cheap labour pool to initiate the expansion of HIV services (Ferguson, 2006, p. 39). The Mufudzi volunteers were then discarded, deemed as no longer usable. They were caught between not having sufficient technical expertise, from the perspective of MISAU and funders, and the need to preserve their altruistic motives from the perspective of Mufudzi administrators. The intervention that was 'taken to scale' itself ended up collapsing under the pressure of the scale-up. In some ways Mufudzi itself suffered from a lack of care, as it was granted far more resources than it could successfully utilise in order to carry out national and global priorities. With insufficient training and oversight, the organisation became collateral damage of the scale-up.

Though the intertwined biography framework highlights the particularities of this context, CHWs and other global health volunteers in diverse contexts across the Global South occupy a similar structural position, a grey zone between formal and informal labour and permanent and temporary employment, where there is neither adequate recognition nor remuneration (Akintola, 2011; Maes, 2012; Nading, 2013; Prince, 2014; Rödlach, 2009; Swartz, 2013; Swidler & Watkins, 2009). This is not an inevitable development, however. Partners in Health's social justice approach to community-based HIV and TB care, positions the health care system as an enabler of social and economic development rather than a drain on the economy (Mukherjee & Eustache, 2007). CHWs are employed and this has been shown to lead to improved health and economic outcomes. A distinguishing feature of this intervention is its continuity, as it has been operating for over 20 years. Low-tech innovations outside the formal health care system strengthening public institutions, services and safety nets remain well-known paths to improved well-being in low-income countries (Ferguson, 2010; Pfeiffer, 2013). CHW programmes may yet prove to be opportunities to synergistically provide medical treatment and poverty-reducing employment.

Funding

This article was written with the support of the Center for Biological Futures at the Fred Hutchinson Cancer Research Center. The research was funded by a Fulbright-Hayes Doctoral Dissertation Research Award, the University of California, Berkeley Center for African Studies, and the University of California, San Francisco School of Medicine.

Notes

1. Names of people and organisations in this paper are pseudonyms.
2. Mufudzi is Chiteve for Shepherd.
3. Fieldwork was conducted over 4 visits for 2 months in 2003, 2 months in 2004, 12 months in 2005–6 and 2 months in 2010.
4. Frelimo is the Portuguese acronym for *Frente da Libertação de Moçambique* (Mozambican Liberation Front), the group that fought the Portuguese for independence and has since been the ruling political party.
5. Renamo is the Portuguese acronym for *Resistência Nacional Moçambicano* (Mozambican National Resistance).

6. The other two initiatives, pastor and youth education and training for HIV/AIDS prevention, are not discussed here.
7. See Maes (2012) for an example of similar dynamic in Ethiopia with a secular organisation.
8. Volunteers visited all suffering from chronic disease in order to avoid visiting only PLWHA and thereby inadvertantly revealing someone's serostatus.
9. Motivations include prosocial values, such as compassion and a desire to reduce suffering, fulfilling civic and religious values of sacrifice and service, desires for better compensation and stable employment, as well as recognition and appreciation, and opportunities for education and self-improvement (Akintola, 2011; Maes, 2012; Maes & Kalofonos, 2013; Rödlach, 2009; Swidler & Watkins, 2009). Also in keeping with this literature, spiritual motivation was commonly cited by volunteers working for secular NGOs providing CHBC in Chimoio and elsewhere in Mozambique, and not exclusively in faith-based organisations.
10. The 'community and other social sectors' are also referenced, but the majority of new services were medical.
11. Problems specific to children were transferred to volunteers who specialised in 'OVC.'
12. The pace and scale of Mufudzi's growth was typical of the trajectory of similar organisations across Africa at the time. See Droggitis and Ooman (2010) and Oomman et al. (2007).
13. Tellingly, OVC work involved no clinical care and no incentive. Swartz (2013) similarly discusses distinct experiences along generational lines for CHWs in South Africa.
14. These amounts were down from the 2006 allotment of 36 kg rice, 18 kg CSB, 6 kg legumes, andd 1.5 L oil. The available food supplements did not keep pace with the increasing number of patients.

References

Agência de Informação Moçambicana (AIM) (2002, May 7). Textáfrica in crisis. Retrieved from http://www.poptel.org.uk/mozambique-news/newsletter/aim231.html#story9

Akintola, O. (2008). Unpaid HIV/AIDS care in Southern Africa: Forms, context, and implications. *Feminist Economics, 14*, 117–147. doi:10.1080/13545700802263004

Akintola, O. (2011). What motivates people to volunteer? The case of volunteer AIDS caregivers in faith-based organizations in KwaZulu-Natal, South Africa. *Health Policy and Planning, 26*, 53–62. doi:10.1093/heapol/czq019

Artur, D. R. (1999). *Cidade de Chimoio: Ensaio histórico-sociológico* [City of Chimoio: A historical-sociological essay]. Chimoio: ARPAC.

Chapman, R. R. (2010). *Family secrets: Risking reproduction in central mozambique*. Nashville, TN: Vanderbilt University Press.

Comaroff, J. L., & Comaroff, J. (1999). *Civil society and the political imagination in Africa: Critical perspectives*. Chicago: University of Chicago Press.

Droggitis, C., & Ooman, N. (2010). *Think long term: How global AIDS donors can strengthen the health workforce in Africa*. Washington, DC: Center for Global Development.

Du Preez, C., & Niehof, A. (2008). Caring for people living with AIDS. A labour of love. *Medische antropologie, 20*, 87–104. Retrieved from http://tma.socsci.uva.nl/20_1/preez.pdf

Ferguson, J. (2006). *Global shadows: Africa in the neoliberal world order*. Durham, NC: Duke University Press.

Ferguson, J. (2010). The uses of neoliberalism. *Antipode, 41*, 166–184. doi:10.1111/j.1467-8330.2009.00721.x

Foley, E. E. (2010). *Your pocket is what cures you: The politics of health in Senegal*. New Brunswick, NJ: Rutgers University Press.

Guerreiro M. S. (2003). Textáfrica está à venda. *Moçambique, 34*, 37–38. Retrieved from http://www.ccpm.pt/revista_34.htm

Hanlon, J. (1991). *Mozambique: Who calls the shots?* Bloomington: Indiana University Press.

Hanlon, J. (1996). *Peace without profit: How the IMF blocks rebuilding in Mozambique*. Portsmouth, NH: Heinemann.

Hanlon, J., & Smart, T. (2008). *Do bicycles equal development in Mozambique?* Rochester, NY: James Currey.

Hansen, K. T. (1997). *Keeping house in Lusaka*. New York, NY: Columbia University Press.

Honwana, A. M. (2002). *Espíritos vivos, tradicões modernas: Possessão de espíritos e reintegração social pos-guerra no sul de Moçambique* [Living spirits, modern traditions:

Spiritual possession and postwar social reintegration in southern Mozambique]. Maputo: Promédia.

Iliffe, J. (2006). *The African AIDS epidemic: A history.* Oxford: James Currey.

Instituto Nacional de Estatística (INE). (2008). *População da Província de Manica, 2007* [Population of Manica province, 2007]. Retrieved from http://www.ine.gov.mz/censo2007/rp/pop07prov/manica

Kalofonos, I. A. (2010). "All I eat is ARVs": The paradox of AIDS treatment interventions in central Mozambique. *Medical Anthropology Quarterly, 24,* 363–380. doi:10.1111/j.1548-1387.2010.01109.x

Kleinman, A., & Hanna, B. (2008). Catastrophe, caregiving and today's biomedicine. *BioSocieties, 3,* 287–301. doi:10.1017/S1745855208006200

Kleinman, A., & Van Der Geest, S. (2009). "Care" in health care. *Medische Antropologie, 21,* 159–168. Retrieved from http://tma.socsci.uva.nl/21_1/kleinman.pdf

Lehmann, U., & Sanders, D. (2007). *Community health workers: What do we know about them?* Geneva: World Health Organization.

Maes, K. (2012). Volunteerism or labor exploitation? Harnessing the volunteer spirit to sustain AIDS treatment programs in Urban Ethiopia. *Human Organization, 71,* 54. Retrieved from http://www.pubmedcentral.nih.gov/articlerender.fcgi?artid=3783341&tool=pmcentrez&rendertype=abstract

Maes, K., & Kalofonos, I. (2013). Becoming and remaining community health workers: Perspectives from Ethiopia and Mozambique. *Social Science & Medicine, 87,* 52–59. doi:10.1016/j.socscimed.2013.03.026

Matsinhe, C. (2006). *Tábula Rasa: Dinâmica da resposta Moçambicana ao HIV/SIDA* [Tabula rasa: Dynamics of the Mozambican response to HIV/AIDS]. Maputo: Texto Editores.

Meyer, B. (2004). Christianity in Africa: From African independent to Pentecostal-charismatic churches. *Annual Review of Anthropology, 33,* 447–474. doi:10.1146/annurev.anthro.33.070203.143835

MISAU. (2004). *National strategic plan to combat STI/HIV/AIDS, health sector, 2004–2008.* Maputo: Author.

MISAU. (2006). *Cuidados domiciliários PVHS e outras doenças crónicas: Guião de operacionalização* [Home-based care of PLWHA and other chronic diseases: Operationalization manual]. Maputo: Author.

Mukherjee, J. S., & Eustache, F. E. (2007). Community health workers as a cornerstone for integrating HIV and primary healthcare. *AIDS Care, 19*(Suppl. 1), S73–S82. doi:10.1080/09540120601114485

Nading, A. M. (2013). "Love isn't there in your stomach": A moral economy of medical citizenship among Nicaraguan community health workers. *Medical Anthropology Quarterly, 27,* 84–102. doi:10.1111/maq.12017

Oomman, N., Bernstein, M., & Rosenzweig, S. (2007). *Following the funding for HIV/AIDS: A comparative analysis of the funding practices of PEPFAR, the global fund and world bank MAP in Mozambique, Uganda and Zambia.* Washington, DC: Center for Global Development.

Pfeiffer, J. (2003). International NGOs and primary health care in Mozambique: The need for a new model of collaboration. *Social Science and Medicine, 56,* 725–738. Retrieved from http://www.ncbi.nlm.nih.gov/entrez/query.fcgi?cmd=Retrieve&db=PubMed&dopt=Citation&list_uids=12560007

Pfeiffer J. (2005). Commodity fetichismo, the holy spirit, and the turn to Pentecostal and African independent churches in central Mozambique. *Culture, Medicine, and Psychiatry, 29,* 255–283. doi:10.1007/s11013-005-9168-3

Pfeiffer, J. (2011). Pentecostalism and AIDS treatment in Mozambique: Creating new approaches to HIV prevention through anti-retroviral therapy. *Global Public Health, 6*(Suppl. 2), S163–S173. doi:10.1080/17441692.2011.605067

Pfeiffer, J. (2013). The struggle for a public sector: PEPFAR in Mozambique. In J. Biehl & A. Petryna (Eds.), *When people come first: Critical studies in global health* (pp. 166–181). Princeton, NJ: Princeton University Press.

Pfeiffer, J., & Chapman, R. (2010). Anthropological perspectives on structural adjustment and public health. *Annual Review of Anthropology, 39,* 149–165. doi:10.1146/annurev.anthro.012809.105101

Pitcher, M. A. (2002). *Transforming Mozambique: The politics of privatization, 1975–2000*. New York, NY: Cambridge University Press.

Prince, R. J. (2014). Precarious projects: Conversions of (biomedical) knowledge in an east African city. *Medical Anthropology*, *33*, 68–83. doi:10.1080/01459740.2013.833918

Rödlach, A. (2009). Home-based care for people living with AIDS in Zimbabwe: Voluntary caregivers' motivations and concerns. *African Journal of AIDS Research*, *8*, 423–431. doi:10.2989/AJAR.2009.8.4.6.1043

Scheper-Hughes, N. (1992). *Death without weeping: The violence of everyday life in Brazil*. Berkeley: University of California Press.

Simon, S., Chu, K., Frieden, M., Candrinho, B., Ford, N., Schneider, H., & Biot, M. (2009). An integrated approach of community health worker support for HIV/AIDS and TB care in Angónia district, Mozambique. *BMC International Health and Human Rights*, *9*, 13–19. doi:10.1186/1472-698X-9-13

Sullivan, N. (2011). Mediating abundance and scarcity: Implementing an HIV/AIDS-targeted project within a government hospital in Tanzania. *Medical Anthropology*, *30*, 202–221. doi:10.1080/01459740.2011.552453

Swartz, A. (2013). Legacy, legitimacy, and possibility: An exploration of community health worker experience across the generations in Khayelitsha, South Africa. *Medical Anthropology Quarterly*, *27*, 139–154. doi:10.1111/maq.12020

Swidler, A., & Watkins, S. C. (2009). "Teach a man to fish": The doctrine of sustainability and its effects on three strata of Malawian society. *World Development*, *37*, 1182–1196. doi:10.1016/j.worlddev.2008.11.002

UNAIDS. (2002). *Report on the global HIV/AIDS epidemic*. Geneva: Author.

UNAIDS. (2010). *Global report: UNAIDS report on the global AIDS epidemic*. Geneva: Author.

Walt, G. (1983). The evolution of health policy. In G. Walt & A. Melamed (Eds.), *Mozambique: Towards a people's health service* (pp. 1–25). London: Zed Books.

Wendland, C. L. (2012). Moral maps and medical imaginaries: Clinical tourism at Malawi's college of medicine. *American Anthropologist*, *114*, 108–122. doi:10.1111/j.1548-1433.2011.01400.x

WHO. (2002). *Community home-based care in resource-limited settings: A framework for action*. Geneva: Author.

Participation, decentralisation and déjà vu: Remaking democracy in response to AIDS?

Nora J. Kenworthy

Nursing and Health Studies Program, University of Washington, Bothell, WA, USA

Participation, decentralisation and community partnership have served as prominent motifs and driving philosophies in the global scale-up of HIV programming. Given the fraught histories of these ideas in development studies, it is surprising to encounter their broad appeal as benchmarks and moral practices in global health work. This paper examines three intertwined, government-endorsed projects to deepen democratic processes of HIV policy-making in Lesotho: (1) the 'Gateway Approach' for decentralising and coordinating local HIV responses; (2) the implementation of a community council-driven priority-setting process; and (3) the establishment of community AIDS councils. Taken together, these efforts are striking and well intentioned, but nonetheless struggle in the face of powerful global agendas to establish meaningful practices of participation and decentralisation. Examining these efforts shows that HIV scale-up conveys formidable lessons for citizens about the politics of global health and their place in the world. As global health initiatives continue to remake important dimensions of political functioning, practitioners, agencies and governments implementing similar democratising projects may find the warnings of earlier development critics both useful and necessary.

Introduction

Community participation has been promoted as a cornerstone of HIV scale-up efforts in recipient communities, touted as a strategy that will simultaneously ensure better biomedical outcomes, solidify citizen support of donor and non-governmental organisation (NGO) initiatives, and reinforce the broader development ideals of good governance, civil society and accountability (Bristol-Myers Squibb, 2009; Kapilashrami & Brien, 2013; The Joint United Nations Program on HIV/AIDS (UNAIDS), 2001). With the rapid and unprecedented scale-up of HIV programmes throughout sub-Saharan Africa, a wide range of donors and international partners embraced community partnerships, the support of civil society organisations and celebrations of the 'local' as guiding philosophies and tools for programme implementation (Birdsall & Kelly, 2007; Edström & MacGregor, 2010; Low-Beer, 2010; Parker, 2011). One of the most long-lasting impacts of global HIV scale-up may be the way in which it has elevated the community to holy ground, while also expecting a great deal more labour and responsibility from citizens than ever before.

These moves are not without precedent. Initiatives that push for good governance, decentralisation and participation have fraught histories in Africa. A significant body of literature has documented and critiqued efforts to decentralise governance and increase citizen participation in development and health initiatives during earlier eras (see, for example, Cooke & Kothari, 2001; Peters, 1996; Ribot & Oyono, 2005). Yet among HIV practitioners and institutions, these goals remain largely untarnished, held to be good in and of themselves. Among researchers, such goals are viewed with more scepticism; in particular, a robust literature is now exploring the character and quality of civil society engagement, in addition to the transnational politics that shape much of HIV policy-making (see, for example, Birdsall & Kelly, 2007; Cassidy & Leach, 2009; Kapilashrami & Brien, 2013; Parker, 2011; Swidler, 2009). Far less research, however, has looked in detail at efforts to increase citizen participation and localise priority-setting for HIV (Campbell, Nair, & Maimane, 2007; Paiva, 2003). As I will argue here, some of these efforts capitalise on the broad appeal and early successes of AIDS activism, but supplant oppositional, citizen-driven mobilisations with top-down task-shifting onto already beleaguered communities. Regardless of their varying success, efforts to build participation and decentralise HIV policy-making are a crucial example of the power of scale-up to remake political worlds – involving changes in citizenship roles, perceptions of political functioning, and relations between the public and the institutions involved in global health programming.

During the advent of HIV programme scale-up in Lesotho, the government and its international partners initiated several programmes designed to (1) decentralise HIV decision-making (the 'Gateway Approach'); (2) elevate the role of local representatives in determining HIV priorities (the 'Essential Services Package' [ESP]); and (3) increase citizen participation in policy dialogues (District and Community AIDS Committees). A closer examination of these efforts is valuable – not in order to tell yet another cautionary tale about the challenges of participation, but instead to tease out the complex tensions between genuine, well-intentioned efforts to make HIV initiatives more deliberative and democratic, and neoliberal approaches that treat 'participation' as good behaviour, 'decentralisation' as unfair devolutions of responsibility without rights and 'civil society' as implementing partners (see, for example, Ferguson & Gupta, 2002). Studying Lesotho's efforts to develop more democratic approaches to HIV policy also provides an opportunity to think more broadly about the complex challenges implicit in the relationship between HIV scale-up, political process and citizen subjectivity. Ultimately, HIV initiatives like the ones described here have broad sociopolitical impacts: even when they do not achieve their stated objectives, they convey far-reaching lessons for citizens about forces of political change and the place of participation in political arenas increasingly shaped by the transnational machinations of global health endeavours.

Old dogmas, new tricks

The prominence of activism in the historical narrative of the HIV pandemic is well known. It is a hard-won legacy, forged by patient movements throughout the North and South, whose efforts challenged scientific expertise and bureaucratic irrationality, becoming models for innovative, grassroots struggles across the globe. Activists' efforts ensured that HIV would be seen not just as a pathogenic disease, but a political one (Bayer, 1992; Berkman, Garcia, Munoz Laboy, Paiva, & Parker, 2005; Epstein, 1996; Parker, 2011; Petchesky, 2003). In the global scramble to expand HIV programmes throughout resource-poor countries, however, the activist politics of AIDS ceded ground to expert-driven efforts to 'administer the epidemic' (Parker, 2000), even as activists were finally granted the treatment access they had long fought to secure.

The massive deployment of resources, technocratic expertise and policies, broadly known as 'HIV scale-up', has revived old development dogmas that complicate the activist legacies of previous eras. The past decade has witnessed a consistent grafting of development strategies onto new global health movements. For example, The Paris declaration on Aid Effectiveness emphasises 'inclusive partnerships' (Organisation for Economic Cooperation and Development [OECD], 2008); and the Ouagadougou Declaration on Primary Health Care and Health Systems in Africa, which emerged from the Paris Declaration, places community ownership, participation and partnerships for health as cornerstones of a new African health agenda (Somanje et al., 2010). Drawing on the language of the original 1978 Alma Ata Declaration, Ouagadougou recognises the importance of 'redistributing authority, responsibility, and financial resources' but nevertheless offers little clarification about to whom, or what, this decentralisation should be aimed (Somanje et al., 2010, p. 12). And a 2001 report from the Joint United Nations Program on HIV/AIDS (UNAIDS) defined decentralisation, multisectoralism, and community partnerships as key aspects of a strategic approach for building 'AIDS-competent societies' in recipient states (2001, p. 1). Much of the dialogue around global health governance reiterates these goals in equally vague terms. But decentralisation, partnership and participation are much older tropes: as histories of development show, these goals are not inherent goods. The vague ways in which they are deployed provides fertile ground for a productive confusion that contributes to further disenfranchisement.

Current efforts at decentralisation represent only the most recent resurgence of its popularity as a development strategy. In fact, the modern origins of decentralisation in Africa can be traced to the institutionalisation of 'indirect rule' by colonial administrators, who promoted 'traditional authorities' as a means of ensuring the subjugation of African populations (Mamdani, 1996; Ribot & Oyono, 2005). According to Mbembe (2001), the perverse power of colonialism was 'administered by a decentralised state apparatus – to be precise, by its agents – through specialized institutions, some of recent origin, some indigenous but reshaped for this purpose' (p. 28). One result of such rule was a reinforcement of a '*régime d'exception*' – an institutionalisation of legal exceptionality that buttresses sovereign power (p. 29; see also Agamben, 1998).

Decentralisation regained popularity during the development initiatives of the 1980s and 1990s. In Ferguson's (1994) analysis of a rural development project in Lesotho, decentralisation was implemented as an 'apolitical administrative reform' (p. 133), while development agencies failed to comprehend the bureaucratic structures of the nation state as actual *political* entities. With the advent of structural adjustment programmes in Africa, decentralisation joined efforts to empty out the civil service, shift resources away from social services, derogate responsibility to non-state entities and 'responsibilise' citizens to meet their own needs in the absence of state protection (Ferguson & Gupta, 2002; Pfeiffer & Chapman, 2010). Citing old colonial patterns of subjugation, Ribot and Omoyo (2005) argue that 'today's decentralizations also appear to be proceeding in ways that risk reproducing old patterns of indirect rule: administratively driven local authorities managing people in the name of self-determination' (p. 206). Though often touted as a measure for localising democracy, decentralisation can be acutely depoliticising, remaking the schizophrenic dualities of colonialism, where claims to decentralise rule enshrine the hegemonic power of an illegitimate ruler or set of rules.

Participation also gained popularity in the development movements of the 1970s, particularly as a strategy for subverting the top-down approaches of rural development projects (Chambers, 1992). Subsequent efforts to build participation often ignored the rich political cultures and histories onto which such projects were grafted, and evaluations of 'participation' often reflected the ideologies and political leanings of implementing agencies (Morgan, 1993). When programmes falter, fault is often found with the structure, character or desires of communities. But, as Lynne Morgan (1993) points out, these forms of 'induced' participation can hardly be compared with spontaneous, citizen-driven activism and its outcomes (p. 5). The close kinship between neoliberalism and decentralisation – what Robins (2008, p. 128) calls the 'downsizing neoliberal state's imperatives of governance-at-a-distance' – was promoted by entities such as the World Bank, which embraced strategies like participation in so far as they offered solutions to the 'political market imperfections' that were undermining democratisation initiatives in developing countries (Keefer & Khemani, 2005). Such strategies reconceptualise citizens as conduits of information between rulers and the ruled in a machinery of efficient and cost-effective state functioning that is decidedly apolitical.

HIV scale-up took participation and community empowerment as central principles. Though scholars put forth important efforts advocating for forms of meaningful community participation and examining its challenges in the context of HIV programming that should not be overlooked (Campbell et al., 2007; Paiva, 2003; Robins, 2008; Seeley, Kengeya-Kayondo, & Mulder, 1992), public discourses of 'participation' and 'empowerment' tended to exacerbate the conceptual fuzziness of these terms (Morgan, 1993; Petchesky, 2003). As a result, HIV 'participation' took on discordant meanings: it could equally indicate, for example, putting on a condom, handing out a condom, endorsing the use of condoms among neighbours, or advocating for or against a condom-based prevention strategy with the government. Many programmatic uses still appear to conflate participation as a patient with participation as a citizen, though the postures and purposes of such forms of participation retain fundamental differences.

Scholars writing about biological and therapeutic citizenship trace biopower into new spaces of global health programming, exploring incursions that not only render bodies and the biological as a primary means and object of politics, but become themselves a prevalent and far-reaching form of governance (see, for example, Biehl, 2007; Fullwiley, 2011; Nguyen, 2008). These accounts are rightfully sceptical of empowerment paradigms: Nguyen (2010) adeptly describes the 'confessional technologies' that HIV patients must learn and deploy in order to successfully access treatment. Discourses of empowerment and participation can act as disciplinary forces on patient subjectivities, constraining rather than widening the scope of possible action. Yet for many of my informants in Lesotho, the problem with HIV programming is not that it reaches too far into their lives, but that HIV represents a retreat of the state, its eclipse by NGOs and donors and its absence from public discourse with citizens – even as it became more and more accountable to external partners (see Kenworthy, 2013). Rather than solely examine the politics of HIV at the level of biological intrusions and interventions, it seems essential to examine the influence of HIV scale-up on the agency and subjectivity of citizens and the forms of public life that they value.

Like many countries, Lesotho struggles to reconcile HIV's global activist legacies with its domestic realities – in particular, the predominant logics of good governance and the lack of vibrant public mobilisations for HIV services. The relevance of Lesotho's efforts to build a more decentralised and participatory HIV response, for the purposes of this paper, is not to be found in any overt shortcomings, but in the pitfalls encountered despite genuine intentions to build a deliberative democracy around HIV programming. The initiatives detailed here demonstrate how conceptual tensions in decentralisation and participation became translated into multivalent struggles over political engagement. It is here – at the interface between discourse, policy, practice and citizen lives – that HIV efforts are conveying important lessons to citizens, local governments and ultimately states, about the new political dynamics of a post-scale-up world.

Methods

In 2008, I embarked on a project to better understand the felt impact of scale-up's sociopolitical changes on the lives of Lesotho's citizens, community activists, patients, health workers and policy-makers. A critical, multisited ethnographic approach was used to answer these questions, involving participant observation and qualitative interviewing in social systems surrounding HIV treatment programmes in diverse sites. As part of the project, extended research was conducted with community councils (CCs), community AIDS councillors, NGO representatives, service providers and individuals involved in policy-making. Data from interviews and participant observation was analysed against extensive archival research and policy analysis. In addition to the above, this article draws on an in-depth analysis and compilation of existing evaluations of some of the policy initiatives described here (Chiyoka, 2009; Chiyoka & Hoohle-Nonyana, 2010; UNAIDS & MoLGC, n.d.).

Lesotho: Scale-up amidst scarcity

Like a number of poorer countries in sub-Saharan Africa, Lesotho's scale-up was late coming, rapid and heavily influenced by external partners and policies. Though Lesotho still claims the world's third highest prevalence rate, 93% of all clinics now offer Highly-Active Antiretroviral Treatment (HAART) across all 10 districts (National AIDS Commisssion [NAC], 2011).[1] Despite the influence of external partners in Lesotho's scale-up of HIV programmes, the country is remarkable for its early and on-going efforts to ensure local ownership of programmes and a decentralised process of programme priority-setting. These aspects of Lesotho's early response make its HIV politics particularly interesting as a case study.

By 2003 and early 2004, Lesotho's leaders realised that demonstrations of political commitment were essential to attracting HIV funding (see Gore et al., 2014), and they embarked on a top-down process of building political will. In 2004, the government released a detailed document detailing their vision and plans for scaling up the national response, titled *Turning a Crisis into an Opportunity* (Kimaryo, Okpaku, Githuku-Shongwe, & Feeney, 2004). A strikingly progressive document, it emphasises the importance of a multisectoral, participatory response attentive to structural determinants of HIV risk. The document outlines plans that focus on social and political metamorphoses to ensure a radical transformation of the health sector and HIV response, rather than only discussing the expansion of biomedical programmes. This was followed by the launch of a nation-wide testing campaign that, while controversial (Human Rights Watch, 2008), made Lesotho an ideal site for HIV programme scale-up for two reasons: it was a concrete demonstration of 'political commitment'; and it provided a ready population of already tested patients to enrol for treatment, at a time when agencies had significant concerns about countries' 'absorption capacity' for HIV funds.

These policy developments laid the groundwork for the three highly interrelated initiatives I wish to explore here: (1) The Gateway Approach, an initiative to promote CCs as 'gateways' for coordinating the local HIV response; (2) the creation of specialised

Community and District Council AIDS Committees (CCACs and DCACs) situated within the local government system; and (3) The Essential HIV/AIDS Services Package, an initiative to involve councils in priority-setting processes for the HIV response and to mentor councils in implementing their own HIV/AIDS activities. My intention here is not to provide a thorough evaluation of any of these initiatives, but rather to understand them as a contested policy terrain upon which divergent ideas about governance, participation, decentralisation, accountability, and ultimately, the politics of epidemic response, played out.

The Gateway Approach

In the same year that Lesotho launched its national testing campaign, the government, in partnership with the German Technical Cooperation (GIZ, previously GTZ) and UNAIDS, announced a new initiative called the Gateway Approach.[2] As a formalisation of the plans for a decentralised HIV response outlined in *Turning a crisis into an opportunity*, this strategy announced that communities – through local CCs – would now serve as the 'Gateway to fighting HIV and AIDS' (German Technical Cooperation [GTZ], 2006). In its original form, the Gateway Approach would engage communities in priority-setting processes to determine HIV-related needs and encourage NGOs and citizens alike to view councils as 'gateways' to intervention – arbiters of whether and how programmes should be run, putting community-determined priorities into practice. CCs would emerge as relevant local-level institutions for coordinating the response according to community need. In this sense, the Gateway Approach was a novel and promising strategy: If any country was going to succeed in utilising HIV scale-up to build, rather than to dismantle, democratic participation and civic action, surely Lesotho seemed committed to providing the fertile conditions for such a development. In addition, it seemed to represent an ambitious vision of how HIV scale-up and grassroots democratisation processes could become mutually beneficial.

From its very inception, however, the Gateway Approach was at the mercy of competing visions of what decentralisation and participation might mean in practice – as the following document from the National AIDS Commission (NAC, 2007) makes clear:

> the Gateway Approach will be the main coordination strategy ... whereby the Local Authorities are the gateways in the holistic response against the epidemic within the district coordination mechanism. The goal of the gateway approach [sic] is to provide a platform for all stakeholders including NAC to successfully implement their strategies ... by involving the communities and their representatives right from the inception ... The approach aims to empower and make the local authorities and other local leaders HIV and AIDS competent and to promote a demand-driven support system at local, district and national levels. (p. 2)

Here, the language of a 'demand-driven', 'holistic' response that directly involves communities comes immediately into conflict with a strategy that aims to use local government to 'implement' the 'strategies' of the national government and plans to 'make' communities 'HIV and AIDS competent'. Without a clear vision or any means of monitoring the policy's implementation, it quickly became unclear which way programmes, priorities and empowerment were moving through the 'gateway' – whether from communities towards NGOs, donors and government, or from those institutions into communities.

In practice, many service providers and partners ignored the aims of the Gateway Approach. In an inversion of the policy's original intent, councils and service providers became gatekeepers through which community members had to pass in order to access powerful agencies and donors. Councils struggled to serve as coordinating institutions, having never solidified a role overseeing NGOs, service providers and donors (Chiyoka, 2009, p. 19). 'The roll-out of the Gateway Approach is yet to be fully understood and "accepted" by all players', an official assessment reported, '[as a result], stakeholders continue to implement their interventions with no consultations or communication with the [councils]' (Chiyoka, 2009, p. 19). Councillors with whom I worked more closely agreed that NGOs would sometimes come to meetings and 'announce' their plans, but rarely engage in meaningful consultations. As one representative explained:

> You don't know who is in charge of what. Between the NGOs and the councils, [the councils] are never sure who is responsible because today [the NGO] comes with one guy, and the next time they come with another guy … and there is no follow-up of issues.

Often it seemed that councils themselves were held responsible for the lack of coordination, as government officials blamed councillors' lack of knowledge, training, and 'capacity'. Invocations of councillors' 'ignorance' were common, even from community members. Mme 'Mamaseko, a nurse, explained:

> We know that money has been given to the councils to help us, but the people in the council are old and ignorant, they are not knowledgeable about HIV … They are supposed to be the 'gateway'. We are familiar with the Gateway, we know that we are supposed to do everything through the council, but we struggle to get anything through them.

Mme 'Mamaseko thought the councils lacked 'relevance' and, because of it, suspected they let HIV money 'go back to the politicians' rather than staying in the community where it was needed. Instead of the council coordinating with actors 'above' the community, the community itself 'struggle[s] to get anything through them' that they need to accomplish.

The perceived weakness of councils in the face of NGOs, donors and politicians also made them prone to accusations of corruption. Mme 'Mats'eliso, a support group leader who worked closely with her council, explained that the Gateway Approach was 'not working out. It doesn't work at all. It never worked'. When I asked why, she explained 'the councilors never took it to *the people*. They were supposed … we were expecting them to take it to the village level, but they implemented it for their own good'. Caught between those who orchestrated the HIV response 'up there' and those who were meant to be their constituents 'down here', councils lacked legitimacy but were viewed with distrust by citizens. Yet Mme 'Mat'seliso was also ready to admit that the council simply became 'rubber stamps' on HIV policies handed down by the government, and commented that civil servants and other agencies 'just overpowered them in their own office … [the councillors] don't have their own voice'. Drawing on an interesting dichotomy between what she saw as the expertise of civil servants and NGO workers and the council as community representatives, she explained that, although she blamed the council for its poor implementation, she also understood its hands were tied because of the power differentials between the council and those with whom it was supposed to work:

> They are just keeping quiet, keeping quiet … because they are scared of them [the government, NGOs, and other agencies] … because they are educated and qualified. *But as villages we are appointing [councillors] because of their integrity, not their qualifications.* [emphasis added]

What she highlights is, in fact, a normative disjuncture – between what is of value to communities, and what is prioritised by HIV scale-up.

The Essential HIV/AIDS Services Package

In the year following the launch of the Gateway Approach, CCs across the country were led in an HIV/AIDS priority-setting process referred to as the 'Essential HIV and AIDS Services Package', or more commonly, the ESP. The process was ostensibly designed to decentralise decision-making and priority-setting on HIV to councils, and was spear-headed by UNAIDS, GIZ, the Ministry of Local Government and Chieftainship, and the National AIDS Commission (NAC), with funding from the Global Fund and, later, the World Bank. The initial phase of the project presented councils with five different categories of 'objectives' in the HIV/AIDS response: 'Prevention through change in sexual behaviour'; 'Access to HIV testing and health services'; 'Prevention of mother to child transmission'; 'Orphans and vulnerable children'; and 'Support for people who are HIV-positive' (Ministry of Local Government and Chieftainship [MOLGC] n.d.). Within each category, councils were instructed to select and rank their top three priorities from predetermined lists of possible interventions, which had been drawn from the National Strategic Plan on HIV and AIDS (the priorities and interventions are listed in Table 1). Each council received a handbook describing the possible interventions in more detail, including specific templates for interventions, ideal outcomes and benchmarks for measuring success (MOLGC n.d.).

After CCs chose priorities, they were given small grants with which to implement their selected interventions, a pilot project to test whether councils could effectively manage projects. Some councils successfully carried out small-scale interventions, such as registering needy patients or orphans, coordinating trainings,[3] or organising condom distributions. Most, however, struggled to conceive of and implement interventions that met donor and government expectations. Some ended up giving out funds to needy families, or buying food or transport for sick patients – 'interventions' that seemed reasonable given community needs, but were difficult to justify to donors, or to account for in budgets (Chiyoka, 2009). Despite these many challenges, however, councils reported that the process had made them feel as if they had been granted the legitimacy to talk about HIV. 'Our communities feel for the first time HIV has been brought to their doorstep', one councillor reported, '[we] now know that the prevention of HIV and care for the affected is not [just] the role of NAC' (Chiyoka, 2009, p. 32).

ESP processes have been used by the UN in other countries to help identify health intervention priorities, more often employed by experts as a tool for evaluating cost-effectiveness and comparing interventions to gauge which offer the best impact for the money (Ensor et al., 2002; González-Pier et al., 2006). Even in Lesotho, ESPs have more recently been utilised as a standardised, externally-selected set of primary health services that should be available through community-based health centres, used as a tool by which donors and global health partners measure health system effectiveness. Though the HIV/AIDS ESP in Lesotho allowed councils to select their own priorities, it is difficult to recognise the process as one that democratised priority-setting. Priorities were pre-selected by funders and experts, with implementation strategies also drawn from National Strategic Plans (which, along with other policy planning documents, are notorious for reflecting global priorities). Councillors scoffed at the limited choices they were offered, saying that the process 'could not accommodate some of the issues' that they felt were most important (Chiyoka, 2009, p. 10). Many councils simply listed additional

Table 1.   Ranked HIV priorities from 128 community councils in Lesotho.

HIV priorities from 128 community councils in Lesotho	First priority (%)	Second priority (%)	Third priority (%)
Objective 1: prevention through change in sexual behaviour			
Male-focused discussions	29.6	20.8	8
Facilitation of regular activities for youth such as football, volleyball, dance groups, drama groups and life skills groups	26.4	18.4	22.4
Distribution of male and female condoms and proper usage education	20	20	10.4
Building the capacity of traditional community leaders in HIV and AIDS and in implementing related initiatives	11.2	14.4	18.4
Parent involvement in shaping the behaviour of children on HIV and AIDS related issues	8	15.2	8.8
Registration of initiation schools and facilitating adherence to best practices within the schools	4	8	18.4
Building the capacity of church leaders in HIV and AIDS and in implementing related initiatives	.8	2.4	8.8
Facilitating the capacity building of business leaders in HIV and AIDS and in the implementation of related activities	0	1.6	4
Objective 2: access to HIV testing and health services			
Support mechanism for critical patients to [access] hospital/health facility (council to agree on the mechanisms)	25.6	27.2	17.6
Registration of chronically ill patients	24.8	20	14.4
Facilitate and ensure provision of HBC supplies and gloves and limited training to registered HBC groups	24	20.8	27.2
Registration of home-based care (HBC) support groups	9.6	11.2	11.2
Facilitate and ensure training of at least one health facility worker per facility to do HIV counselling and testing	8.8	8.8	12
Facilitate provision of testing kits to trained community HIV&AIDS counsellors	7.2	12	11.2
Advocacy for provider-initiated testing at health care facilities	0	0.8	4
Objective 3: prevention of mother-to-child transmission			
Provide training to at least on health facility worker per facility to do PMTCT and testing and ART/PEP support	36	18.4	16
Train CHWs to test and support prevention of mother-to-child transmission	33.6	28.8	24
Establish referral system for emergency delivery for mothers	16	29.6	36.8
Conduct door-to-door/community education campaigns and male involvement on PMTCT + exclusive breastfeeding	16	22.4	21.6
Objective 4: orphans and vulnerable children			
Registration of OVC	38.4	17.6	8
Ensure that registered orphans and OVCs have access to basic services such as education, nutrition and food security and health care	33.6	37.6	20.8
Capacitate and empower councilors, chiefs and community members in protection of OVC and ensure access to required services	16	26.4	45.6
Facilitate counselling services for orphans and OVC including support/play therapy	12.8	16.8	24.8

Table 1 (*Continued*)

HIV priorities from 128 community councils in Lesotho	First priority (%)	Second priority (%)	Third priority (%)
Objective 5: support for people who are HIV+			
Sponsoring HIV+ facilitators to do door-to-door, community gatherings and small group meetings /speeches/discussions on living positively with HIV/AIDS, stigma and discrimination	30.4	32	24
Placement of one 'expert' or HIV+ patient at each health facility	27.2	14.4	14.4

Note: Percentages of councils ranking each priority as primary, secondary, or tertiary within five categories of objectives.

interventions that they felt were equally important, and these self-chosen priorities show striking patterns of similarity, reflecting pressing and under-acknowledged needs faced by communities: acute food insecurity; a concern about vulnerable populations overlooked by formulaic HIV policies (like 'herdboys'[4]); and educational and training needs for groups and individuals less often reached with HIV messaging (UNAIDS & MoLGC n.d.). These priorities are outlined in Table 2.

In addition, some of the pre-determined interventions most commonly selected by councils reflected broader gaps and deficits in the health system, such as mechanisms for transporting critically ill patients, and the need for additional health worker training (see Table 1). Unfortunately, these priorities, though important to councils, were later dismissed by national stakeholders and the ESP organisers as 'not within the scope of [Community Council] work and therefore ill-advised' (Chiyoka, 2009, p. 23). It was 'generally agreed' that council-selected priorities were 'not … entirely realistic [or] sustainable', as they were the responsibility of the Ministry of Health (Chiyoka, 2009). As a result, the ESP process implicitly taught councils that such priorities were out of reach, and that advocating for them was beyond their mandate. It subtly reinforced their

Table 2. Additional community council HIV priorities.

Additional community council HIV priorities	Number of councils listing priority
HIV education needs of special groups	99
Herdboys	38
Traditional healers	15
Support groups	13
Public servants (teachers, council, police)	12
Elderly	11
Disabled	10
Agricultural/nutritional needs of patients, orphans, affected families	55
Income generation or vocational training for vulnerable – especially orphans	14
Need for first aid kits/gloves in homes of sick and public places	10
Develop traditional/herbal medicines to treat HIV	5
Human rights and gender equality campaigns	4
Other improvements in clinic service/infrastructure	4
Need to train men in home-based care	2

subordinate position, and conveyed that the scope of councils' influence and their realm for activism was highly constrained.

Ultimately, donors baulked at renewing the council grants for priority implementation, in part because financial accounting had been so poor. Accusations of corruption and mismanagement were rampant. Those in government took this as evidence that future projects should not solicit community leadership, an observation that would further solidify centralised, expert-driven policy-making. One civil servant involved in the project suggested, upon reflecting on the outcomes of the ESP, that efforts be made to replace currently elected councillors with retired Members of Parliament (MPs) and civil servants who had the expertise he felt was necessary to make councils effective as policy-makers. Such sentiments reveal on-going tensions between participatory approaches as moral practice, and pragmatic realisations that technocratic expertise and non-democratic process is the most efficient means by which to achieve the goals of HIV scale-up.

Citizens were also sceptical of the results of this democratic experiment. Expectations were high, and many citizens presumed that councils had received large grants for implementation; in reality, councils were working with micro-grants of a few thousand dollars, and within the constraints of pre-determined interventions. In a dynamic that I would see repeated over and over again within communities when one institution or organisation received funding support, the perceived failure of the council to establish meaningful improvement opened up social fissures fuelled by distrust, disappointment and suspicions of corruption, as is discussed below.[5]

Community and district AIDS councils

Following the ESP, AIDS committees were established in conjunction with councils at district and community levels. By the end of 2010 it was reported by NAC that almost 96% of CCACs were functional (NAC, 2007, p. 12). The purpose of this initiative was to establish a local, standing body responsible for coordinating the HIV response in communities. It was hoped that these bodies, whose representatives were drawn from many sectors and groups relevant to the HIV response (clinicians, PLWHA representatives, traditional healers, support group representatives, expert patients) would be more knowledgeable about HIV and better able to coordinate with NGOs, clinics and NAC, to continue working on the priorities set forth in the ESPs. Trained coordinators were also deployed to all districts as Community Council Support Persons (CCSPs) to help build skills and capacity among committees.

In 2010, I attended a national meeting to assess the implementation of CCACs and DCACs; in attendance were committee members and councillors from across the country. Though members were enthusiastic about their positions and expressed sincere commitments to addressing HIV in their communities, the general outlook was far from positive. Members were not clear on their roles or responsibilities, lacked basic knowledge about HIV despite training efforts, and repeatedly insisted that they had no idea how to fulfil roles as 'coordinators' of the response. In discussions at the meeting, it emerged that many communities perceived the committees as hurriedly put together, with little forethought about the selection of representatives. Both committee members and their intended constituents were unaware of the purpose of their role as representatives. One meeting attendee explained:

> I don't even know where the idea itself came from that such committees should be established … They went to the clinic and they told the nurse, 'we are establishing a

committee of the council, we need a person living with HIV, can you give us someone living with HIV?' … Even the nurse did not know what that person was going to do on the committee …The only thing they [said] is that they are establishing a committee, but it wasn't clear what this committee would be working on … or what their role would be on the committee.

Thus, while hoping to bring democratic decision-making and participatory processes to a local level, AIDS committees' confusion about their roles and mission, and their token representation of ill-defined interest groups, further muddied the local political terrain of HIV and AIDS responses.

Though AIDS committees were intended to bolster the coordination between local government, service providers, citizens and national government, official documents explaining their mandate emphasised localised implementation. They would design and carry out small projects, collect data, submit reports on activities to national entities, raise and budget funding, and develop and carry out monitoring and evaluation activities in their areas (Chiyoka & Hoohle-Nonyana, 2010). Not surprisingly, committees lacked the specialised skills necessary to do much of this work, despite well-intentioned training and capacity-building efforts. But CCSPs and other policy-makers tended to blame members' lack of ability on 'illiteracy', 'ignorance' and poor education among members, even though Lesotho has very high literacy rates.

Despite these limitations, committee members remained committed to fulfilling their 'advocacy' and 'coordination' roles by indexing HIV needs in their communities and trying to address those needs with limited support. Though many remained unaware of strategies for engaging in law or policy reform, and felt this was not a legitimate part of their duties, members were very active in mobilising support for needy patients from neighbours and other community members. Without training on how to solicit funding or support from donors and NGOs, and without a clear mandate for working with such entities, councillors and committee members tended to appeal primarily to constituents for financial assistance during funerals, school meetings, *pitsos* (community meetings called by the chief) and church services.

In spite of their significant efforts, DCACs and CCACs remained marginal players in HIV efforts, often serving as labour for implementations in which they had little voice, but still being held accountable by communities for HIV outcomes. As one example of the double bind they occupied, NGOs would frequently approach the council or its committees, asking them to provide lists of potential beneficiaries in the community – orphans and vulnerable children (OVCs), caretakers, or sick patients – to whom they could provide support. So they solicited the help of support groups and volunteers to go through villages collecting names, talking to those in need of assistance. Names would be written down, needs catalogued. And expectations of future assistance were reasonable. Many times these names would be turned into data that made its way into grants or requests for funding – if assistance materialised, it frequently appeared years later, and was disbursed along the lines of revised priorities. For those who collected the names, it seemed a ruse: in response to one NGO that repeatedly requested information on OVCs, a community leader explained, 'We keep calling the *pitsos*, calling the children and they take their names, but they are just toying with the orphans…we are now so discouraged'. For those who hoped to receive services, it was not a stretch of the imagination to assume that their councillors had failed them, or pocketed the assistance that never seemed to materialise. 'They promised us, as people living with HIV', one patient said, distraught, after another NGO's disappearance, 'that we would be given money … we felt that maybe this disease of ours was important ... we were told ... they could help us to get payments. And they *lied*'. In this way, initiatives that purport to decentralise and build partnership can in fact undermine community leaders' standing and legitimacy, while making them increasingly accountable to external partners or national priorities rather than their own constituents.

Negotiating the right to govern

As institutions caught between NGOs, funders, initiatives and recipient communities, CCs and AIDS committees occupy an awkward position, lacking the power to adequately influence responses to the epidemic, but remaining an important symbol of partnership for NGOs and donors. In observing the on-going relations between councils and NGOs, government officials, funders and clinic staff, it became clear that councils were most often used to endorse new or existing programmes with the community, to identify and triage potential recipients in their local areas and to organise *pitsos* so NGOs could recruit individuals for new programmes, disseminate information, or conduct educational initiatives. It was not lost on Lesotho's citizens that the original intent of the Gateway Approach was being inverted. As early as 2006, when Bill and Melinda Gates visited Lesotho, a local newspaper printed a picture of the couple with the caption, 'The Gateway to treatment', a play on their name that emphasised donors' real influence over HIV programming (Lekhetho, 2006).

Even though many donors and NGOs seem extremely sincere in their commitment to community partnerships, and view engagement with communities as a healthy democratic alternative to working with (at times) autocratic governments, the lived experience of citizens, committee members and councillors tends to be far different. Exchanges with NGOs were perceived as unequal, stressful and, at times, dishonest. Councillors and citizens reported that 'these people' just came and went, 'disappearing' for long periods of time. As described above, the constant movement of NGOs and programmes in and out of council areas causes considerable problems for communication and mutual accountability. When questions or problems arose, representatives had no one they could contact, no means of getting in touch with the programme's managers. They were also unable to follow-up with programmes or initiatives that had been promised but had not materialised.

As one example, while I was working in a peri-urban clinic, some impoverished patients were on an NGO-supported food aid programme. One month, the food aid stopped suddenly; patients went hungry, and faced the terror of unexpected shortages. Patients continued to come to the clinic each month, lining up to wait for food to be delivered; each month they left disappointed and without answers. Clinic workers and local councillors were unable to help, as they themselves did not know how to contact the NGO, and noted that even from month to month different workers would deliver the food. As patients watched the inaction of their local leaders, frustration mounted and rumours of theft or corruption filtered through social networks. Many months later, I heard it mentioned at a national policy meeting that the programme had ended, having only had temporary funding for food packages. There are multiple lessons here: as the council's true powerlessness was revealed, citizen trust waned and perceived corruption mounted. The tendency of external NGOs and partners to always seem as if they have 'disappeared' is significant for citizen subjectivities, as is their perceived inaccessibility. Finally, the temporality of many programmes – their shifting priorities, and the overlapping and competing mandates of different NGOs – poses acute challenges for accountability to citizens.

The ease with which projects or NGOs can usurp the power of councils is also striking, even when councillors clearly understand their mandates. As I sat with one council over a period of months, I watched in shock as it struggled to regain legitimacy with citizens after an American volunteer working with a nearby NGO reappointed the representatives of a local political committee, and arbitrarily imposed and collected a head tax to pay for one of the NGO projects (see Kenworthy, 2013). More often, however, NGOs in the towns in which I worked played a more proximate role to the communal tensions they left in their wake. By elevating councils to positions of responsibility without altering the cultures of practice through which organisations and donors carry out projects creates acute political problems at village and communal levels. In doing so, projects intended to improve participation and decentralise democratic practice end up incrementally eroding the very bedrock of political society and communal trust.

Implications for the future

Architects of the programmes I discuss here might be tempted to fix such problems by further clarifying council and committee mandates or providing additional training. To do so, however, ignores the deeply fraught histories of ill-defined strategies for improved governance. As conceived and carried out in the context of Lesotho's scale-up, such strategies deploy a conceptual fuzziness from which donors and national governments benefit, even when they fail to achieve their stated objectives. Despite common patterns of resistance to decentralisation efforts among mid-level bureaucrats, national leaders can see considerable benefits from such schemes. While they retain unquestionable power over budgets and policy development, decentralisation and participation schemes allow leaders to shift responsibility for implementation to local entities. For communities, participation comes with significant and unexpected costs, as they may find themselves less able to hold government accountable for lacking services, and find that their own 'ignorance' is blamed for poor outcomes. As outcomes are increasingly tied to the development of so-called 'HIV competent societies' in Lesotho, it is the presumed incompetence of citizens that offers a scapegoat for donors and governments alike when programmes do not succeed. Meanwhile, donors and NGOs continue promoting a strategy that is seen as a moral practice in global health efforts, such that participatory approaches provide positive outcomes even when more objective measures of results are remarkably poor.

As particularly ahistorical endeavours, global health projects take up the mantels of participation, decentralisation and community partnership with little heed for the fraught histories of these approaches. Yet those who have studied development and its various reincarnations must feel a keen sense of déjà vu. In a seminal article on the discourses of development, Hintjens (1999) argues that 'in recycling the language of grassroots social movements, aid agencies have jettisoned most of the radical practices associated with such language in particular settings' (p. 385). The appropriation of democratic sentiments by international agencies and campaigns masks what is often an entrenched reticence to cede power to citizens in recipient states – or even, for that matter, to view them as citizens, rather than 'participants'. As Sarah White (1996) argues in her critique of participation in development projects, participatory approaches 'may be the means through which existing power relations are entrenched and reproduced' (p. 6). Other critics go so far as to call participation a 'new tyranny' (Cooke & Kothari, 2001). Indeed, the conceptual meanings of these terms were emptied out long before global health embraced them. They were then deployed in the service of global and programmatic goals: as Ribot and Oyomo (2005) write, in Africa 'public and private are conflated by many practitioners who believe that democracy and decentralization are about letting anyone who is local make decisions and by believing that NGOs and other community groups represent the public' (p. 208).

Given the political history of HIV – and its legacies of engaged, even transformative activism – the appropriation of the language of deliberative, decentralised democracy by powerful donors, national governments and transnational NGOs has been especially insidious. What is enlightening about the efforts described here is that even very well-meaning intentions to deepen democratic processes in HIV programming were under-mined when orchestrated from above, in a country without a vibrant activist history, and amidst a broader political environment dominated by powerful HIV institutions and policies.

HIV scale-up efforts, and now, global health programmes, constitute powerful social forces within recipient countries. One of the lasting legacies of HIV scale-up may be what it teaches citizens and communities about the roles they can and cannot play in both domestic and international politics. If the experiences of citizens with the 'democratising' projects described above are any indicators, it is likely that citizens are not fooled by the language of participation, decentralisation and community partnership when it does not translate into meaningful – and more equal – roles in global health planning. Though democracy has come to be viewed with increasing suspicion (both among social theorists and Lesotho's citizens), wholly dispensing with initiatives that attempt to deepen democratic participation may be far too drastic. To do so would be to ignore the powerful desires of citizens in places like Lesotho to have more, rather than less, of a voice in policy decisions. But we cannot expect more equitable participation and policy-making to spontaneously spring forth from citizens or 'the community' in Africa's recipient states, because they are informed by policy that they are empowered. Instead, we must expect more equitable means and measures of practicing global health from powerful donors, NGOs, bilateral funding institutions and international organisations. Rather than speak about democracy, we must speak about power: the fix will arise not from changes or clarifications of procedural rules or technical mandates, but out of the recognition of truly undemocratic inequities in global health practice. To continue to use the language of democratisation in initiatives that fail to address fundamental inequities between communities and institutions is to conceal the undemocratic tendencies in largely well meaning global health approaches.

Acknowledgements

I am most grateful to numerous colleagues and informants in Lesotho who allowed me to access data, attend meetings, and sit in on council proceedings. Earlier versions of this benefitted from the feedback and input of Richard Parker, Ron Bayer, Mamadou Diouf, Kim Hopper, and Rosalind Petchesky, as well as two anonymous reviewers. I would like to thank the Lesotho Ministry of Health and Social Welfare for research clearance, and the National University of Lesotho for research support.

Funding

This material is based upon work supported by the National Science Foundation under [Grant No. 1024097], the US Fulbright IIE program, the American Association of University Women American Fellowship, and the Leitner Family Foundation.

Notes

1. Unfortunately, <70% of those in need of HAART were able to access it in 2010, and further expansion has been stymied by funding shortfalls (Médecins Sans Frontières, 2011; NAC, 2010).
2. In Sesotho, the Gateway Approach is often referred to as *Khoro*, which means an entrance, or a mountain pass.
3. Many trainings were, sadly, implemented by hiring Ministry of Health officials to come speak to communities or councils at exorbitant rates. For some councils, this took up much of their budget.
4. Herdboys are young men – some as young as 8 or 9 – who spend long periods of time tending livestock away from home, with little access to education or services.
5. Similar patterns of social fissure in Lesotho are observed by Turkon (2008), Coplan (1994), and perhaps most prominently, Ferguson (1994).

References

Agamben, G. (1998). *Homo sacer: Sovereign power and bare life*. Stanford, CA: Stanford University Press.
Bayer, R. (1992). *AIDS in the industrialized democracies: Passions, politics, and policies*. New Brunswick, NJ: Rutgers University Press.
Berkman, A., Garcia, J., Munoz Laboy, M., Paiva, V., & Parker, R. (2005). A critical analysis of the Brazilian response to HIV/AIDS: Lessons learned for controlling and mitigating the epidemic in developing countries. *American Journal of Public Health, 95*, 1162–1172. doi:10.2105/AJPH.2004.054593
Biehl, J. (2007). *Will to live: AIDS therapies and the politics of survival*. Princeton, NJ: Princeton University Press.
Birdsall, K., & Kelly, K. (2007). *Pioneers, partners, providers: The dynamics of civil society and AIDS funding in southern Africa*. Johannesburg: CADRE/OSISA.
Bristol-Myers Squibb. (2009). *Secure the future manual: Seven steps to involve the community in HIV/AIDS treatment support programmes*. New York, NY: Author.
Campbell, C., Nair, Y., & Maimane, S. (2007). Building contexts that support effective community responses to HIV/AIDS: A South African case study. *American Journal of Community Psychology, 39*, 347–363. doi:10.1007/s10464-007-9116-1
Cassidy, R., & Leach, M. (2009). *AIDS, citizenship and global funding: A Gambian case study*. [Institute of Development Studies Working Paper No. 325]. Brighton: University of Sussex.
Chambers, R. (1992). *Rural appraisal: Rapid, relaxed and participatory*. [Institute for Development Studies Discussion Paper No. 311]. Brighton: University of Sussex.
Chiyoka, W. (2009). *External review of the essential HIV & AIDS services package*. Maseru: National AIDS Commission and Ministry of Local Government and Chieftainship.
Chiyoka, W., & Hoohle-Nonyana, N. (2010). *Capacity assessment report for District AIDS Committees (DACs) and Community Council AIDS Committees (CCACs)*. Maseru, Lesotho: Government of Lesotho and National AIDS Commission.
Cooke, B., & Kothari, U. (Eds.). (2001). *Participation: The new tyranny*? New York, NY: Zed Books.
Coplan, D. B. (1994). *In the time of cannibals: The word music of South Africa's Basotho migrants*. Chicago, IL: University of Chicago Press.
Edström, J., & MacGregor, H. (2010). The pipers call the tunes in global aid for AIDS: The global financial architecture for HIV funding as seen by local stakeholders in Kenya, Malawi and Zambia. *Global Health Governance, 4*(1), 1–12.
Ensor, T., Dave-Sen, P., Ali, L., Hossain, A., Begum, S. A., & Moral, H. (2002). Do essential service packages benefit the poor? Preliminary evidence from Bangladesh. *Health Policy and Planning, 17*, 247–56. doi:10.1093/heapol/17.3.247

Epstein, S. (1996). *Impure science: AIDS, activism, and the politics of knowledge*. Berkeley, CA: University of California Press.

Ferguson, J. (1994). *The anti-politics machine: 'Development,' depoliticization, and bureaucratic power in Lesotho*. Minneapolis, MN: University of Minnesota Press.

Ferguson, J., & Gupta, A. (2002). Spatializing states: Toward an ethnography of neoliberal governmentality. *American Ethnologist*, *29*, 981–1002. doi:10.1525/ae.2002.29.4.981

Fullwiley, D. (2011). *The enculturated gene: Sickle cell health politics and biological difference in West Africa*. Princeton, NJ: Princeton University Press.

German Technical Cooperation. (2006). *The gateway approach: Mainstreaming HIV and AIDS using local authorities*. Maseru, Lesotho: Author.

González-Pier, E., Gutiérrez-Delgado, C., Stevens, G., Barraza-Lloréns, M., Porras-Condey, R., Carvalho, N., ... Salomon, J. A. (2006). Priority setting for health interventions in Mexico's System of Social Protection in Health. *Lancet*, *368*, 1608–1618. doi:10.1016/S0140-6736(06)69567-6

Gore, R. J., Fox, A. M., Goldberg, A. B., & Bärnighausen, T. (2014). Bringing the state back in: Understanding and validating measures of governments' political commitment to HIV. *Global Public Health*. Advance online publication. doi:10.1080/17441692.2014.881523

Hintjens, H. (1999). The emperor's new clothes: A moral tale for development experts? *Development in Practice*, *9*, 382–395. doi:10.1080/09614529952873

Human Rights Watch. (2008). *A testing challenge: The experience of Lesotho's universal HIV counseling and testing campaign*. New York, NY: Human Rights Watch and Aids and Rights Alliance for Southern Africa.

Kapilashrami, A., & Brien, O. O. (2013). The global fund and the re-configuration and re-emergence of 'civil society': Widening or closing the democratic deficit? *Global Public Health*, *7*, 437–451. doi:10.1080/17441692.2011.649043

Keefer, P., & Khemani, S. (2005). Democracy, public expenditures and the poor. *The World Bank Research Observer*, *20*(1), 1–27. doi:10.1093/wbro/lki002

Kenworthy, N. J. (2013). *What only heaven hears: citizens and the state in the wake of HIV scale-up in Lesotho* (Doctoral dissertation). Columbia University, New York.

Kimaryo, S. S., Okpaku, J. O., Githuku-Shongwe, A., & Feeney, J. (2004). *Turning a crisis into an opportunity: Strategies for scaling up the national response to the HIV/AIDS pandemic in Lesotho*. New Rochelle, NY: Third Press.

Lekhetho, N. (2006, July 21). Billionaire's boost in drive against Aids. *Public Eye*, p. 1. Maseru, Lesotho.

Low-Beer, D. (2010). Social capital and effective HIV prevention: Community responses. *Global Health Governance*, *4*(1), 1–18.

Mamdani, M. (1996). *citizen and subject: Contemporary Africa and the legacy of late colonialism*. Princeton, NJ: Princeton University Press.

Mbembe, A. (2001). *On the postcolony*. Berkeley: University of California Press.

Médecins Sans Frontières. (2011, December). *Reversing HIV/AIDS? How advances are being held back by funding shortages*. Médecins Sans Frontières Briefing Note, Paris.

Ministry of Local Government and Chieftainship. (n.d.). *Guidelines for implementation of interventions in the Essential HIV and AIDS Services Package*. Lesotho: Author, pp. 1–44.

Morgan, L. M. (1993). *Community participation in health: The politics of primary care in Costa Rica*. New York, NY: Cambridge University Press.

National AIDS Commission. (2007). *Coordination framework for the national response to HIV and AIDS*. Maseru, Lesotho: Author.

National AIDS Commission. (2010). *UNGASS country report, Lesotho: Status of the national response to the 2001 Declaration of Commitment on HIV and AIDS*. Maseru, Lesotho: Author.

National AIDS Commission. (2011). *Report on the national response to HIV and AIDS*. Maseru, Lesotho: Author.

Nguyen, V.-K. (2008). Antiretroviral globalism, biopolitics, and therapeutic citizenship. In S. J. Collier & A. Ong (Eds.), *Global assemblages: Technology, politics and ethics as anthropological problems* (pp. 124–144). Malden, MA: Blackwell.

Nguyen, V.-K. (2010). *The republic of therapy: Triage and sovereignty in West Africa's time of AIDS*. Durham, NC: Duke University Press.

Organization for Economic Cooperation and Development. (2008). *The Paris declaration on aid effectiveness and the Accra agenda for action*. Paris: Author.

Paiva, V. (2003). Beyond magic solutions: Prevention of HIV and AIDS as a process of 'psychosocial emancipation'. *Interface*, *6*(11), 25–38. doi:10.1590/S1414-32832002000200003

Parker, R. G. (2000). Administering the epidemic: HIV/AIDS policy, models of development, and international health. In L. Whiteford & L. Manderson (Eds.), *Global health policy, local realities: The fallacy of the level playing field* (pp. 39–56). Boulder, CO: Lynne Rienner.

Parker, R. G. (2011). Grassroots activism, civil society mobilization, and the politics of the global HIV/AIDS epidemic. *Brown Journal of World Affairs*, *17*(2), 21–37.

Petchesky, R. (2003). *Global prescriptions: Gendering health and human rights*. New York, NY: Zed Books.

Peters, P. (1996). 'Who's local here?': The politics of participation in development. *Cultural Survival Quarterly*, *20*(3), 22.

Pfeiffer, J., & Chapman, R. (2010). Anthropological perspectives on structural adjustment and public health. *Annual Review of Anthropology*, *39*(1), 149–165. doi:10.1146/annurev. anthro.012809.105101

Ribot, J. C., & Oyono, P. R. (2005). The politics of decentralization. In B. Wisner, C. Toulmin, & R. Chitiga (Eds.), *Towards a new map of Africa* (pp. 205–228). London: Routledge.

Robins, S. (2008). *From revolution to rights in South Africa: Social movements, NGOs & popular politics after apartheid*. Rochester, NY: James Currey.

Seeley, J. A., Kengeya-Kayondo, J. F., & Mulder, D. W. (1992). Community-based HIV/AIDS research—whither community participation? Unsolved problems in a research programme in rural Uganda. *Social Science & Medicine*, *34*, 1089–1095. doi:10.1016/0277-9536(92)90282-U

Somanje, H., Kirigia, J. M., Nyoni, J., Bessaoud, K., Trapsida, J., Ndihokubwayo, J. B., … Sambo, L.. (2010). The Ouagadougou declaration on primary health care and health systems in Africa: Achieving better health for Africa in the new millennium. *The African Health Monitor*, *12*, 11–21.

Swidler, A. (2009). Dialectics of patronage: Logics of accountability at the African AIDS – NGO interface. In D. C. Hammack & S. Heydenmann (Eds.), *Globalization, philanthropy and civil society* (pp. 192–220). Bloomington, IN: Indiana University Press.

Turkon, D. (2008). Commoners, kings, and subaltern: Political factionalism and structured inequality in Lesotho. *Political and Legal Anthropology Review*, *31*, 203–223. doi:10.1111/ j.1555-2934.2008.00022.x.Page

UNAIDS. (2001). *Local responses to HIV/AIDS: A strategic approach toward an AIDS-competent society*. Geneva: Author.

UNAIDS, & MoLGC. (n.d.). *Community council plans, essential HIV and AIDS services package*. Maseru, Lesotho: MoLGC.

White, S. C. (1996). Depoliticising development: The uses and abuses of participation. *Development in Practice*, *6*(1), 6–15. doi:10.1080/0961452961000157564

Elusive accountabilities in the HIV scale-up: 'Ownership' as a functional tautology

Daniel E. Esser

School of International Service, American University, Washington, DC, USA

Mounting concerns over aid effectiveness have rendered 'ownership' a central concept in the vocabulary of development assistance for health (DAH). The article investigates the application of both 'national ownership' and 'country ownership' in the broader development discourse as well as more specifically in the context of internationally funded HIV/AIDS interventions. Based on comprehensive literature reviews, the research uncovers a multiplicity of definitions, most of which either divert from or plainly contradict the concept's original meaning and intent. During the last 10 years in particular, it appears that both public and private donors have advocated for greater 'ownership' by recipient governments and countries to hedge their own political risk rather than to work towards greater inclusion of the latter in agenda-setting and programming. Such politically driven semantic dynamics suggest that the concept's salience is not merely a discursive reflection of globally skewed power relations in DAH but a deliberate exercise in limiting donors' accountabilities. At the same time, the research also finds evidence that this conceptual contortion frames current global public health scholarship, thus adding further urgency to the need to critically re-evaluate the international political economy of global public health from a discursive perspective.

Introduction

Throughout the past two decades, the separate but often interchangeably used concepts of 'national ownership' and 'country ownership' have become essential 'buzzwords and fuzzwords' (Cornwall & Eade, 2010) in international development discourse. By signing the 2005 Paris Declaration for Aid Effectiveness, donor countries converged on the promotion of 'ownership' of policies and programmes by recipient country governments as a central component of a continuously emerging aid effectiveness paradigm (de Renzio, Whitfield, & Bergamaschi, 2008). Notably, this convergence happened despite 'no consensus on just how broad ownership needs to be (or ought to be)' (Best, 2007, p. 480) in a given recipient country, as well as concerns that it 'is obviously not a scientific concept' (Booth, 2012, p. 538). Indeed, some analysts have gone as far as labelling ownership 'an article of faith' (Riddell, 2007, p. 370) and a 'donor obsession' (McKinley, 2008, p. 95). Development assistance for health (DAH), an increasingly well-funded sector of international development, has been no exception. Although in

2011, DAH rose 'at a slower rate than before the [global] recession' (Institute for Health Metrics and Evaluation [IHME], 2011, p. 9), it 'has been sustained at levels of spending that would have been inconceivable a decade ago' (IHME, 2012, p. 9). Against the backdrop of this groundswell of international resources to tackle health-related challenges, the notion of 'ownership' features prominently in the strategies of both public and private donors aiming to help curb the spread of AIDS and create better treatment options for those living with HIV in the global South. Yet, even though the theoretical case for 'ownership' derived from principal-agency theory is compelling (e.g., Khan & Sharma, 2003), attempts to empirically investigate its practical relevance for achieving more efficient and effective DAH have been hindered by the aforementioned conceptual ambiguity. A problem first pointed to in the late 1990s (e.g., Leandro, Schafer & Frontini, 1999), numerous scholars and donor agencies have since proposed supposedly broadly applicable definitions; however, none have gained traction. Instead, a cacophony of claims asserting the importance of 'ownership' has persisted in parallel with a multiplicity of conceptualisations, so much so that Buiter (2007) urged scholars and practitioners to drop the term from their vocabulary altogether. Indeed, the discourse analysis of a comprehensive sample of relevant sources carried out in this article will demonstrate that assertions of its importance have been based almost exclusively on either theoretical or normative arguments. Sources that do analyse qualitative data from specific settings suggest that purported observations of increased 'ownership' cannot, in fact, be equated with real shifts in political leverage from donors towards recipients. Despite its definitional deficiency and the scarcity of replicable empirical studies which, at least in part, results from it, why has 'ownership' become such a salient concept?

This article examines the underlying causes of the term's rise to prominence. It hypothesises that the absence of conceptual clarity is a functional component of the contemporary international political economy of DAH, brought about neither by deliberate collusion among donors (e.g., conspiracy) nor happenstance but rather as a rational outcome of competing interests amid skewed bargaining positions favouring donors. The ensuing investigation treats the HIV scale-up – 'a game changer that has irreversibly changed perceptions of and approaches to global health', according to De Cock, El-Sadr, and Ghebreyesus (2011, p. S61) – as a case study to illustrate the logic at play, both internationally and within countries. Based on comprehensive reviews of the literature on 'ownership' in international development discourse and specifically in the context of the HIV scale-up of the past decade, the article demonstrates how different conceptualisations of 'ownership' have continuously reframed policies, programming and increasingly global public health scholarship since the early 1990s. The article offers reflections on the utility and apparent deliberateness of donors rallying around an ostensibly insubstantial concept and concludes that the latter's salience is not only a reflection of power relations in contemporary DAH but, in fact, an ongoing exercise to limit donors' accountabilities internationally and, in the case of public agencies, also nationally.

Method

Literature on 'ownership' in international development discourse was reviewed based on previous research including – but not limited to – scholarship by influential authors on this topic, such as de Renzio (2006), Best (2007), Mawdsley (2007), Cornwall and Eade (2010), Eyben (2010) and Booth (2011, 2012). A more targeted search for relevant literature on 'national ownership' and 'country ownership' in the context of HIV/AIDS programming was then carried out by entering three combined search terms into seven electronic databases, listed here in alphabetical order: Cambridge Journals Online, IngentaConnect, Oxford University Press Journals, ProQuest Research Library, Wiley Interscience, ScienceDirect, and Taylor & Francis Group Journals Online. The three combined search terms were 'HIV' AND 'ownership', 'HIV' AND 'national ownership' and 'HIV' AND 'country ownership'. The stopping point for each search in each database was two results pages (with 10 results displayed per page) after the last relevant hit had been identified. This approach rendered a total of 54 scholarly articles published between 1999 and 2013 classified as relevant. Following a closer reading of all sources included in the sample, four of these 54 articles were subsequently dropped due to insufficient relevance.

Emergence and gradual depoliticisation of 'ownership' since 1992

The term 'national ownership' can be traced back to literature from the early 1990s on education in the context of international development. Kenneth King (1992) noted that there had been a trend in this field to favour those education policies over donor-dictated projects that were 'sustainable, equitable, locally owned and executed, and supportive of good policies in the education sector as a whole'. He went on to predict 'that both the projects and the policies need to be nationally owned. Which means, ideally, conceptualised, costed and executed nationally. Not just agreed to and tolerated, as perhaps happened with a number of earlier aid projects'. 'Ownership' in his view thus denoted a lead role for implementing countries throughout both programming and project cycles. A report authored later in the same year under the leadership of Gerry Helleiner (1992) similarly promotes 'ownership' of development initiatives by recipient govern-ments, declaring that the relative influence of the International Monetary Fund (IMF) and World Bank on African programmes had grown too large. In a 1995 report (Helleiner, Killick, Lipumba, Ndulu, & Svendsen, 1995), Helleiner and colleagues offered several concrete recommendations for how to translate the concept into aid practice, specifically to the case of Tanzania. For instance, they defined 'national ownership' as the recipient government's ability to control the administration, operations and strategies of develop-ment programmes. They also viewed outside technical assistance as an imposition and called on donors to cease practices that undermine the public control of operations. According to the report (p. 29), 'national ownership' also comprised the 'right' of the Tanzanian government 'to prepare the first drafts of future [Policy Framework Papers], Letters or Intent and Letters of Development Policy, and that [international funding institutions] should honor that right'. Finally, the report emphasised the importance of the proactive setting of national priorities, which required the Tanzanian government to engage in 'consultation with the wider public, civil society and the donor community [and to] be far more vigorous in seeking to impose the resulting policy and project priorities on the donors' (p. 29). 'Ownership' thus denoted a quintessentially political struggle, namely the wrestling of power from the hands of donors and the subsequent transfer of agency into recipient governments' hands based on varying degrees of societal consultation. This was emphasised as recently as 2009 by the Organisation for Economic Co-operation and Development (OECD, 2009, p. 11) in a progress report on the 2005 Paris Declaration in which the organisation called ownership 'the most overtly political of the five Paris Declaration commitments: strengthening partners' ownership represents a shift of power in the aid relationship, while underlining the need for mutual accountability'. And yet, throughout the last 10 years, donors have expanded and supplanted it in ways that distance it from its definitional origin and increasingly hide its political dimension.

It is important to note that the theoretical case for greater 'ownership' is indeed compelling. Due to information asymmetries and imperfect monitoring, 'agents' contracted by 'principals' to carry out complex projects, such as the implementation of a national anti-retroviral therapy scheme, are less likely to engage in diversion of funds if their interests are aligned with those of the funder (Khan & Sharma, 2003). However, while this argument is solid in both theory and mathematical models, it does little to provide guidance since the need for 'ownership' is evoked most commonly where stakeholders sense its absence. Thus, Dijkstra (2013) concludes her study of budget support in Nicaragua by asserting that, in practice, '[d]onors will only be prepared to respect ownership where there is a minimum of preference alignment' (p. 121). At the same time, the assumption that 'donors can only advise and support but not buy or induce' (Koeberle, 2003, p. 257) reforms in recipient countries, as stated in a paper published in the *World Bank Research Observer*, denies the inter-governmental politics of forging 'ownership' – one of the central concerns and hallmarks of the post-Paris development effectiveness agenda (Fritz & Menocal, 2007) – by imposing ex-post rather than ex-ante conditions on recipient governments (Adam, Chambas, Guillaumont, Jeanneney, & Gunning, 2004).

In the wake of the adoption of the Millennium Development Goals in 2000, the politics of language have played a central role in inserting 'ownership' into the policy mainstream. Prior, Hughes, and Peckham (2012) remind us that '[I]t is in language that policy is made', and the institutionalisation of donor agencies' language of 'ownership' in the Paris Declaration represents a typical example of a 'coordinative discourse among policy actors' (Schmidt, 2008, p. 310). Such 'discourses determine what is considered acceptable and appropriate' (Joachim, 2007, p. 25; see also Gardner & Lewis, 2000; Motion & Leitch, 2009; St. Clair, 2006) while at the same time excluding alternative approaches (Deacon, 1999). Concurring with the rising importance of private sector funders, especially in the field of DAH, as well as ongoing corporatisation of aid relations more broadly as a result of outsourcing of development work to private companies, key terms in international aid increasingly overlap with the vocabulary of business. Although not inherently problematic, changing discourses both reflect and frame policy and programming. Jerve (2002), for instance, has argued that the relabeling of aid recipients as 'partners' lies at the heart of depoliticising 'ownership' as it obscures an inherent 'trade-off between partnership and ownership' (p. 389) that is reinforced by the incentive structures governing the giving and receiving of aid. The World Bank's country-specific poverty reduction strategy paper (PRSP), one of the primary national development strategy documents, provides a telling example. According to the World Bank, they are to be developed 'in partnership and consultation not only with donors, but also with representatives of domestic civil society and poor people themselves to ensure both national ownership and that development resources benefit the poor' (Abrahamsen, 2004, p. 1456, cited in Poirier, 2006). For this purpose, the Bank calls for 'the active participation of civil society at all levels and lays emphasis on the evaluation of poverty reduction performance' (Poirier, 2006). Although Dijkstra (2005) does not adopt Jerve's proposition of a trade-off between partnership and 'ownership', she presents evidence from Latin America suggesting that PRSPs:

> are written because donors want them to be written, and domestic ownership of the strategies is limited. Participation processes are held because the donors want them to be held, but the elected Parliaments are barely involved, the agenda is restricted to technical issues and the participation process exercises hardly any actual influence. (Dijkstra, 2005, p. 23; see also Jones, 2012)

Near-identical dynamics have been reported from Ghana where the 'government formulated development strategies with a view of pleasing the donors but with little intention to alter conventional patterns of everyday politics' (Woll, 2008, p. 74), thus providing further illustration of a 'misguided interpretation [by donors] of poverty reduction as a technical, rather than a political, project' (Canagarajah & van Diesen, 2011, p. S152).

'Missing politics' did eventually arise as an issue of concern among donors and informed an increasingly sharp conceptual distinction between 'national ownership' and 'country ownership'. Whereas the former is focused on securing political buy-in from recipient countries' political elites and bureaucratic apparatuses, the latter invokes the notion of either mediated or unmediated democratic priority-setting. For instance, the United Nations Development Programme's (UNDP) Working Group Report on National Ownership found 'participation' to be the term that best captured the real meaning of ownership and urges for active participation by 'civil society, [...] individuals [...] who are not necessarily represented by institutionalised consortia [and] voices of the poor/ vulnerable' (UNDP, n.d.). Notably, critiques of this more explicitly political take on 'ownership' have focused on contextual challenges while falling short of a systemic critique. Responding to an 'encompassing ownership discourse [that] persists at the strategic level' (Faust, 2010, p. 530), Wollack and Hubli (2010) have proposed that 'the greater the country's democratic deficits, the less effective the country's government is likely to be in expressing country ownership on behalf of its citizens' (p. 41). While logically correct, the argument implies that recipient countries with relatively well-functioning democracies undergo effective deliberative processes of preference formation. But do they? The assumption that democratic systems, short of referendums, provide de facto legitimisation of programme-level decisions via 'civil society' involvement is as questionable as the concurrent argument that relatively young democracies in the global South are capable of organising popular participation around every major donor-financed initiative, as several authors (Eberlei, 2001; Fritz & Menocal, 2007; McKinley, 2008; Seballos & Kreft, 2011) have suggested. Conflicts of interest around resource allocation undoubtedly exist (Kim, Kim, & Kim 2013), and at least when compared to other political systems, democratic polities seem most capable of diffusing resulting tensions. The point here, however, is that the ideal of 'country ownership', if defined as popular legitimisation at the level of programmes, is a problematic proposition which could be more reflective of the UN's as well as 'Washington's love affair with "civil society"' (Booth, 2011, p. S14), i.e., an idealisation of democracy, rather than actual political realities both nationally and globally. Indeed, it appears that donors' incentives remain stacked against wider participation in recipient countries since the latter risks interfering with a timely disbursement of funds – which, after all, is donor agencies' primary efficiency benchmark vis-a-vis their own principals (Shankland & Chambote, 2011).

This critique of 'country ownership' should not imply that 'national ownership' – in which aid providers presumably look to political leaders and senior bureaucrats in recipient countries for guidance (Chandy & Kharas, 2011) – is a less problematic concept. Frictions in this conceptualisation are just as acute, both within recipient governments (Hayman, 2009) and between recipient governments and donor agencies. The organisation that forged the Paris Declaration admitted even prior to this 2005 landmark that '[t]he lack of capacity at the middle management levels [...] pose an inherent challenge for donors pursuing [...] ownership' (OECD, 2003, p. 128). Facing multiple reporting systems set up by donor agencies (Ikhide, 2004), middle management systems in recipient country governments are often unable to execute and report on policy priorities and resulting programmes, thus severing the link between senior-level political commitments to 'national ownership' and actually implementable public policy. Nonetheless, donor agencies have leveraged 'ownership' to demand that 'recipient governments must take responsibility for a consensus reached between themselves and their development partners, as well as responsibility for the implementation and success or failure of the agreed set of policies and strategies' (Mouelhi & Rückert, 2007, p. 286). Donors just pretend that recipient governments are not agents of the principal but, in fact, free actors on a global market for aid. However, this notion of aid squarely contradicts both theoretical propositions of 'ownership', as explained above, and the nature of aid as self-interested donations from richer to poorer countries that hinge on the 'insertion of a set of policies' (Anders, 2008, p. 197) purported to facilitate allegedly mutually desirable outcomes. Resulting policy sets are in many cases substantively identical despite marked contextual differences (Mawdsley, 2007) but 'governments understand what they need to say and do in order to enjoy continued access to foreign assistance' (de Renzio, 2006, p. 635) irrespective of whether specific policies and programmes actually promise desirable results. Donors, in turn, despite 'proclaim[ing] in unison the importance of national ownership of the development process by recipient countries' (Blunt, Turner, & Hertz, 2011, p. 180), ultimately put their own accountabilities first:

> While many aid agency officials start out with a commitment to ownership defined as control over policies, as soon as there is some disagreement over policy choices they tend to fall back on a definition of ownership as commitment to their preferred policies. (de Renzio et al., 2008, p. 2)

Moreover, as a result of the Paris Declaration's simultaneous emphasis on results-based management, reiterated in the Declaration's follow-up compacts signed in Ghana (2008) and South Korea (2011), stricter prioritisations on behalf of donor governments limit 'the time and space [for recipient governments] to come up with their own solutions' (de Renzio et al., 2008, p. 1), thus narrowing the policy space for those expected to own the process (Sjöstedt, 2013).

'Ownership' in the midst of the HIV scale-up

Once the need for 'ownership' had been established discursively in development policy, broadly conceived, it also began to permeate DAH. Arguably among the first mentions specifically in the context of DAH, Costello and White (2001) urged 'national ownership for family health (by lobbying for expenditure increases, and by attracting good staff back into national institutions)' (p. 102). As part of the 'debate in the global health community on how best to accelerate positive health outcomes', proponents among political elites in recipient countries were quick to argue that 'ownership is the surest way for developing countries to chart their own course of development and overcome the challenges they face in building effective and productive states' (Ghebreyesus, 2010, p. 1127 in *The Lancet*). This statement by the then-Minister of Health (now Minister of Foreign Affairs) of Ethiopia provides a telling illustration of how elites in recipient countries interpreted 'ownership' primarily as political capital to enlarge national control over policies and programmes rather than as a donor-driven strategy to forge in-country commitment. Addressing McCourt's (2003) concern that such '[c]ommitment is a classic "black box", a cloudy concept habitually invoked in reform post-mortems: there was a reform programme, we tried to implement it, but we failed because "commitment" was not forthcoming' (p. 1016), Fox, Goldberg, Gore, and Bärnighausen (2011) have argued more recently that 'political commitment' by central governments reaches across 'expressed, institutional and budgetary' (p. S5) dimensions. Yet, while presenting a framework for measuring such commitment in the case of reduced HIV incidence in developing nations, they do not provide an actual application.

Aside from such conceptual forays, most applications of 'ownership' in DAH and specifically in HIV policies and programmes have focused on notions of 'country ownership' rather than 'national ownership', reflecting deliberate decisions within the AIDS community to emphasise the central role of civil society in this context.[1] Indeed, 'country ownership' has even been termed one of the 'keystones of [...] health development assistance' (Goldberg & Bryant, 2012, p. 531) for the most important bilateral donor, the US government. At the same time, global policy-makers have reinforced the notions that 'ownership' requires an integration of proposed programmes into already existing national strategies and priorities and that public–private partnerships are pivotal in this context (World Health Organisation [WHO], 2006).[2] This discourse is reflective of a trend in DAH and HIV programming more specifically, namely a persistent emphasis on 'partnerships' and 'country compacts' (Shorten, Taylor, Spicer, Mounier-Jack, & McCoy, 2012). This approach, however, ignores Jerve's (Shorten et al., 2012) concern that notions of 'partnership' and 'ownership' stand in conceptual tension and thus risks eclipsing the role of politics rooted in diverging incentive structures for donors and recipients of DAH. At the same time, whereas international development scholars writing on ownership-related challenges have pointed to several conceptual problems plaguing the notion of 'ownership', as discussed in the previous section of this article, most of the public health literature has actually applied the term descriptively rather than analytically, let alone critically – a discourse which, as I will demonstrate, is particularly salient in contributions to the leading medical journal, *The Lancet*.

Yet a critical look seems both warranted and timely. Among the first to review the promise of 'ownership' in DAH, yet without a specific focus on HIV/AIDS, Sridhar (2009) lamented that 'implementation has lagged far behind their endorsement' (p. 1364). More recently, Hunsmann (2012) has pointed to donors' persistent neglect of 'HIV prevention policies result[ing] from a politically negotiated aggregation of competing, frequently non-optimising rationalities' (p. 1477). 'In order to keep up appearances of national ownership and to avoid administrative obstruction', Hunsmann (2012) recalls from primary research on the lack of evidence-based HIV policy-making in Tanzania, 'several donors describe how they (at times desperately) look for counterparts within national administrations who will allow them to smooth the implementation of their programmes' (p. 1481). In addition, vertical programmes such as those focusing on preventing the spread of HIV by definition run counter to achieving systemic reform: 'Development agendas of recipient countries are highly influenced by donors, and instead of prioritising a horizontal development of public health structures, these privilege vertical targeting centred on particular diseases' (Bidaurratzaga-Aurre & Colom-Jaén, 2012, p. 227).

In light of these challenges, Sridhar and Batniji (2008) have argued that so long as partnerships focus on improving coordination among donors for vertical interventions, the relative bargaining power of recipient governments will effectively be weakened rather than strengthened. Such partnerships increase cohesion among donors while doing little or nothing at all to capacitate recipient governments in more effectively engaging with or confronting donors' priorities. While correct, this argument does not necessarily imply that partnerships that also involve actors and agencies in recipient countries are more likely to overcome this power disparity. The critical issue here is which actors are included, which ones are excluded and how fluid or rigid this selection pattern proves to be over time. For instance, private sector funders such as the Bill and Melinda Gates Foundation were readily captured by the proposition of 'ownership through partnership' with in-country 'stakeholders', and one of the guiding principles for the Global Fund for Aids, Tuberculosis and Malaria (GFATM), which the Gates Foundation supported early on, has been that funding proposals be submitted by so-called Country Coordinating Mechanisms (CCMs) composed of members of recipient governments as well as local experts, including at least one presumed representative of 'civil society'. Notably, however, there are no standard requirements specifying *how* the civil society representative(s) shall be chosen, other than mandating that selection be 'based on a documented, transparent process', with in-country consortia determining the details of such processes (GFATM, 2013). Adding to this ex-ante procedural vagueness, Kerr, Kaplan, Suwannawong, Jürgens, and Wood (2004) explained in a commentary published in *The Lancet* that while generally desirable:

> [s]uch partnerships [...] can also create barriers to access to the available funding, which is why the Global Fund has produced criteria for non-CCM applications. Specifically, such applications can be considered when from a country that has no legitimate government, is in conflict or facing a natural disaster, or has suppressed or never established partnerships with civil society and nongovernmental organisations (NGOs). (p. 11)

In other words, the preference of both the AIDS community and private donors to seek 'partnerships' in the spirit of 'country ownership' rather than 'national ownership' is, in reality, undermined by donors' incentive to disburse funds even if the legitimacy of in-country preference formulation is dubious at best. This observation is in line with related macro-level research on persistent mismatches between private DAH flows and recipients' priorities (Esser & Keating Bench, 2011) and illustrates why the belief that private donors tailor their disbursements more in line with needs and less with overriding foreign policy objectives is false (MacKellar, 2005; see also Shiffman, 2008; Sridhar & Batniji, 2008). And yet, the track record of government donors is hardly more impressive in this regard. In the case of the US President's Emergency Plan for AIDS Relief (PEPFAR), 'funding allocations were remarkably consistent despite epidemiological and health systems' differences across Mozambique, Uganda and Zambia' (Biesma et al., 2009, p. 242). This observation mirrors Mawdsley's (Biesma et al., 2009, p. 242) findings described above and once again illustrates that recipient country preferences are followed only to the extent to which they do not conflict with donors' priorities, irrespective of whether the latter are driven by programmatic or foreign policy considerations (Esser, 2009; see also Brugha et al., 2004). Similar to case-based circumventions of CCMs, where governments have either been politically too weak or timid to interfere or judged to be either uncooperative and insufficiently capacitated, 'new [DAH] donors, such as PEPFAR and the Gates Foundation, disburse funds directly to NGOs, thus making it difficult for ministries to plan their efforts' (Sridhar, 2009, p. 1371). This undermining of cross-sector priority-setting from the tail end is the antithesis of what 'country ownership' was originally meant to achieve. Instead of investments into building diverse civil societies around sexual and reproductive health over time, for instance, donors have responded to the Paris Declaration's emphasis on results by shoring up a select group of NGOs (Seims, 2011) – 'partnerships' with these NGOs remain at the centre of HIV programming.

Analogous dynamics can be observed with regard to different types of technical assistance. In a 2007 article in *The Lancet*, AbouZahr, Adjei, and Kanchanachitra (2007) argued as follows:

> One of the difficulties with global estimation efforts is that they sometimes fail to generate ownership on the part of those in a position to effect change at a country level. Ownership means more than passive consultation from technical experts to national focal points. In developing estimates of HIV prevalence, a proactive approach has been taken to ensure country involvement. The estimation and projection package and spectrum AIDS modules, developed with support from WHO and UNAIDS, are used by countries themselves [...]. This approach has helped greatly, not only to ensure acceptance of the results but also to strengthen basic data collection because all countries receive training and capacity building on a regular basis. However, the process is costly and time-consuming and can be perceived as diverting resources away from the delivery of interventions. (p. 1043)

Here again, an instrumentalisation of 'ownership' in the interest of global health donors becomes apparent. Although aiming to move beyond 'passive consultation', countries are asked to carry out data collection with tools developed on their behalf by donor and development agencies in the global North. Such involvement as data gatherers 'helped greatly' with respect to increasing buy-in and is justified despite the higher cost. Yet was any attention paid to what recipient countries actually wanted out of the process? Apparently this was not the case.

Contradicting the intention of 'country ownership', such arguments and practices of de facto denial of recipient countries' leadership in HIV programming also create political momentum for enforcing an ex-post conditionality in the guise of 'ownership', especially in bilateral aid relations. The US Global Health Initiative, for instance, 'explicitly breaks with past behaviour and promotes local involvement by embracing the notion of "country ownership"', as Goldberg and Bryant (2012, p. 2) explain. Characterising this move as 'a capacity building strategy that shifts the leadership of and responsibility for health promotion efforts onto the partner country and its organisations on the ground', they warn that 'a huge influx of development funding will soon be allocated to a new concept, "country-owned capacity building", that is not clearly understood by practitioners or researchers alike' (Goldberg & Bryant, 2012, p. 2). Definitional confusion around 'ownership' thus continues. A complete inversion of its original meaning and intent, 'ownership' has even been used as a semantic proxy for (and potential threat of) gradual defunding. For example, in a recent article in *Health Affairs*, Collins, Isbell, Sohn, and Klindera (2012) urged that:

> the US government should carefully manage and support the transition of HIV/AIDS programs to country 'ownership,' [which implies] moving from national dependence on external support to countries funding their HIV responses by themselves. [...] Country ownership of AIDS responses has been imperfectly realized in Africa, underscoring the need for intensified US health diplomacy to encourage greater national investments in HIV and other health services. (p. 1581)

Writing in *The Lancet*, Reich and Takemi (2009) have similarly pointed to an 'obvious trade-off [...] between country ownership [...] and independent assessments' (p. 512) and have suggested that '[d]espite a growing trend for performance-based disbursement, agencies are still vulnerable to political pressure from recipient countries' (Reich and Takemi, 2009, p. 512) – without, however, providing evidence of recipient countries effectively exerting such pressure on donors. In sum, 'country ownership' is no longer about recalibrating the locus of power in priority-setting for development assistance in order to achieve greater leverage for recipient countries; rather, it has become a disciplinary tool for those concerned that true 'ownership' cannot be achieved as long as aid is flowing and that only a reduction in aid might eventually produce 'owned' policies. The conceptual inversion produces an even starker imbalance between donors and recipients as it allows the former to retain their original negotiating power while shifting political responsibility towards the latter. Such discursive adjustments, which feed on the definitional ambiguity described earlier in this article, raise the question of intentionality.

'Ownership' as a functional tautology

Public and private donor agencies' desire for more accountable development 'partners' in the global South is as politically understandable as it is managerially justifiable. Why should they continue pouring resources into either recipient governments' or local NGOs' coffers without demanding that these resources be used both efficiently and effectively? At face value, donors' reinterpretation of 'ownership' as denoting greater expectations confronting recipients rather than a wider array of choices for the latter thus appears reasonable. But is it? As long as donors' influence in bilateral, multilateral and global agenda-setting falls between outright imposition and option-excluding framing (Rasche & Esser, 2006), it is hard to see why recipient countries or local organisations should carry full responsibility for programme implementation since, in Brown's words, '[c]oncessional aid flows are arguably inimical to "national ownership" in any meaningful sense of the term' (Brown, 2004, p. 239). As much as a reduction of tensions between the ideals of national autonomy and international accountability is desirable for better development outcomes, recommendations along the lines of 'emphasis[ing] actions to ensure that complementarity between them is achieved' (Germain, 2011, p. 141) seem far-fetched. Any participation of donors in actively forging 'ownership' is politically risky, and those doing so are likely to be 'seen as partisan, non-transparent and unaccountable' as they make decisions on whom to include and with whom to coalesce (Eyben, 2010, p. 392). While illustrating a fundamental dilemma of foreign aid policy and practice, this reality – which is reinforced by direct budget support falling out of favour due to the drive for more easily demonstrable aid effectiveness – increases public donor agencies' reluctance to listen to and engage constructively in recipient countries' local politics with a view to maximising health gains. Instead, DAH has become an instrument of donor countries' foreign policies yet again:

> [G]lobal health investment is an important component of the [US] national security 'smart power' strategy, where the power of America's development tools – especially proven, cost-effective health care initiatives – can build the capacity of government institutions and reduce the risk of conflict before it gathers strength. (White House, 2009; see also Feldbaum, Lee, & Michaud, 2010)

Finally, in addition to overarching foreign policy and security concerns, political considerations *within* donor countries in times of recurrent fiscal crises provide yet another rationale for retaining 'ownership' as a central concept in DAH discourse. By stressing that it carries the dual advantage of promising better outcomes and creating possibilities for 'building capacity' in 'partner' countries, public agencies maintain breathing space in case of both executive and legislative scrutiny while simultaneously positioning themselves advantageously vis-à-vis competing line ministries in pursuit of non-aid (and therefore, arguably, non-security) objectives, which shores up their leverage in budget negotiations. As a result, the concept of 'ownership', void of actual meaning as it is, emerges as a discursive tool available to donor agencies to reduce their accountabilities both internationally and domestically, which increases their tactical elbowroom and thus helps them gain an edge over external recipients as well as internal political rivals.

Acknowledgements

Michael Bader, Kim Blankenship, Rachel Sullivan Robinson, Jeremy Shiffman, Sharon Weiner, Nina Yamanis and two anonymous reviewers provided very helpful comments on different drafts of the manuscript. Nora Kenworthy, Richard Parker and the *GPH* editorial team offered crucial guidance as well. Julie J. Altier and Galant Au Chan made important intellectual contributions to an earlier version of this project. Jed B. Byers, Shelby Jergens and Mac Krzyzewski provided outstanding research assistance; Byers also copyedited the manuscript. All remaining errors are the author's responsibility.

Funding

Thanks are due to American University's School of International Service for a summer grant in support of the research.

Notes

1. I thank one of the anonymous reviewers for pointing this out.
2. Another insight shared by one of the anonymous reviewers, which I gratefully acknowledge.

References

AbouZahr, C., Adjei, S., & Kanchanachitra, C. (2007). From data to policy: Good practices and cautionary tales. *The Lancet*, *369*, 1039–1046. Retrieved from http://www.ebscohost.com/academic/academic-search-premier

Abrahamsen, R. (2004). The power of partnerships in global governance. *Third World Quarterly*, *25*, 1453–1467. doi:10.1080/0143659042000308465

Adam, C., Chambas, G., Guillaumont, P., Jeanneney, S. G., & Gunning, J. W. (2004). Performance-based conditionality: A European perspective. *World Development*, *32*, 1059–1070. doi:10.1016/j.worlddev.2004.01.004

Anders, G. (2008). The normativity of numbers: World Bank and IMF conditionality. *PoLAR: Political and Legal Anthropology Review*, *31*, 187–202. doi:10.1111/j.1555-2934.2008.00021.x

Best, J. (2007). Legitimacy dilemmas: The IMF's pursuit of country ownership. *Third World Quarterly*, *28*, 469–488. doi:10.1080/01436590701192231

Bidaurratzaga-Aurre, E., & Colom-Jaén, A. (2012). HIV/AIDS policies in Mozambique and the new aid architecture: Successes, shortcomings and the way forward. *The Journal of Modern African Studies*, *50*, 225–252. doi:10.1017/S0022278X12000031

Biesma, R. G., Brugha, R., Harmer, A., Walsh, A., Spicer, N., & Walt, G. (2009). The effects of global health initiatives on country health systems: A review of the evidence from HIV/AIDS control. *Health Policy and Planning*, *24*, 239–252. doi:10.1093/heapol/czp025

Blunt, P., Turner, M., & Hertz, J. (2011). The meaning of development assistance. *Public Administration and Development*, *31*, 172–187. doi:10.1002/pad.592

Booth, D. (2011). Aid, institutions and governance: What have we learned? *Development Policy Review*, *29*, S14. doi:10.1111/j.1467-7679.2011.00518.x

Booth, D. (2012). Aid effectiveness: Bringing country ownership (and politics) back in. *Conflict, Security & Development*, *12*, 537–558. doi:10.1080/14678802.2012.744184

Brown, D. (2004). Participation in poverty reduction strategies: Democracy strengthened or democracy undermined? In S. Hickey & G. Mohan (Eds.), *Participation: From tyranny to transformation? Exploring new approaches to participation in development* (pp. 237–251). London: Zed Books.

Brugha, R., Donoghue, M., Starlin, M., Ndubani, P., Ssengooba, F., Fernandes, B., & Walt, G. (2004). The global fund: Managing great expectations. *The Lancet*, *364*, 95–100. Retrieved from http://www.ncbi.nlm.nih.gov/pubmed/15234862

Buiter, W. H. (2007). 'Country ownership': A term whose time has gone. *Development in Practice*, *17*, 647–652. doi:10.1080/09614520701469856

Canagarajah, S., & van Diesen, A. (2011). The poverty reduction strategy approach six years on: An examination of principles and practice in Uganda. *Development Policy Review*, *29*(S1), S135–S156. doi:10.1111/j.1467-7679.2011.00523.x

Chandy, L., & Kharas, H. (2011). Why can't we all just get along? The practical limits to international development cooperation. *Journal of International Development*, *23*, 739–751. doi:10.1002/jid.1797

Collins, C., Isbell, M., Sohn, A., & Klindera, K. (2012). Four principles for expanding PEPFAR's role as a vital force in US health diplomacy abroad. *Health Affairs*, *31*, 1578–1584. doi:10.1377/hlthaff.2012.0204

Cornwall, A., & Eade, D. (Eds.). (2010). *Deconstructing development discourse: Buzzwords and fuzzwords*. Bourton on Dunsmore: Practical Action Publishing.

Costello, A., & White, H. (2001). Reducing global inequalities in child health. *Archives of Disease in Childhood*, *84*(2), 98–102. doi:10.1136/adc.84.2.98

Deacon, B. (1999). Social policy in a global context. In A. Hurrell & N. Woods (Eds.), *Inequality, globalization, and world politics* (pp. 211–47). Oxford: Oxford University Press.

De Cock, K. M., El-Sadr, W. M., & Ghebreyesus, T. A. (2011). Game changers: Why did the scale-up of HIV treatment work despite weak health systems. *Journal of Acquired Immune Deficiency Syndromes*, *57*(Suppl 2), S61–S63. doi:10.1097/QAI.0b013e3182217f00

de Renzio, P. (2006). Aid, budgets and accountability: A survey article. *Development Policy Review*, *24*, 627–645. doi:10.1111/j.1467-7679.2006.00351.x

de Renzio, P., Whitfield, L., & Bergamaschi, I. (2008). *Reforming foreign aid practices: What country ownership is and what donors can do to support it*. Briefing Paper, Global Economic Governance Programme, University of Oxford, Oxford.

Dijkstra, G. (2005). The PRSP approach and the illusion of improved aid effectiveness: Lessons from Bolivia, Honduras and Nicaragua. *Development Policy Review*, *23*, 443–464. doi:10.1111/j.1467-7679.2005.00296.x

Dijkstra, G. (2013). Governance or poverty reduction? Assessing budget support in Nicaragua. *The Journal of Development Studies*, *49*, 110–124. doi:10.1080/00220388.2012.713468

Eberlei, W. (2001). *Institutionalized participation in processes beyond the PRSP*. Eschborn: Gesellschaft fuer Technische Zusammenarbeit.

Esser, D. E. (2009). More money, less cure: Why global health assistance needs restructuring. *Ethics & International Affairs*, *23*, 225–234. doi:10.1111/j.1747-7093.2009.00214.x

Esser, D. E., & Keating Bench, K. (2011). Does global health funding respond to recipients' needs? Comparing public and private donors' allocations in 2005–2007. *World Development*, *39*, 1271–1280. doi:10.1016/j.worlddev.2010.12.005

Eyben, R. (2010). Hiding relations: The irony of 'effective aid'. *European Journal of Development Research*, *22*, 382–397. doi:10.1057/ejdr.2010.10

Faust, J. (2010). Policy experiments, democratic ownership and development assistance. *Development Policy Review*, *28*, 515–534. doi:10.1111/j.1467-7679.2010.00496.x

Feldbaum, H., Lee, K., & Michaud, J. (2010). Global health and foreign policy. *Epidemiologic Reviews*, *32*, 82–92 doi:10.1093/epirev/mxq006

Fox, A. M., Goldberg, A. B., Gore, R. J., & Bärnighausen, T. (2011). Conceptual and methodological challenges to measuring political commitment to respond to HIV. *Journal of the International AIDS Society*, *14*(Suppl 2), S5. doi:10.1186/1758-2652-14-S2-S5

Fritz, V., & Menocal, R. (2007). Developmental states in the new millennium: Concepts and challenges for a new aid agenda. *Development Policy Review*, *25*, 531–552. doi:10.1111/j.1467-7679.2007.00384.x

Gardner, K., & Lewis, D. (2000). Dominant paradigms overturned or 'business as usual?' Development discourse and the white paper on international development. *Critique of Anthropology*, *20*, 15–29. doi:10.1177/0308275X0002000106

Germain, A. (2011). Ensuring the complementarity of country ownership and accountability for results in relation to donor aid: A response. *Reproductive Health Matters*, *19*, 141–145. doi:10.1016/S0968-8080(11)38595-3

GFATM. (2013). *Guidelines and requirements for country coordinating mechanisms*. Geneva: Author. [GFATM online publication]. Retrieved from http://www.theglobalfund.org/documents/ccm/CCM_Requirements_Guidelines_en/

Ghebreyesus, T. A. (2010). Achieving the health MDGs: Country ownership in four steps. *The Lancet, 376*, 1127–1128. doi:10.1016/S0140-6736(10)61465-1

Goldberg, J., & Bryant, M. (2012). Country ownership and capacity building: The next buzzwords in health systems strengthening or a truly new approach to development? *BMC Public Health, 12*, 531. doi:10.1186/1471-2458-12-531

Hayman, R. (2009). From Rome to Accra via Kigali: 'Aid effectiveness' in Rwanda. *Development Policy Review, 27*, 581–599. doi:10.1111/j.1467-7679.2009.00460.x

Helleiner, G. K. (1992). Structural adjustment and long-term development in sub-Saharan Africa. In F. Stewart, S. Lall, & S. Wangwe (Eds.), *Alternative development strategies in sub-Saharan Africa* (pp. 48–78). New York, NY: St. Martin's Press.

Helleiner, G., Killick, T., Lipumba, N., Ndulu, B., & Svendsen, K. (1995). *Report of the group of independent advisers on development cooperation issues between Tanzania and its aid donors.* Copenhagen: Royal Danish Ministry of Foreign Affairs.

Hunsmann, M. (2012). Limits to evidence-based health policymaking: Policy hurdles to structural HIV prevention in Tanzania. *Social Science & Medicine, 74*, 1477–1485. doi:10.1016/j.socscimed.2012.01.023

IHME. (2011). *Financing global health 2012: Continued growth as MDG deadline approaches.* Seattle, WA: Author.

IHME. (2012). *Financing global health 2011: The end of the golden age?* Seattle, WA: Author.

Ikhide, S. (2004). Reforming the international financial system for effective aid delivery. *World Economy, 27*, 127–152. doi:10.1111/j.1467-9701.2004.00593.x

Jerve, A. M. (2002). Ownership and partnership: Does the new rhetoric solve the incentive problems in aid? *Forum for Development studies, 29*, 389–407. doi:10.1080/08039410.2002.9666216

Joachim, J. M. (2007). NGOs and UN agenda setting. In J. M. Joachim (Ed.), *Agenda setting, the UN, and NGOs: Gender violence and reproductive rights* (pp. 15–33). Washington, DC: Georgetown University Press.

Jones, S. (2012). Innovating foreign aid – progress and problems. *Journal of International Development, 24*, 1–16. doi:10.1002/jid.1758

Kerr, T., Kaplan, K., Suwannawong, P., Jürgens, R., & Wood, E. (2004). The global fund to fight AIDS, tuberculosis and malaria: Funding for unpopular public-health programmes. *The Lancet, 364*, 11–12. doi:10.1016/S0140-6736(04)16610-5

Khan, M. S., & Sharma, S. (2003). IMF conditionality and country ownership of adjustment programs. *The World Bank Research Observer, 18*, 227–248. doi:10.1093/wbro/lkg007

Kim, E. M., Kim, P. H., & Kim, J. (2013). From development to development co-operation: Foreign aid, country ownership, and the developmental state in South Korea. *The Pacific Review, 26*, 313–336. doi:10.1080/09512748.2012.759263

King, K. (1992). The external agenda of aid in internal educational reform. *International Journal of Educational Development, 12*, 257–263. doi:10.1016/0738-0593(92)90002-4

Koeberle, S. (2003). Should policy-based lending still involve conditionality? *The World Bank Research Observer, 18*, 249–273. doi:10.1093/wbro/lkg009

Leandro, J. E., Schafer, H., & Frontini, G. (1999). Towards a more effective conditionality: An operational framework. *World Development, 27*, 285–300. doi:10.1016/S0305-750X(98)00127-2

MacKellar, L. (2005). Priorities in global assistance for health, AIDS, and population. *Population and Development Review, 31*, 293–312. doi:10.1787/725643456002

Mawdsley, E. (2007). The millennium challenge account: Neo-liberalism, poverty and security. *Review of International Political Economy, 14*, 487–509. doi:10.1080/09692290701395742

McCourt, W. (2003). Political commitment to reform: Civil service reform in Swaziland. *World Development, 31*, 1015–1031. doi:10.1016/S0305-750X(03)00044-5

McKinley, T. (2008). Economic policies for growth and poverty reduction: PRSPs, neoliberal conditionalities and 'post-consensus' alternatives. *IDS Bulletin, 39*(2), 93–103. doi:10.1111/j.1759-5436.2008.tb00450.x

Motion, J., & Leitch, S. (2009). The transformational potential of public policy discourse. *Organization Studies, 30*, 1045–1061. doi:10.1177/0170840609337940

Mouelhi, M., & Rückert, A. (2007). Ownership and participation: The limitations of the poverty reduction strategy paper approach. *Canadian Journal of Development, 28*, 277–292. doi:10.1080/02255189.2007.9669206

OECD. (2003). Joint assessment of ownership and partnership in Tanzania, comparative review of the aid programmes of Denmark, Finland, Ireland and Japan. *DAC Journal*, *4*, 111–176. doi:10.1787/journal_ dev-v4-art29-en

OECD. (2009). *Aid effectiveness: A progress report on implementing the Paris Declaration*. Paris: Author.

Poirier, S. (2006). *How 'inclusive' are the World Bank's poverty reduction strategies? An analysis of Tanzania and Uganda's health sectors*. Project submitted in partial fulfillment of the requirements for the degree of Master of Arts, Simon Fraser University, Vancouver.

Prior, L., Hughes, D., & Peckham, S. (2012). The discursive turn in policy analysis and the validation of policy stories. *Journal of Social Policy*, *41*, 271–89. doi:10.1017/S0047279411 000821

Rasche, A., & Esser, D. E. (2006). From stakeholder management to stakeholder accountability: Applying habermasian discourse ethics to accountability research. *Journal of Business Ethics*, *65*, 251–267. doi:10.1007/s10551-005-5355-y

Reich, M. R., & Takemi, K. (2009). G8 and strengthening of health systems: Follow-up to the Toyako summit. *The Lancet*, *373*, 508–515. doi:10.1016/S0140-6736(08)61899-1

Riddell, R. C. (2007). *Does foreign aid really Work*? New York, NY: Oxford University Press.

Schmidt, V. A. (2008). Discursive institutionalism: The explanatory power of ideas and discourse. *Annual Review of Political Science*, *11*, 303–326. doi:10.1146/annurev.polisci.11.060606.135342

Seballos, F., & Kreft, S. (2011). Towards an understanding of the political economy of the PPCR. *IDS Bulletin*, *42*(3), 33–41. doi:10.1111/j.1759-5436.2011.00220.x

Seims, S. (2011). Improving the impact of sexual and reproductive health development assistance from the like-minded European donors. *Reproductive Health Matters*, *19*(38), 129–140. doi:10.1016/S0968-8080(11)38578-3

Shankland, A., & Chambote, R. (2011). Prioritising PPCR investments in Mozambique: The politics of 'country ownership' and 'stakeholder participation'. *IDS Bulletin*, *42*(3), 62–69. doi:10.1111/j.1759-5436.2011.00223.x

Shiffman, J. (2008). Has donor prioritization of HIV/AIDS displaced aid for other health issues? *Health Policy and Planning*, *23*, 95–100. doi:10.1093/heapol/czm045

Shorten, T., Taylor, M., Spicer, N., Mounier-Jack, S., & McCoy, D. (2012). The international health partnership plus: Rhetoric or real change? Results of a self-reported survey in the context of the 4th high level forum on aid effectiveness in Busan. *Globalization and Health*, *8*(13), 1–13. doi:10.1186/1744-8603-8-13

Sjöstedt, M. (2013). Aid effectiveness and the Paris Declaration: A mismatch between ownership and results-based management? *Public Administration and Development*, *33*, 143–155. doi:10. 1002/pad.1645

Sridhar, D. (2009). Post-accra: Is there space for country ownership in global health? *Third World Quarterly*, *30*, 1363–1377. doi:10.1080/01436590903134981

Sridhar, D., & Batniji, R. (2008). Misfinancing global health: A case for transparency in disbursements and decision making. *The Lancet*, *372*, 1185–1191. doi:10.1016/S0140-6736(08) 61485-3

St. Clair, A. L. (2006). Global poverty: The co-production of knowledge and politics. *Global Social Policy*, *6*, 57–77. doi:10.1177/1468018106061392

UNDP. (n.d.). *Working group report on national ownership*. New York, NY: Author, mimeo.

White House. (2009). Statement by the President on global health initiative. Office of the Press Secretary [press release]. Retrieved from http://www.whitehouse.gov/the_press_office/Statement-by-the-President-on-Global-Health-Initiative

WHO. (2006). *Health workforce issues and the Global Fund to fight AIDS, Tuberculosis and Malaria: An analytical review*. Geneva: Author.

Woll, B. (2008). Donor harmonisation and government ownership: Multi-donor budget support in Ghana. *European Journal of Development Research*, *20*, 74–87. doi:10.1080/0957881070 1853215

Wollack, K., & Hubli, K. S. (2010). Getting convergence right. *Journal of Democracy*, *21*(4), 35–42. doi:10.1353/jod.2010.0007

Evidence and AIDS activism: HIV scale-up and the contemporary politics of knowledge in global public health

Christopher J. Colvin

Division of Social and Behavioural Sciences and the Centre for Infectious Disease Epidemiology and Research (CIDER), School of Public Health and Family Medicine, University of Cape Town, Cape Town, South Africa

The HIV epidemic is widely recognised as having prompted one of the most remarkable intersections ever of illness, science and activism. The production, circulation, use and evaluation of empirical scientific 'evidence' played a central part in activists' engagement with AIDS science. Previous activist engagement with evidence focused on the social and biomedical responses to HIV in the global North as well as challenges around ensuring antiretroviral treatment (ART) was available in the global South. More recently, however, with the roll-out and scale-up of large public-sector ART programmes and new multi-dimensional prevention efforts, the relationships between evidence and activism have been changing. Scale-up of these large-scale treatment and prevention programmes represents an exciting new opportunity while bringing with it a host of new challenges. This paper examines what new forms of evidence and activism will be required to address the challenges of the scaling-up era of HIV treatment and prevention. It reviews some recent controversies around evidence and HIV scale-up and describes the different forms of evidence and activist strategies that will be necessary for a robust response to these new challenges.

Introduction

On a recent visit to the Cape Town Heart Museum, I learned that after Christiaan Barnard performed the world's first heart transplant in South Africa, to much national chest thumping and great global acclaim, he only performed 10 more over the next 6 years. Barnard was by all accounts a careful and thorough researcher and clinician. His first heart transplant was preceded by years of basic and clinical research and dozens of heart transplants in dogs to get him and his team ready for the first human transplant. His first patient lived for 18 days, his second for 18 months and his longest living patient from those first years stayed alive for 23 years.

In the rest of the world, however, news of his life-saving feat inaugurated a veritable heart transplant rush, with nearly 100 being performed in a number of countries by poorly prepared surgical teams in the 12 months after Barnard's first surgery. While Barnard's survival rates were very high in these first years (limited mainly by the then unsolved problem of rejection), those of other teams were dismally low and only a few years later, the annual number of transplants globally had dropped to 18.

While Barnard's overall approach was cautious, part of the reason the first heart transplant was done in South Africa rather than the USA – where many of the surgical and medical techniques were rapidly being developed, and where Barnard had recently trained – was that the ethical and policy contexts in South Africa around research and clinical practice were significantly more accommodating to this kind of experimental enterprise. Forceful criticisms soon came, however, from his colleagues for acting without sufficient evidence or consensus in the medical community. The Cape Town Heart Museum contains several display cases of letters and telegrams from ordinary citizens condemning Barnard for his 'ghoulish' act, claiming that he had blood on his hands.

I thought a lot about these historical events while reviewing contemporary debates in the scientific literature on the development and scale-up of new HIV treatment and prevention interventions. While some elements of the debates around HIV science are unique to this particular epidemic, there are nonetheless a number of revealing resonances between the controversies around scaling up new medical technologies: the fraught tension between researcher, clinician and bioethical perspectives on how fast the envelope of scientific knowledge should be stretched; the multi-disciplinary character – and thus evidentiary challenges – of clinical practice; the variation across countries in clinical and research regulatory regimes; the important role of professional competition and national prestige; and the popular rhetoric of accusing those one disagrees with of having 'blood on their hands'.

In Barnard's case, vigorous debates about the research evidence base on which he justified his surgical exploits were largely confined to his professional colleagues. HIV, on the other hand, is widely recognised as having prompted one of the most remarkable intersections ever of illness, science and activism in the popular sphere. While patient involvement and advocacy in the health sciences was not new at the time (Wachter, 1992), AIDS activists, many themselves HIV-positive, managed from the very early years of the epidemic to work their way forcefully into the tightly guarded worlds of scientific knowledge production and health policy development (Epstein, 1996). AIDS activism was aimed not only at broad social stigma and discrimination and state neglect and oppression of those with HIV – it also squarely engaged with the worlds of the basic and clinical sciences of HIV, of pharmaceutical production and pricing regulation, and of health policy-making's translation of evidence into new forms of practice.

The production, circulation, use and evaluation of empirical scientific 'evidence' in particular played a central part in activists' engagement with AIDS science. 'Expert patients' were trained up on the existing evidence base and told to use this knowledge-as-power in their engagement with health care workers (HCWs) and the wider community. Activists critiqued the poor state of the early evidence base on HIV (especially clinical and pharmaceutical science) and prompted a dramatic increase in funding for further research. They challenged regulatory processes that they argued fetishised certain forms of evidence and processes of scientific review that unnecessarily delayed access to life-saving treatment. They connected with each other and with academic researchers through transnational advocacy networks (Marx, Halcli, & Barnett, 2012), and in the process marshalled reams of highly technical epidemiological, virological and health economics evidence from around the world for legal and political campaigns against governments and drug companies. They helped foster the creation of a new range of HIV surveillance mechanisms and databases, contributed to the growth (and critique) of global clinical trial research, and catalysed countless academic journals, research centres and conferences aimed at generating evidence to be used in the response to HIV and AIDS.

This history of activist engagement with evidence can be divided roughly into three phases: (1) the early response in the global North to the terrifying new epidemic, leading up to the development of combination antiretroviral therapy, (2) a subsequent phase focused on making antiretroviral treatment (ART) available in those Southern countries that had generalised epidemics, struggling health systems and health budgets that were outmatched by the high prices for ARVs in the North and (3) the current phase that finds many countries concerned with sustaining longer-term treatment and prevention efforts such as the scale-up and maintenance of public-sector ART programmes and new multi-dimensional prevention efforts in the form of 'combination prevention' interventions. To some degree, there are challenges of evidence that are shared across these phases. Drug development started as soon as the epidemic was identified and continues today, as do the political debates about the pace and cost of drug development. Research on why behavioural interventions may succeed or fail in preventing transmission or why people with HIV may or may not remain adherent to treatment has always been a mainstay of the response to the epidemic.

There are important ways, however, in which the political stakes and the epidemiological and health system challenges are distinct between these three phases as well. The first phase was shaped by the fact that the epidemic was understood at the time as a largely concentrated epidemic in the global North with no known treatment that attracted tremendous social stigma. Fighting stigma against the disease and the marginalised populations it was connected to, and developing some form of effective treatment were the priorities shaping activist mobilisations of evidence during this period. The second phase was defined by the fight for affordable treatment access for those countries in the global South with generalised epidemics in the heterosexual population. Stigma of course remained a serious issue during this phase, as did the problem of HIV infection in marginalised communities. The central thrust of activist engagement with science in this period, however, revolved around convincing drug companies and/or governments to lower drug prices and encouraging sometimes prejudiced donors to fund ART programmes in poor countries with already struggling health systems and small health budgets.

The activist challenge in the current phase is a product of both the victories during the second phase in introducing ART programming in the global South as well as the global financial crisis and recession. It centres around questions of how to scale up a large-scale, long-term and sustainable treatment and prevention response in a context of restricted global health funding and urgent competing public health priorities such as chronic diseases, maternal and child health and climate change. Developing a sustainable and effective ART programme in the public sector is, for many countries, a formidable undertaking and involves technical, social and political problems not previously or adequately addressed. Equally challenging is designing, implementing, managing and evaluating combination prevention efforts that work simultaneously at the biological, behavioural and structural scales. These efforts will require the development of new concepts and theoretical frameworks in the basic, clinical and social sciences as well as new activist strategies for mobilising this evidence in ways that maintain the earlier eras' productive dialectics of research, practice, advocacy and policy.

This paper reviews some of these new forms and mobilisations of evidence that will be required in this third phase of the fight against HIV. The next section reviews two recent controversies and explores some of the challenges of developing scientific evidence and mobilising it to support scale-up. It is followed by a section that considers the constellation of forms of evidence that will be necessary for a robust response to HIV scale-up. The final section considers how these new forms of evidence will require new political strategies to activate them. It also discusses the extent to which these developments both grow out of and may in turn affect the broader politics of global health in a post-ART, post-financial crisis world.

Recent controversies in HIV treatment and prevention programme scale-up

Given the new priorities and challenges of this next era of the response to HIV, and the intense knowledge production and activist energies that still attend to HIV and AIDS, there is no shortage of controversies in the scientific and activist literature over new treatment and prevention initiatives and the nature of evidence that exists or not to support their scale-up. This section briefly reviews two of these – one involving treatment and the other prevention – and considers some of the common themes that have emerged in these debates.

One of the most celebrated of recent ideas in treatment and prevention is the 'test and treat' approach, where people who are diagnosed with HIV infection are offered immediate access to lifelong ART, regardless of their CD4 count or clinical presentation. There are a number of variations on this idea, one of which is 'Option B+' within Prevention of Mother to Child Transmission (PMTCT) programmes. B+ aims to refocus efforts on preventing maternal deaths from HIV by offering lifelong ART to any pregnant woman testing positive for HIV (UNICEF, 2012). This approach has been rolled out in Malawi, and preliminary results of the national programme are just becoming available (CDC, 2013). Early indications are that B+ has dramatically increased ART coverage for pregnant women in a short period of time (over seven-fold in the space of 1 year), but it should be noted that Malawi's B+ intervention involved not only a change in ART protocols for pregnant women but also national training for all HCWs, task shifting to provide the necessary human resources, a new national surveillance infrastructure and quarterly visits from a national task team to each PMTCT site (CDC, 2013).

Critics of B+ have argued that there are a range of concerns about the evidence supporting B+ that should cause other countries to hesitate before rolling out similar programmes. These critics have asked about: the potential impact on families and communities of significantly different treatment access for pregnant women; the long-term and as yet unknown risks and benefits of starting ART early in disease progression; the effects of this new initiative on access for others seeking ART in the health system; the impact of lifelong ART for pregnant women on horizontal transmission; the impact of unresolved barriers to adherence on resistance and disease progression; the opportunity costs with respect to other health priorities; the validity of the 'economies of scope' argument that combination prevention/treatment will have synergistic effects, and the retention rates that would be required to make the cost–benefit analysis come out in favour of B+ (Coutsoudis et al., 2013). A recent systematic review conducted on health system barriers and enablers to maternal ART bore out a number of these concerns and raised additional ones about the ability of weak health systems to manage the effective coordination of adult HIV services, PMTCT services and antenatal services and retain women in care over the long term (Colvin, Konopka, & Chalker, 2013).

While the debate over B+ is brewing but has not yet played out in dramatic fashion in the scientific literature and popular press, the debate over microbicides has been more public. Microbicides are part of a 'pre-exposure prophylaxis' approach (PrEP) to prevention that gives women control over a form of HIV prevention. Taken orally or applied vaginally in gel form, microbicides can be used by women without their partner's knowledge and there was hope that this prevention technology would provide a way for women to take some control over their exposure to infection. Researchers reported in 2010 that the CAPRISA 004 trial of a tenofivir-based gel had demonstrated an overall reduction in incidence of 39% in women, with 54% reductions seen in 'high-adherers' (Abdool Karim et al., 2010). These results were widely reported as a breakthrough in HIV prevention for women, and there soon came significant pressure from activists, clinicians, researchers and patient groups for the rapid roll-out of this new intervention.

Regulatory approval of the gel, however, would require a second trial to confirm the initial results, and advocates were concerned that the time required to conduct such a trial would unnecessarily assign 'thousands of women to a known inferior treatment' (Stein & Susser, 2010, p. 3). Despite calls for an exception to be made, it soon became clear that the results of further similar trials that were already in the field (e.g. the iPrEx, FEM-PrEP and VOICE trials) would be necessary before proceeding with rolling out the gel. Activists set about preparing the ground for these expected confirmatory results by preparing for 'fast-track' regulatory review and expanding the pipeline for production and distribution of the gel (AVAC: Global Advocacy for HIV Prevention, 2010).

When the FEM-PrEP and VOICE trials both reported no effect between the intervention and placebo arms in their trials, however, the prevention community was taken aback (MTN, 2012; Van Damme et al., 2012). Poor adherence to the interventions has been identified as the likely cause of the lack of effect, but this is yet to be confirmed. Critics argued that while other trials appear to have demonstrated the pharmacological *efficacy* of PrEP, poor adherence nonetheless represents a critical weakness in the *effectiveness* of the intervention, especially given the fairly well-supported trial context. They argued that further research was warranted on ways to increase women's adherence to the regimen. While PrEP has now been approved by the Food and Drug Administration in the United States, on the strength of positive results in other trials, there remains ambiguity around it as a recommended protocol or for standard of care in future prevention trials (Haire et al., 2013).

These debates over the nature, meaning and mobilisation of scientific evidence for new treatment and prevention approaches are not limited to these two cases. We have recently seen similar controversies over medical male circumcision (Ncayiyana, 2011; Wamai et al., 2011), treatment as prevention (Mills, Nachega, & Ford, 2013), nurse-initiated and managed ART (Georgeu et al., 2012), and the timing of treatment for TB/HIV co-infection (Boulle et al., 2010). Indeed, these kinds of debates have been a central thread running throughout the history of AIDS science and activism. There are some common issues that run throughout these debates. Table 1 summarises some of these issues in the form of key questions asked of or about the evidence.

Key forms of evidence for the era of ART and combination prevention

The diversity of questions in Table 1 should highlight how complicated the production and mobilisation of evidence can be. There are many kinds of evidence at stake in the complicated process of scale-up, present often in varying degrees of quality and quantity, and of uncertain relationship to each other when it comes to assessing the evidence 'for' or 'against' a particular option. It should also be clear that our need for different forms of evidence extends far beyond just the 'gold standard' randomised controlled trial (RCT), even though the results of these trials tend to garner most of the attention.

Table 1. Common issues in controversies around evidence for HIV treatment and prevention programmes.

Key question	Explanation
When do we have enough evidence?	When is the quality and quantity of evidence sufficient to make a policy decision? And who decides on the answer to this question? What scientific and policy processes might allow walking the very fine-line between forging ahead too quickly (and putting people at serious risk) and delaying too long (and keeping life-saving interventions unnecessarily out of reach)?
Why do people not follow the intervention (and does that matter)?	What are the behavioural, social and structural reasons that people do not participate in treatment or prevention efforts in the way intended? Should our evidence-making be focused around showing efficacy (i.e. proof of principle, in a controlled setting) or demonstrating effectiveness (in the real world), and who decides where this focus should lie?
Have implementation factors been adequately taken into account?	Are the costs, health system constraints and issues of community acceptability part of the evidence base? If so, how should we weigh up this evidence against the effectiveness evidence we might get from a trial? How much is it possible to know, with precision, about these implementation factors?
Should we privilege individual or community benefits when assessing the evidence?	What are the tensions between medical, human rights and public health perspectives on the problem? Can we use evidence to address them or are these ultimately political/philosophical questions? Or both?
How do we handle the known unknowns and unknown unknowns?	How do we factor in the fact that there will always be elements of the problem, either anticipated or not anticipated, about which we have no evidence available? How should we specify and assess 'potential long-term risks' in relation to known risks?
What is the relationship between evidence and policy?	To what extent does evidence of effectiveness and sustainability really factor into policy decisions? To what extent should it? What other factors are at play? How should the various forms of evidence relate to each other in this process? Again, who decides?

In this section, I map out what I see as the key forms of evidence that will need to be produced and mobilised if we are to engage effectively with the challenges of HIV treatment and prevention scale-up. The forms of evidence we need are diverse and cannot be ranked by a single or rigid 'hierarchy' of evidence of the kind so central to evidence-based medicine's (EBM) approach to scientific knowledge. The notion of a hierarchy can be useful when considering narrowly defined research objectives. RCTs, for example, are demonstrably better at assessing drug efficacy than interviews; ethnography is demonstrably better at understanding cultural perceptions and assumptions than population surveys. But the task of scale-up will require addressing a vast and diverse set of research questions, each of which will have forms of evidence that are more useful and robust than others.

Ogden, Gupta, Fisher, and Warner (2011) described this complex constellation of necessary evidence succinctly when they argued that evidence needed to be 'multi-level, multi-modal, multi-method and multi-disciplinary' (p. S291). They were talking about evidence around HIV prevention, but the same can be said for the enterprise of producing scientific knowledge on treatment and prevention programmes, especially ones 'at scale' or across scales. This section maps the forms of evidence that would ideally flourish in an effective response to the policy and practice challenges of this new era of HIV scale-up. Table 2 summarises these key forms.

Improved evidence about the health system and more robust surveillance data about the impact of health interventions (and other factors) on population health (Point 1 in Table 2) are perhaps the most obvious forms of evidence that emerge as important in the era of scaling-up. The field of health system research is itself fairly new and working to establish itself as about substantially more than just health service research (Sauerborn, Nitayarumphong, & Gerhardus, 1999). Delivering ART at the coalface of service delivery requires a large, complicated and dynamic health system to provide logistics, infrastructure, finance, information, education, regulation, technology and human resources. We need rich evidence that takes the health system as a whole as its context and considers the effectiveness of treatment and prevention interventions from this broader perspective. Similarly, routine surveillance of ART programme data (both process and outcome data) as well as other health and health system variables is critical if we are to get a dependable bird's eye view of the current state of and recent changes in population health. Some initiatives, like the IeDEA collaboration, have begun developing regional databases of ART cohorts in public sector programmes, but more of this kind of initiative is needed (Wandeler et al., 2012).

For the last 10 years or so in public health, and indeed for longer if one looks in the critical social science literature, there have been pleas to pay more attention to, the social determinants of health, the social drivers of HIV or the structural forces shaping the

Table 2. Key forms of evidence for HIV treatment and prevention scale-up.

(1) Better health systems and surveillance evidence

(2) More evidence on the social and structural determinants of health and HIV/AIDS

(3) Renewed attention to evidence on the 'middle range' (meso-level, micro-sociology and interactionism, practice-oriented and phenomenological designs)

(4) Use of evidence from EBM, including RCTs and systematic reviews, but incorporating more expansive and more pragmatic designs and meaningfully integrating process evaluation components

(5) Basic science, behavioural, operational and translational research as a critical contextual evidence for RCTs and other interventional designs

(6) Careful use of modelling evidence and 'big data'

(7) Health economics evidence, including costing studies (cost, cost effectiveness, cost-benefit, opportunity costs), health financing studies, macroeconomics and health studies, from a variety of conceptual frameworks (deficit-oriented, needs-based, asset-based, capabilities-based)

(8) Features that cross-cut the evidence base: multi-level/scalar, multi-sectoral and multi-disciplinary, context-responsive and integrating time as a dynamic variable

epidemic (Mykhalovskiy & Rosengarten, 2009; Ogden, Gupta, Warner, & Fisher, 2011; Seeley et al., 2012; Point 2 in Table 2). This is generally set in contrast to the preponderance – and hegemonic authority – of evidence available in the domains of individual biology and behaviour. Combination prevention and lifelong ART both involve much more than just behaviour change and the delivery of technologies through the health system. These social and structural determinants of health, and of HIV in particular, exert a powerful mediating influence on individual agency and can represent critical barriers to or enablers of effective uptake of prevention and treatment.

That said, however, there is also increasing recognition that between the poles of individual-level evidence and evidence of the structural determinants of health, there exists a large and critical terrain of inter-personal, community and social interaction about which we also need strong evidence (Kippax, Stephenson, Parker, & Aggleton, 2013; Point 3 in Table 2). Between individuals and structures, there is an entire world of 'middle-range' phenomenon that is fundamental to understanding how treatment and prevention regimens are interpreted and engaged with (Knauft, 2006). It is in this domain where most of the dynamism and complexity of social responses to HIV are to be found and where most of the potential interventions to support treatment and prevention might be targeted.

Much of this dynamism and complexity is not to be found in the HIV world's most dominant microcosm of evidence – EBM. EBM is an approach to evidence review and synthesis that aims to provide a set of procedures for transparently and systematically assessing the quality of studies and strength of findings of specific research questions and synthesising these findings into an overall judgement on the state of scientific knowledge about a particular question (Mykhalovskiy & Weir, 2004; Solomon, 2011). While the broad aims of EBM are broadly unproblematic – transparent and systematic reviews of evidence on a narrow research question are generally better than ones that are not – the procedures of EBM can be overly narrow and rigid, driven by a technicist fantasy that if one just apply the correct protocol, the right answer will reveal itself.

As argued above, policy and practice questions are much broader and more complicated than narrow research questions, and EBM is poorly suited by itself to provide the sole evidence for these bigger challenges. RCTs and systematic reviews, the twin stars of EBM, will continue to provide essential evidence for HIV scale-up, but our approach to EBM also needs to change and apply its core strengths (systematic methods for identifying bias in research and synthesising a body of evidence) to a wider set of study designs and in a more flexible and pragmatic way. This process of change is already under way within the heart of the EBM enterprise, the Cochrane Collaboration, which recently published the first ever systematic review of qualitative evidence to be included in the 'Cochrane Library' (Glenton et al., 2013a, 2013b). Though this development marks a fairly radical departure from the portrait of EBM orthodoxy drawn by most of its critics, there is still much to be done in making the EBM project better suited to responding to the complex questions of HIV prevention and treatment programmes.

While RCTs will continue to provide critical evidence on the specific questions they are designed to answer, a broad and useful portfolio of evidence also requires robust findings from a wide range of other domains, including basic science, behavioural science, operational research and translational research (Point 5 in Table 2). This body of evidence provides critical contextual and explanatory evidence for the findings of RCTs and other intervention study designs. And they provide the foundation on which to design and implement HIV prevention and treatment interventions in the first place.

Given the complexity of the policy and practice questions described above, and the fact that research disciplines have to work within both the ethical and material constraints of empirical research, modelling has come to occupy a prominent role in evidence for HIV programming (Point 6 in Table 2). Modelling studies have looked at the effect of sexual networks on HIV transmission, at the potential impact of treatment-as-prevention strategies, and at the likely comparative health and health economic outcomes of different prevention strategies (Eaton, Hallett, & Garnett, 2011). Modelling can be a powerful tool for generating hypotheses and for addressing research questions that would be difficult to answer through empirical research. However, modelling is also highly sensitive to the initial assumptions of which models are based and great care has to be exercised in both producing and assessing the output of models (Hallett, 2012). A related area of evidence that has not yet made a big contribution to HIV research but might in the future is the world of so-called 'big data' (Mayer-Schonberger & Cukier, 2013). Massive datasets, such as those that might be held within national health information systems, medical insurance schemes and social networking could eventually play a similar role to modelling research by identifying trends that would otherwise not be visible and fostering hypotheses about patterns in these datasets.

Most HIV scale-up challenges involve the production and long-term maintenance of delivery systems, whether in the community, the health system or the market. If understanding how systems work (Point 1) is one of the most salient challenges in HIV scale-up, understanding how they can be resourced is a central component of that problem (Point 7 in Table 2). Evidence from health economics has been important in HIV research but most often in its most narrow form – costing, cost-effectiveness and cost–benefit studies. As I argued above with respect to EBM, this costing evidence provides crucial information, but we need greater diversity of health economics evidence including evidence on health financing, microeconomics and health behaviours, and the interrelationships between macroeconomics and health outcomes. Importantly, we also need more of the research to come from a variety of conceptual frameworks, ones that move beyond the deficit-based approaches of classical economics and include needs-based, asset-based and capabilities-based approaches (Seckinelgin, 2012). Understanding the long-term opportunities and challenges of the scale-up of HIV treatment and prevention programming will require these much richer forms of health economics evidence.

All of the above points have so far focused on the different kinds of evidence necessary for effective HIV scale-up. I want to turn now to some general features that all of these forms of evidence will need to share, ones that reflect the complexity of the task at hand. They will all need to be able to work at multiple levels or scales, be responsive to the impact of context on their findings, integrate input from multiple sectors and multiple disciplines, and make use of time as a dynamic variable (Point 8 in Table 2). The importance of working at multiple scales and levels has already been discussed above in a number of ways as a critical feature of this evidence base. The importance of local context and individual-level experience is often something to which lip-service is paid, but substantive incorporation of context and experience into research designs is still weak and usually undertaken after the fact in post-hoc analyses. Also in short supply are research designs that produce evidence in multiple sectors (e.g. HIV/AIDS, maternal and child health, education, housing) and from multiple disciplines (e.g. epidemiology, sociology, engineering).

Finally, time is a critical element that needs to be integrated in a much more central and complex fashion in the production of HIV evidence. HIV scale-up is by definition an enterprise that unfolds in the long term. However, too much of the research we have either does not model the effect of time at all – by only asking the question 'Does it work?' – or it only incorporates time in the sense of 'sustainability' – by asking the question, 'How long can we keep it working?' The challenge of time in HIV scale-up is not how to sustain interventions in the long-term that show promise in the short-term. It is rather how to design interventions that are responsive and resilient to the fact that changes that occur over time are always dynamic and unpredictable. Research on the experience of chronic diseases has made this point well – chronicity is not the rigid and inevitable persistence of a particular state of being (Manderson & Smith-Morris, 2010). Rather, it is something that is experienced as episodic and uneven, and as something that is always subject to broader short- and long-term changes in the life-course and the contexts of those suffering chronic disease. Much of the thinking in HIV research, however, has not moved beyond a static notion of prevention and treatment, as something that needs to be 'implemented' and then 'maintained' for the long-term (Nixon, Hanass-Hancock, Whiteside, & Barnett, 2011).

The politics of evidence after scale-up: the mundane, the democratic and the critical

While the complex array of evidence outlined above would speak to most of the key evidentiary challenges of HIV scale-up, it risks remaining merely a technical exercise and laundry list of useful forms of knowledge if it is not guided by a particular political urgency and strategy. Knowledge production and mobilisation does not – and should not – happen in isolation of the political field but is rather shot through with the political in a variety of ways. This final section considers how activism and evidence-making might most usefully intersect in this third phase of the HIV response.

Activist mobilisation of scientific knowledge during earlier eras in the epidemic was framed and energised through the lens of crisis and emergency. During the first period, the so-called 'plague years' when HIV represented a terrifying death sentence, activists demanded awareness efforts and effective prevention strategies, more rapid treatment research, and social solidarity with stigmatised and marginalised populations. During the second period, the struggle for treatment access in the South, activists called for global regulation of pharmaceutical pricing and changes in prejudiced donor attitudes that steered money away from poor African countries and their citizens who were considered unable to effectively implement life-saving ART.

In both periods, the urgent spectre of needless death and suffering happening or just about to happen framed activist efforts. In the era of HIV scale-up, however, these deaths are delayed and the problems reframed. No longer are corporate giants, ignorant aid policy-makers or neglectful states framed as the main culprits. Instead, the struggle for effective prevention and lifelong treatment centres around much more diffuse and ambiguous notions like ongoing community acceptability; individual adherence practices in the context of chronic care and competing health and social demands; migration and continuity of care; the human resources crisis in health; increasing drug resistance and the evolution of pricing mechanisms for next-generation medications; issues of drug supply and formulation; and health financing schemes for long-term sustainability of ART.

In many Northern countries, where ART has been accessible for a number of years, treatment has not quite 'killed activism' (Robins, 2005), but it has certainly transformed it. In many of these contexts, however, the 'scale-up' of HIV treatment initiatives often entailed the provision of ART to thousands or tens of thousands of people within the context of large, relatively well-functioning, well-resourced health systems. The problems that emerged in these settings were not so much whether the health system could handle ART but whether the marginalised groups who experienced the greatest burden of HIV would be able to access this care and whether gains in prevention efforts with 'key populations' at greater risk would be lost as time passed.

In many of the Southern countries that have recently begun scaling-up treatment and combination prevention, however, the numbers of people who need ART represent a significant portion of the population, in settings where health systems already struggle to keep up with basic primary health care needs. In these contexts, the policy and practice questions that evidence will be asked to address will not be 'what treatments are effective?' or 'can ART can be provided effectively in poor countries by nurses at the primary level?', but rather, 'how can HIV programmes, health systems, individuals and communities be supported in the long-term to sustain a complex, dynamic and always shifting treatment and prevention response?'

This new set of questions brings new political challenges as well. Below, I outline three strategies for activist engagement with evidence in this phase. The first strategy is to engage more fully with the 'mundane' as a political problem and terrain. In the context of HIV scale-up, activists must decide how to mobilise their base and key allies, elicit moral outrage, pursue political and legal strategies, and generate a public narrative or frame for this new struggle that has some traction. They must do this in relation to a set of challenges that are not particularly headline-grabbing, ones that are not directly tied to imminent (or at least readily visible) suffering or death, and ones for which there is not a convenient and discrete set of villains. And they must do it in a global health funding environment that has rapidly contracted and in a global health policy context that has decided that other health problems like maternal and child health and chronic diseases should merit a greater proportion of money and attention than they had during the heyday of the global response to HIV/AIDS.

While the results of name-branded RCTs of acronymed interventions – MaxART for TasP, VOICE for PrEP, and so on – have typically commanded a great deal of attention in activist and popular imaginations, AIDS activists have in fact never been shy about engaging with the more mundane aspects of HIV intervention evidence including dosing and formulation recommendations, drug supply chain issues, health financing and drug pricing policies, etc.

Often, however, their engagement with these forms of evidence has happened 'backstage', in technical meetings to prepare affidavits for litigation, or in policy briefs for meetings with key global health actors. Activist-academic links have been important in this regard, and activists' ability to collate, interpret and make use of this more mundane information has led to notable victories (Colvin & Heywood, 2010). Again, though, the role of evidence in securing these victories is often less recognised or celebrated than the role of political protest and media engagement.

The Treatment Action Campaign (TAC) in South Africa has managed to continue and extend this trend in the current era. It has increasingly focussed on monitoring and evaluating the day-to-day operational aspects of ART scale-up. During a recent crisis, for example, in the supply of ARVs caused by HR disputes at one drug depot in the Eastern Cape Province, TAC, along with Médecins Sans Frontières (MSF, or Doctors without Borders) and other partners, hired temporary workers to handle the backlog and deliver drugs to facilities. They also set up a hotline and monitoring service to better detect stock outs of essential drugs at specific clinics. They now plan to develop a nationwide monitoring system:

> To improve essential drug supply monitoring, the RHAP [Rural Health Advocacy Project], the Southern African HIV Clinicians' Society, SECTION27, TAC and MSF plan to set up a drug stock-out monitoring system. The aim is to centralise reporting on supply ruptures from patients and health staff into a national database, to identify clinics requiring emergency supplies. (TAC, 2013)

Mundane then clearly does not mean unimportant. These drug stock-outs were indeed emergencies for those left without the medication they needed. But these events took place at a level and a domain of the health system that is not the usual province of activists. And they involved a set of complicated health system challenges that do not necessarily have straightforward or dramatic solutions. Nonetheless, they were able to build a visible coalition of activists, academics, clinicians, lawyers and state officials to respond to a particular crisis in one small part of the country, and in the process, set in motion plans for a new source of national operational evidence about the scale-up.

One important element of the example from TAC above is its mobilisation of civil society actors in the production and application of evidence for scale-up. In the absence of effective government management of supply chains and health information, this loose coalition came together to mount its own intervention and develop its own evidence. This was not meant to be a displacement of the government's roles and responsibilities; nor was it intended to substitute for expert academic knowledge production. It did, however, represent a democratisation of the relationship between evidence-making and the public. The democratisation of evidence, both in terms of access and production, is the second political strategy around evidence I would like to advocate.

Zackie Achmat, one of the founders of TAC, has taken this strategy of engaging with evidence around the daily administration of the state further in a new organisation called *Ndifuna Ukwazi* (NU, literally 'I Want to Know' but glossed by the NGO as 'Dare to Know;' www.nu.org.za). NU engages trainee-activist 'fellows', partner non-governmental organisations and communities in a range of activities designed to build literacy and active engagement among ordinary members of the public in technical legal, financial and medical domains. In contrast to the back-room technical consultations between expert activists and academic experts that characterised earlier periods, NU tries to deepen the 'democratisation of the AIDS response' (Sidibe, 2011). It also tried to extend the lessons learned in the AIDS response beyond HIV and into other political struggles. While similar to the 'expert patient' strategy and treatment literacy initiatives TAC used in previous years, this new approach focuses not only on training people to understand an evidence base but also in ongoing citizen engagement with, and even production of, the routine forms of information and evidence deployed in the daily administration of the state.

This approach is similar to strategies used by activists working in other domains, including self-census for access to housing and sanitation, community audits of health facilities and people's budgets (Robins, 2003). Indeed, many of the key challenges and strategies with respect to evidence that are faced by AIDS activists in this latest phase are shared by other activists in global public health. The need to work on multiple levels, scales and timeframes; to respond to intersecting crises; to think about systems and structures in ways that enable effective intervention; and to engage in the conversation about scientific evidence and its relationship to policy on an equal footing with the other stakeholders around the table – all of these are critical challenges more generally for the political mobilisation of scientific evidence in global health.

Again, democratising the production of and access to health evidence does not entail reducing government responsibilities or ignoring expert academic contributions. The role of scientific institutions in producing evidence and state institutions in stewarding and applying the evidence base should remain central. So too should the activist's mandate to hold both scientific and state institutions to account for their obligations to produce and use evidence effectively and equitably. But there are signs, far beyond the field of HIV, that the democratisation of information is a critical political fact of life and potent political instrument in a world globally cross-cut by social media, cheap laptops, cloud computing, smartphones and 'big data'.

Finally, activists will need to move beyond some of the conventional kinds of 'data-driven advocacy' described above (Baral & Phaswana-Mafuya, 2012) and promote the production and deployment of new forms of evidence that are 'critical' in perspective and independent of existing institutional and hegemonic modes of knowledge production. Too often, activists join with those in the biomedical mainstream in framing evidence as something that can and should stand apart from politics, as if the 'answer' is in the data. On the one hand, as Nathan Geffen (2013) argues, activists need 'clear' scientific evidence and internationally recognised guidelines in order to bring pressure on governments to provide services to its citizens. On the other hand, however, if they rely only on state-sanctioned forms of 'knowledge [created] for governing healthcare' (Mykhalovskiy & Rosengarten, 2009) such as 'evidence-based norms and standards', activists may find themselves increasingly co-opted in both a discourse and a practice of evidence that reproduces some of the worst elements of the status quo.

Being 'critical' about the production of scientific knowledge does not (necessarily) mean being dismissive of foundational epistemological claims of contemporary science. Rather it means framing the complicated process of knowledge production and application as a series of decisions that are always both technical and political. It involves asking why certain questions get asked and others do not (or why they get asked in certain ways). Or why certain groups are included as participants, producers or consumers in scientific research and others excluded. Or why certain forms of evidence such as clinical trials are privileged and others such as social research or life histories are marginalised. This kind of critical questioning needs to extend even into the detailed methodological choices that go into making evidence, including issues like the relative merits and uses of efficacy versus effectiveness research designs, the complex strategies for sampling effectively and avoiding bias, and the ways in which complex bodies of evidence are synthesised and then communicated to a wide audience.

This work of a critical science of HIV is not new – these are the kinds of questions that activists have asked from the very early days of the epidemic. But they are the kinds of questions that are becoming harder to ask and answer in an era when HIV scale-up is increasingly understood as a messy set of technical problems, mundane tasks of health financing, long-term maintenance of behaviour change, supply chain management and careful realignment of primary health care services.

In HIV scale-up, and indeed in global health more generally, we need to find ways of doing both things at once – meeting the urgent need to 'know more' about the world's health problems and make effective use of this evidence, while also responding to the just as urgent demand for ways to complicate conventional ways of 'knowing' that tend to leave out so much of what is in fact critical to understand.

Acknowledgements

The thinking behind this paper emerged from a number of different projects around HIV and knowledge production that I have conducted with a wide range of academics, scientists, policy-makers, activists and community members in South Africa and elsewhere. I am grateful to all of them for their insights and engagement. I am also grateful to the two anonymous reviewers of an earlier version of this manuscript for their very helpful comments.

Funding

Time to work on this paper was partially supported by the Eunice Kennedy Shriver National Institute of Child Health & Human Development of the National Institutes of Health [award number R24HD077976]. The content is solely the responsibility of the author and does not necessarily represent the official views of the National Institutes of Health.

References

Abdool Karim, Q., Abdool Karim, S. S., Frohlich, J. A., Grobler, A. C., Baxter, C., Mansoor, L. E., … Taylor, D. (2010). Effectiveness and safety of tenofovir gel, an antiretroviral microbicide, for the prevention of HIV infection in women. *Science, 329*, 1168–1174. doi:10.1126/science.1193748

AVAC: Global Advocacy for HIV Prevention. (2010). *A cascade of hope and questions: Understanding the results of CAPRISA 004*. New York, NY: Author.

Baral, S., & Phaswana-Mafuya, N. (2012). Rewriting the narrative of the epidemiology of HIV in sub-Saharan Africa. *SAHARA-J: Journal of Social Aspects of HIV/AIDS, 9*(3), 127–130. doi:10.1080/17290376.2012.743787

Boulle, A., Clayden, P., Cohen, K., Cohen, T., Conradie, F., Dong, K., … Wilson, D. (2010). Prolonged deferral of antiretroviral therapy in the SAPIT trial: Did we need a clinical trial to tell us that this would increase mortality? *South African Medical Journal, 100*, 566, 568, 570–561.

CDC. (2013). Impact of an innovative approach to prevent mother-to-child transmission of HIV–Malawi, July 2011-September 2012. *MMWR Morbidity and Mortality Weekly Report, 62*, 148–151. Atlanta, GA: Centers for Disease Control and Prevention.

Colvin, C. J., & Heywood, M. (2010). Negotiating ARV prices with pharmaceutical companies and the South African government: A civil society/legal approach. In E. Rosskam & I. Kickbusch (Eds.), *Negotiating and navigating global health: Case studies in global health diplomacy* (pp. 351–372). Hackensack, NJ: World Scientific.

Colvin, C. J., Konopka, S., & Chalker, J. (2013). *A systematic review of health system barriers to and enablers of ART for pregnant and postpartum women with HIV*. Washington, DC: Management Sciences for Health and USAID.

Coutsoudis, A., Goga, A., Desmond, C., Barron, P., Black, V., & Coovadia, H. (2013). Is option B+ the best choice? *Lancet, 381*, 269–271. doi:10.1016/S0140-6736(12)61807-8

Eaton, J. W., Hallett, T. B., & Garnett, G. P. (2011). Concurrent sexual partnerships and primary HIV infection: A critical interaction. *AIDS and Behaviour, 15*, 687–692. doi:10.1007/s10461-010-9787-8

Epstein, S. (1996). *Impure science: AIDS, activism, and the politics of knowledge*. Berkeley: University of California Press.

Geffen, N. (2013). World Health Organization guidelines should not change the CD4 count threshold for antiretroviral therapy initiation. *South African Journal of HIV Medicine, 14*(1), 6–7.

Georgeu, D., Colvin, C. J., Lewin, S., Fairall, L., Bachmann, M. O., Uebel, K., … Bateman, E. D. (2012). Implementing nurse-initiated and managed antiretroviral treatment (NIMART) in South Africa: A qualitative process evaluation of the STRETCH trial. *Implementation Science, 7*, 66. doi:10.1186/1748-5908-7-66

Glenton, C., Colvin, C. J., Carlsen, B., Swartz, A., Lewin, S., Noyes, J., & Rashidian, A. (2013a). Barriers and facilitators to the implementation of lay health worker programmes to improve access to maternal and child health: Qualitative evidence synthesis (protocol). *The Cochrane Library, 2*. doi:10.1002/14651858.CD010414

Glenton, C., Colvin, C. J., Carlsen, B., Swartz, A., Lewin, S., Noyes, J., & Rashidian, A. (2013b). Barriers and facilitators to the implementation of lay health worker programmes to improve access to maternal and child health: Qualitative evidence synthesis. *Cochrane Database of Systematic Reviews, 10*, CD010414. doi:10.1002/14651858.CD010414.pub2

Haire, B., Folayan, M. O., Hankins, C., Sugarman, J., McCormack, S., Ramjee, G., & Warren, M. (2013). Ethical considerations in determining standard of prevention packages for HIV prevention trials: Examining PrEP. *Developing World Bioethics*, *13*(2), 87–94. doi:10.1111/dewb.12032

Hallett, T. (2012). *What mathematical models can tell us about prevention packages*. Washington, DC: PEPFAR.

Kippax, S., Stephenson, N., Parker, R. G., & Aggleton, P. (2013). Between individual agency and structure in HIV prevention: Understanding the middle ground of social practice. *American Journal of Public Health*, *103*: 1367–1375. doi:10.2105/AJPH.2013.301301

Knauft, B. M. (2006). Anthropology in the middle. *Anthropological Theory*, *6*, 407–430. doi:10.1177/1463499606071594

Manderson, L., & Smith-Morris, C. (2010). *Chronic conditions, fluid states: Chronicity and the anthropology of illness*. New Brunswick, NJ: Rutgers University Press.

Marx, C., Halcli, A., & Barnett, C. (2012). Locating the global governance of HIV and AIDS: Exploring the geographies of transnational advocacy networks. *Health and Place*, *18*, 490–495. doi:10.1016/j.healthplace.2012.02.006

Mayer-Schonberger, V., & Cukier, K. (2013). *Big data: A revolution that will transform how we live, work, and think*. New York, NY: Houghton Mifflin Harcourt.

Mills, E. J., Nachega, J. B., & Ford, N. (2013). Can we stop AIDS with antiretroviral-based treatment as prevention? *Global Health: Science and Practice*, *1*(1), 29–34. doi:10.9745/GHSP-D-12-00053

MTN. (2012). *MTN statement on decision to discontinue use of tenofovir gel in VOICE, a major HIV prevention study in women*. Pittsburgh, PA: Microbicide Trials Network.

Mykhalovskiy, E., & Rosengarten, M. (2009). HIV/AIDS in its third decade: Renewed critique in social and cultural analysis: An introduction. *Social Theory and Health*, *7*, 187–195. doi:10.1057/sth.2009.13

Mykhalovskiy, E., & Weir, L. (2004). The problem of evidence-based medicine: Directions for social science. *Social Science and Medicine*, *59*, 1059–1069. doi:10.1016/j.socscimed.2003.12.002

Ncayiyana, D. J. (2011). The illusive promise of circumcision to prevent female-to-male HIV infection – not the way to go for South Africa. *South African Medical Journal*, *101*, 775–776.

Nixon, S. A., Hanass-Hancock, J., Whiteside, A., & Barnett, T. (2011). The increasing chronicity of HIV in sub-Saharan Africa: Re-thinking 'HIV as a long-wave event' in the era of widespread access to ART. *Global Health*, *7*, 41. doi:10.1186/1744-8603-7-41

Ogden, J., Gupta, G. R., Fisher, W. F., & Warner, A. (2011). Looking back, moving forward: Towards a game-changing response to AIDS. *Global Public Health*, *6*, S285–S292. doi:10.1080/17441692.2011.621966

Ogden, J., Gupta, G. R., Warner, A., & Fisher, W. F. (2011). Revolutionising the AIDS response. *Global Public Health*, *6*, S383–S395. doi:10.1080/17441692.2011.621965

Robins, S. (2003). Grounding 'globalisation from below': 'Global citizens' in local spaces. In D. Chidester, W. G. James, & P. Dexter (Eds.), *What holds us together: Social cohesion in South Africa* (pp. 242–273). Johannesburg: HSRC Press.

Robins, S. (2005). *From 'medical miracles' to normal(ised) medicine: AIDS treatment, activism and citizenship in the UK and South Africa* (IDS Working Papers). Brighton: Institute for Development Studies, Sussex University.

Sauerborn, R., Nitayarumphong, S., & Gerhardus, A. (1999). Strategies to enhance the use of health systems research for health sector reform. *Tropical Medicine & International Health*, *4*, 827–835. doi:10.1046/j.1365-3156.1999.00497.x

Seckinelgin, H. (2012). The global governance of success in HIV/AIDS policy: Emergency action, everyday lives, and Sen's capabilities. *Health and Place*, *18*, 453–460. doi:10.1016/j.healthplace.2011.09.014

Seeley, J., Watts, C. H., Kippax, S., Russell, S., Heise, L., & Whiteside, A. (2012). Addressing the structural drivers of HIV: A luxury or necessity for programmes? *Journal of the International AIDS Society*, *15*(1), 1–4. doi:10.1186/1758-2652-15-1

Sidibe, M. (2011). *Letter to partners 2011*. Geneva: UNAIDS.

Solomon, M. (2011). Just a paradigm: Evidence-based medicine in epistemological context. *European Journal for Philosophy of Science*, *1*, 451–466. doi:10.1007/s13194-011-0034-6

Stein, Z., & Susser, I. (2010). *Transparency, accountability and feminist science: What next for microbicide trials?* Cape Town: AIDS Legal Network and ATHENA Network.

TAC. (2013). *Systematic problems in drug supply have to be addressed now to avert future crisis TAC Electronic Newsletter*. Cape Town: Treatment Action Campaign.

UNICEF. (2012). *Options B and B+: Key considerations for countries to implement at equity-focused approach*. New York, NY: Author.

Van Damme, L., Corneli, A., Ahmed, K., Agot, K., Lombaard, J., Kapiga, S., … Taylor, D. (2012). Preexposure prophylaxis for HIV infection among African women. *New England Journal of Medicine, 367*, 411–422. doi:10.1056/NEJMoa1202614

Wachter, R. M. (1992). AIDs, activism, and the politics of health. *New England Journal of Medicine, 326*(2), 128–133. doi:10.1056/NEJM199201093260209

Wamai, R. G., Morris, B. J., Bailis, S. A., Sokal, D., Klausner, J. D., Appleton, R., … Banerjee, J. (2011). Male circumcision for HIV prevention: Current evidence and implementation in sub-Saharan Africa. *Journal of the International AIDS Society, 14*, 49. doi:10.1186/1758-2652-14-49

Wandeler, G., Keiser, O., Pfeiffer, K., Pestilli, S., Fritz, C., Labhardt, N. D., … Ehmer, J. (2012). Outcomes of antiretroviral treatment programs in rural Southern Africa. *Journal of Acquired Immune Deficiency Syndrome, 59*, e9–e16. doi:10.1097/QAI.0b013e31823edb6a

Up-scaling expectations among Pakistan's HIV bureaucrats: Entrepreneurs of the self and job precariousness post-scale-up

Ayaz Qureshi

Department of Anthropology, School of Oriental and African Studies, University of London, London, UK

Existing research has documented how the expansion of HIV programming has produced new subjectivities among the recipients of interventions. However, this paper contends that changes in politics, power and subjectivities may also be seen among the HIV bureaucracy in the decade of scale-up. One year's ethnographic fieldwork was conducted among AIDS control officials in Pakistan at a moment of rolling back a World Bank-financed Enhanced Programme. In 2003, the World Bank convinced the Musharraf regime to scale up the HIV response, offering a multimillion dollar soft loan package. I explore how the Enhanced Programme initiated government employees into a new transient work culture and turned the AIDS control programmes into a hybrid bureaucracy. However, the donor money did not last long and individuals' entrepreneurial abilities were tested in a time of crisis engendered by dependence on aid, leaving them precariously exposed to job insecurity, and undermining the continuity of AIDS prevention and treatment in the country. I do not offer a story of global 'best practices' thwarted by local 'lack of capacity', but an ethnographic critique of the transnational HIV apparatus and its neoliberal underpinning. I suggest that this Pakistan-derived analysis is more widely relevant in the post-scale-up decade.

Introduction

Existing research has documented how the expansion of HIV programming has produced new subjectivities, bringing into being the subjects of its policies through the provision of interventions for them. In Africa and Brazil, lives lived with HIV are being transformed into the political category of People Living with HIV/AIDS (Biehl, 2007; Nguyen, 2010; Robins, 2004). In Nepal, myriad practices of sexual exchange are being isolated from their moral economies and brought out as 'hidden commercial sex work' (Pigg, 2002). In India, *meyeli chhele* (girlish boys) are being interpellated as 'men who have sex with men' (Khanna, 2009). This paper contends that it is not only among the subjects of HIV programming, but also among the HIV bureaucracy that changes in politics, power and subjectivities may be seen. Anthropological literature of a 'new ethnography of aid' has emphasised the role of intermediary actors – bureaucrats, clinicians, technicians, non-governmental organisation (NGO) staff and health workers – as 'brokers and translators' in the social life of projects, who translate global policy into their own ambitions, interests and values (Harper, 2011; Mosse, 2005; Mosse & Lewis, 2006; Pigg, 2002). This paper contributes to this literature by tracing the impact of the changes in global policy regimes, such as HIV scale-up and scale-down, on individual bureaucrats at a subjective level. It is not only the 'brokers and translators' who refigure the global policy objectives to suit their interests and values, but changes in the global policy regimes also affect transformations in the subjectivities of these intermediary actors. The recent decade of HIV scale-up has been characterised by increasingly technocratic, top-down initiatives, which have generated thousands of jobs in the emerging administrative apparatus (Pisani, 2008; Rowden, 2009). In Pakistan, traditional government offices have been transformed into flexible bureaucracies (Qureshi, 2014), and the denizens of those offices have been turned into the enterprising but anxious subjects of neoliberalism.

Pakistan is believed to have more than 130,000 HIV-positive people, although less than 6000 are registered with the treatment facilities (National AIDS Control Programme [NACP], 2012; UNAIDS, 2013). A vast majority remain undiagnosed due to extreme stigma in health services and the wider society. While this represents less than 1% of the population, Pakistan has been classified by UN agencies as at 'high risk' of a generalised epidemic (NACP, 2010). This is because the country has among the highest numbers of injecting drug users (IDUs) in the world (UNODC, 2013), and recent surveys among the 'high risk groups' indicate prevalence rates of up to 50% among IDUs in some cities, with overall prevalence rates of 37.8% for IDUs, 7.2% for *hijra* (transgender) sex workers, 3.1% for male sex workers and 0.8% for female sex workers (HIV and AIDS Surveillance Project [HASP], 2011). Although Pakistan's HASP has not collected prevalence data for labour migrants to date, the NACP is in the process of drawing up guidelines for doing so, following feedback from HIV treatment centres that the majority of HIV-positive people registered are returnee labour migrants from the Persian Gulf as well as the wives and children of migrants (Qureshi, 2013b).

Throughout 1990s, the donor funding for HIV, despite lobbying from civil society, was sporadic and loosely monitored, constituting only 20% of the total HIV-related outlay (Zaidi, 2008). However, in 2003, the World Bank sponsored a public–private partnership called the Enhanced HIV and AIDS Control Programme, by convincing the Finance Minister to invest in 'scaling-up' the HIV response as it was, in their opinion, a development problem rather than a health problem alone. The Finance Minister, who was a former city banker from Washington and had recently arrived in the country to serve in the technocratic-military regime of General Musharraf, took a favourable view of the Bank's development policies (Zaidi, 2008). The Ministry of Health (MoH) was sidelined in the negotiations with the Bank as the Ministry of Finance dominated proceedings. The Bank-infused federal government replaced the NACP manager, a senior health bureaucrat, with a junior staff who had proven herself to be receptive to Bank's guidance and expertise. Under the terms of this World Bank soft loan, the role of the government was effectively reduced to that of a purchaser of services and the manager of the contracts. Elsewhere I have argued that the 'new managerialism of international development' (Mosse, 2005) turned Pakistan's AIDS control into a 'hybrid bureaucracy' (Qureshi, 2013a).

The new scaled-up version of the national and provincial AIDS control programmes (ACP) offered big market-based salaries and incentives, which attracted government servants from other departments as well as a range of contractual employees from the 'market' – highly paid western-educated experts and market-based consultants—who brought with them their particular styles of management and work cultures. For instance, by July 2010, the NACP categorised its total 68 employees as follows: 38 'basic pay scale employees', seconded from various government departments; 10 'market-based employees', working on short-term renewable contracts and the 20 'donor-supported employees', whose salaries came directly from United Nations Population Fund (UNFPA), United Nations Children's Fund (UNICEF) and Family Health International (FHI). Technical assistance from a fleet of freelance consultants – 'bands of hunters and gathers' as Jock Stirrat (2000) has called them – was another common feature of the day-to-day life and work at the ACPs.

There is a literature on Pakistan's response to HIV, which has evaluated it in terms of its success or failure in implementing donor-funded projects, and has criticised the Pakistani state as unable to properly implement global 'best practices', and therefore, as in need of 'capacity building' (e.g. see Hawkes, Zaheer, Tawil, O'Dwyer, & Buse, 2012; Hussain, Kadir, & Fatmi, 2007; Karim & Zaidi, 1999; Mayhew et al., 2009; Zaidi, 2008; Zaidi, Mayhew, & Palmer, 2011). However, this paper takes a different approach. Rather than concluding that global policy regimes are hamstrung by the lack of capacity of the Pakistani state, or by related problems of corruption, inefficiency, red tapism and lack of political will, I explore the moral embeddedness of the HIV bureaucracy – following classic studies in the anthropology of bureaucracy, which have critiqued the idea of the Weberian rational bureaucracy (see Crozier, 1964; Sennett, 2006; Shore & Wright, 1997). I suggest that the life of the government departments in which I worked can be illuminated by anthropological work on neoliberal work cultures, drawing from Paul du Gay (1994) on the 'enterprise model' of government, Nadesan and Trethewey (2000) and Peter Kelly (2006) on the 'entrepreneurial self', and Michael Feher (2009) on the 'governance of human capital'. These authors provide the grounds for a conceptualisation of the changing subjectivities of bureaucrats in the decade of HIV scale-up, drawing from psychoanalytic theory.

This paper draws on my ethnographic fieldwork carried out from June 2010 to September 2011 for doctoral research on the politics of Pakistan's response towards HIV – a multi-sited organisational ethnography (Hastings, 2013). The fieldwork coincided with a recession in international donor funding for HIV in Pakistan, especially the rollback of the World Bank-financed Enhanced Programme. I travelled to different cities to interview national and provincial health bureaucracy and AIDS control officials, representatives of donor agencies and NGO/community-based organisation (CBO) bosses and workers, members of civil society and representatives of people living with AIDS. I took part in World AIDS Days-related activities, training workshops for fieldworkers, the launching ceremonies of research reports and guidelines for practitioners and dissemination seminars of bio-behavioural survey results. I carried out participant observation at a large number of high-level internal meetings between government's AIDS control officials and the representatives of their partner organisations. As a research internee at the ACP, I was assigned a line manager, given a desk of my own and obliged to work with a team of colleagues on specific projects. I spent 15 months sharing and observing their everyday work and life in this organisation. In the following, I present an extended case study of a single employee with regards to his dealings with other colleagues and his anxieties concerning his future in the post-scale-up phase in the HIV sector. In doing so, I deploy participant observation 'to locate everyday life in its extralocal and historical context' (Burawoy, 1998, p. 4), to illuminate some of the entrepreneurial relations that were being engendered at the ACP under the World Bank-financed Enhanced Programme and what they entailed for employees who had moulded themselves into enterprising selves. The point is not to demonstrate problems in the practices of individuals, but to explore the work culture that pervaded the institution.

'Entrepreneurial self'

Peter was the de facto manager of the ACP, known to his colleagues and partners in the HIV sector as the 'main guy' there. While the incumbent ACP managers were political appointees, he was the technical expert who took lead in meetings, negotiated the finer details of programmatic interventions, prepared multimedia presentations and wrote speeches for them. With a master's degree from a prestigious British University and a good knowledge of HIV epidemiology, excellent communication skills and command over technical matters, he had built extensive networks in the HIV sector. Superficially, he complained that his colleagues in the ACP depended too much on him. 'Why do you run to me for everything? Is there no one else in this office? How many things can I look into?' he would reprimand his juniors. Yet, nothing went unnoticed by him. Sometimes, he seemed to enjoy being looked up to from all directions. He boasted that he could give presentations on the spur of the moment, could tell the contents of a document just by a cursory look at the first few lines, and that only he was capable of intellectual discussions with external experts. In short, he was sought after by everyone and he could fit all caps. He boasted that he had 'at least two to three job offers at any time', but he did not leave the ACP because 'the government relies too much on me' – so much so that 'the health secretary has personally requested me not to leave'. This he confided to almost every visitor to his office cabin, which was adjacent to mine.

When a junior colleague, Rabia, who worked in a donor-supported position under his supervision shared that she considered quitting the ACP due to non-payment of her salaries over past few months, Peter made it clear to her that she was replaceable from the 'market'. 'We will find someone else to fill your place', he told her firmly while also assuring her that he would look into the bureaucratic hitches that were apparently responsible for the delays in the payment of her salary. A few days later, when she stopped coming to the office, he tried to trivialise her concerns and ridiculed her decision in front of other colleagues. 'If the delay in her salary was such a big issue that she could not trust the ACP', he said dismissively, 'I offered her a bank cheque from my own account which she could have kept as a guarantee and returned when her salary was released, but she didn't accept it'. He was particularly annoyed because she left despite his persuasion along the following lines:

> No matter how good a package NGOs might offer you, no NGO compares the platform you have here. You are very lucky to be here at the time when the Global Fund project is about to start. Imagine yourself in two years – you will be like us! If you decide to leave, we will find someone. But I'm telling you this because we are colleagues and we get along well: this is *not* a good time to leave here. Take my example, when our ship was sinking [i.e. when the ACP was in jeopardy because of low levels of external funding]: everyone left, but I stayed on.

The role of managers in the 'enterprise model' of organisational life, according to Paul du Gay (1994), is to foster enterprise among their subordinates, 'leading them to the promised land of self-realization by encouraging them to make a project of themselves, to work on their relations with employment and on other areas of their lives in order to develop a style of life and relation to self that will maximize the worth of their existence to themselves' (p. 644). While both managers and workers are amenable to 'entrepreneurial reconstitution', the former are charged with 'reconstituting the conduct and self-image of employees; with encouraging them to acquire capacities and dispositions that will enable them to become enterprising persons' (du Gay, 1994). I could see Peter trying to do this, on one hand, by showing Rabia the entrepreneurial possibilities that she could explore if she stuck to her current job – 'imagine yourself in two years time...' – and on the other, by making it very clear that she could easily be replaced if she kept insisting that the backlog in her salary be dealt with or threatened to quit the job. He gave her his own example, emphasising that his relation with her as her manager was intimate rather than distant and formal – 'I am telling you this because we get along well...' This calculatingly charismatic management is in contrast to the remote or officious manager of a traditional bureaucracy, and it reflects the new culture that emerged at the ACP under the Enhanced Programme, with its neoliberal underpinnings. Entrepreneurship came to dominate, but not outright replace, the bureaucratic proceduralism of the postcolonial 'paper government' in this department (cf. Hull, 2012).

Rabia had developed different ideas about her role at the ACP. She confided in me that she could not 'bear the idleness' in the 'government sector'. She said she had 'learnt nothing' in this job because she was given only secretarial work, and that it was time for her now to 'come out of the coordination roles and make some upward progress to programme management roles'. Apparently she already had a job offer from an international NGO, which would give a good pay package and a programme management role. While Peter was a good example of a manager in the emerging 'enterprise model' of organisational life at the ACP, Rabia personified the 'entrepreneurial Self' that Peter Kelly (2006) has identified as the emerging 'Subject' of neoliberalism – 'a *free, prudent, active* Subject [with] *rational, autonomous, responsible* behaviour and disposition' – as the medium through which neoliberalism has emerged to govern the state, economy and civil society (p. 18, *original emphasis*). The HIV sector of the scale-up decade, and the NGOs more broadly, were no exception to this transformation of government employees into prudent subjects, becoming the conduits for the proliferation this encompassing mode of governance.

Human capital and self-appreciation

Michel Feher (2009) has drawn a parallel between corporate governance in the neoliberal world of globalised unregulated financial markets, and the governance of human capital. According to him, 'insofar as our condition is that of human capital in a neoliberal environment, our main purpose is not so much to profit from our accumulated potential as to constantly value or appreciate ourselves – or at least prevent our own depreciation' (p. 27). The way in which employees at the ACP treated themselves as human capital were shown to me a few days into my internship at the ACP when I met Maya in Peter's office. She introduced herself as a physician, who ran her own clinic, taught in a medical school and did research consultancies on infectious diseases. This diversity of occupations was deliberate; according to her, 'my bills are paid by clinical practice, through teaching I want to remain in touch with academia, and the research consultancies on infectious disease complement my PhD plans'. A few days later, I heard Peter upset with her for ignoring his advice on how much to quote as her consultancy fee; 'you should have quoted at least US$400 if not US$500. Send them an email now and tell them that you were in a different frame of mind when you quoted US$250, and that you want to revise it to US$400'. This way, he continued, 'they' might agree to at least US $350 per day. Maya must have panicked, and asked if he had seen the Terms of Reference (TORs) for the consultancy. Peter, who had now calmed down, burst into laughter and said that it was actually him who had written those TORs.

The ACP often hired external consultants for technical and logistical support. The selection procedures varied depending on the donors, but in most cases Maya was selected without any competition because the new flexible work culture of the Enhanced Programme allowed for shelving the old bureaucratic procedures in the name of 'efficiency'. Organising seminars, meetings, training, and workshops was sourced out almost exclusively to her. She carried out this work most of the time from Peter's office – he would often vacate his seat for her. He would make phone calls on her behalf to organise these events. Because of his position at the ACP, he knew people whom she either did not know or had no access to. He used his influence to get things done for her even though she was paid hefty sums for doing just those things. He also involved his subordinates, like Rabia, to 'facilitate' the consultant, which often meant that they ended up doing the work for which she was paid.

Maya cultivated an air of importance about herself. She had eloquent speech, mixing English, Urdu and a rather masculine form of Punjabi – 'code switching' (Gumpertz, 1982) – which enabled her to command any conversation. She also appeared, wearing a doctors' white gown, in commercial adverts on television, advising mothers to use a brand of antiseptic soap to keep their children safe from germs. She was a sort of celebrity among the mix of rather modest old-fashioned government bureaucrats and young NGO-style, market-based employees at the ACP. Compared with her personal charms and a diversity of occupations, it was Peter's position at the ACP that he employed to enhance and maintain his influence in the HIV sector. Together they secured consultancies in her name and together they completed them. Playing to their respective strengths, this duo could put up performances that were not possible for either of them alone. At times when she was frustrated with the amount of work or complained about lack of cooperation from other corners, he calmed her down by promising to get things done all by himself, or by changing the topic to buying a new car, shopping and holidaying.

He set lenient TORs in her contracts, making sure that there were no problems in the release of payments, often spreading the total amount over fewer instalments and substantial portion paid in advance. He used his influence in donor agencies to expedite payments. 'Our payment will be transferred into your account very soon', he told her on phone on one occasion, and explained that out of the three instalments, two would be transferred within a week and the remaining one some time later. She asked if he preferred his share to be transferred into his account right away or he would like to wait until the full amount was first received in her account. The reply was '*Daal daina jab dil kare, abhi daal do ya baad mien daal daiana*' that is, 'send it [in my account] whenever you like, now or later'.

To sustain and to improve the chances of Maya's position as the ACP's favourite consultant, it was very important to raise 'stocks' in the 'human capital' that she was. Feher (2009) defines human capital as 'a set of skills and capabilities that is modified by all that affects me and all that I affect ... It refers to all that is produced by the skill set that defines me' (p. 26). There is an uncomfortable parallel between exchange relations of an individual as 'human capital' and the extended order of capitalist markets – of all sorts, where the performance of exchange relations is characterised by the 'possibility and promise of greed, deception, monopoly, winners and losers, inequalities' (Kelly, 2006, p. 29). The kind of trust displayed in the above transaction between Maya and Peter was very important in their entrepreneurial relationship. He was set to benefit from 'investing' in her. He made sure that she attended most of the HIV stakeholders meetings at the ACP even though she hardly ever contributed in formal discussions. She was not only 'on the scene' but he actively introduced her to important people among donors, NGOs and government policy circles, promoting her as the best consultant in Pakistan on infectious diseases, especially HIV. At the same time, he did not let his 'investment' in her go unaccounted by her, and he reminded her repeatedly that it was because of him that they secured consultancies in her name. For example, he told her on one occasion in his office cabin that he had deliberately asked an international consultant, who she had worked with on a joint project, to give feedback on her performance in the presence of a senior UN official; 'so that he [the official] knows how well you perform [do your work]'. For Peter, investing in Maya, in this way, was a kind of 'self-appreciation' (Feher, 2009) through investment in another.

An anxious subject

Peter appeared to justify the idealised entrepreneurial identity, where, as Nikolas Rose (1996) observes, 'modes of life that appear philosophically opposed – business success and personal growth, image management and authenticity – can be brought into alignment and achieve translatability through the ethics of the autonomous, choosing, psychological self' (p. 157). In Peter, making money for himself – as hinted at above in the unscrupulous joint ventures with Maya – and letting others take their 'share' from the Enhanced Programme had attained translatability with the notion of serving the country, as long as the funds continued to flow uninterrupted by infighting or allegations of corruption against each other. As he commented to me, 'ultimately the money comes to Pakistan and the country benefits – at the end of the day some good does happen' – even though, I thought, some people make a fortune out of, what Li (2010) calls, the 'stealthy violence' of filling ones pockets with aid money for the poor, which consigns large numbers to lead 'short and limited lives' by dispossessing them (p. 67). However, the promise of this 'entrepreneurial self' 'remain(s) empty because of the unsurpassable gap between the hegemonic symbolic identities and everyday social performances' (Nadesan & Trethewey, 2000, p. 245), as I describe below.

The Enhanced Programme completed its 5 years in 2009. It was extended for one more year, while the plan for the second phase was being finalised by the government. The World Bank committed to finance this second phase as well, as quoted on their website: 'the Bank is committed to supporting the government programme over the next phase focusing particularly on increasing service coverage of most at risk groups in all major urban centres, improving access and quality of treatment and care, and strengthening monitoring and evaluation' (p. 5 Pakistan HIV July 2010, WB website, downloaded on 25 November 2010). However, by July 2010, a rumour emerged that the Bank was going to stop financing HIV prevention in Pakistan. This was neither confirmed nor denied by the Bank. In August 2010, the government issued a general appeal to all donors to prioritise relief and rehabilitation of the victims of country's worst floods ever. This gave the Bank an 'escape hatch' into a 'humanitarian triage'. However, no one believed that the floods were the real reason for its withdrawal from the HIV sector. According to a popular rumour, the Bank was not interested in HIV in the first place, and that it had financed the first phase of the Enhanced Programme only to 'improve their own balance sheets' by pushing a 'soft' loan to General Musharaf's regime, which was favourably poised towards neoliberal ideals, in desperate need of international recognition and partnership, and keen to project a positive, soft and progressive image abroad by investing in HIV prevention among marginalised populations at home.

The federal government tried to persuade the Bank to continue financing HIV prevention. But by the end of 2010, it was widely understood that the Bank was not going to extend any further loan for the Enhanced Programme. The government itself had no money for HIV because of other competing agendas; and, marking the end of the HIV scale-up decade, bilateral donors of Pakistan were reluctant to continue investing in this sector. Due to the association of HIV with immoral and dirty 'risk groups', the government had never treated it as a priority for spending from its own pool of resources, though it welcomed foreign aid and loans in this regard. The imminent devolution of the MoH to the provinces, as a result of a constitutional amendment in April 2010, further compounded the situation. Those vertical health programmes that could not bring in enough funds from external donors faced a possible shutdown or at least a merger with other programmes. Therefore, the ACP would not only be scaled-down as a result of the Bank's withdrawal from the HIV sector – pointing to the precariousness of the scale-up decade – but it also faced a possible shutdown.

What would become of the employees like Peter who had pinned all their hopes on the second phase of the Enhanced Programme in this government department, which was practically run on donor money? Amidst these rumours, emotions ran high among the employees and heated debates ensued in the small cabins among colleagues at the ACP. On one such occasion, the discussions between Peter and Maya drifted to a comparison between running HIV prevention NGOs, and providing technical consultancy services in HIV sector; that is, which of the two was a more profitable business, running an NGO or working as a consultant? While Maya did most of the listening, Peter furiously criticised NGOs for pocketing money in their service delivery projects whereas the technical people, like himself and Maya, could do nothing but helplessly watch others make a fortune out of the donor money. 'We know what they deliver and what happens in their detoxification and rehabilitation centres', said Peter, referring to the alleged misappropriation of funds and exploitation of clients by a big NGO for IDUs, which was a hot topic among the government employees at that time (Qureshi, 2014). He went on to whisper that in the Enhanced Programme, the NGO had adopted a 'mobile drop-in centre model' instead of setting up needle and syringe exchange centres in cheap rentable buildings in the target localities, which was the existing model. This was done deliberately to justify purchasing 12 expensive vehicles as mobile drop-in centres, from the project money, which then became the exclusive property of the NGO. He also commented contemptuously that 'all one needs to run HIV prevention projects among MSM is to mobilize half a dozen *hijrae* (transgendered people), set up a drop-in centre and distribute some condoms... Millions of rupees can be made from these projects'. The 'truckers' project' was a good example for that. He shared emphatically with Maya, 'none of the 12 drop-in centres that the NGO (contracted under the Enhanced Programme) set up at truck stops was bigger than the size of my office cabin and all they did was to keep some condoms and few sexually transmitted infections (STIs) medicines. That's all... The project was worth more than six *crore* rupees!' He concluded to Maya in a manner of self-criticism; 'people like us, you know, who are on the technical side, are happy with our salaries only. We never think about other ways of earning money'. Perhaps what they earned was far less than a successful NGO boss.

Driven by dissatisfaction, Peter appeared to fit the description of the 'Lacanian subject', always plagued by the anxiety that his *jouissance* was never enough; a subject that is always driven by a sense that there is something *more*, not fully known but it is there and the subject wants it (Fink, 1997). As the rumour about the withdrawal of the World Bank from the HIV sector and the repercussions for the ACPs intensified, Peter contemplated, for the first time, quitting his job and setting up a private consultancy firm, inviting me to join him. He thought he had built good connections in the donor community to find work for this proposed firm. There was no dearth of examples of those in the public health sector who had trodden the same path before him. But after a careful appraisal of his own situation – his 'human capital' – he gave up the plan. He could not yet trust the extent of his networks. The gap between what he aspired to and what he could do in his everyday social performances was becoming unsurpassable. The whole business of setting up a consultancy firm proved to be a 'fantasy' that he held onto in the face of his imminent failure as a bureaucratic subject in a rapidly 'scaling-down' HIV sector. Fantasy, in the Lacanian sense, is not an object of desire or a desire of objects but it is the 'setting of desire' (Homer, 2005, pp. 88–90), a 'space' that 'functions as an empty surface, a kind of screen for the projection of desire' (Žižek, 1992, p. 8).

He could not hold onto this fantasy for much longer, as it did not end his anxieties. He had worked very hard to build a career for himself at the ACP. Perhaps he never felt confident enough to leave this place, even when he had offers from elsewhere which he boasted as proof of his ability. But now the prospects of continuity were scuppered by the scale-down in funding. What options did he have? Did he regret sticking to one place for so long, instead of diversifying his occupations like Maya, or moving out to work in NGOs, like Rabia? Like many other colleagues, he started hunting for jobs, keeping these hunts secret, but he was not happy with the selection criteria and process of recruitments in NGOs and donor agencies. For instance, he applied for vacancies at a bilateral donor organisation and a UN agency after putting a lot of time and effort on the applications. Before the final interview, all candidates were made to do colossal amounts of paperwork, were required to give multimedia presentations, group tasks and aptitude tests. In his opinion, this was all unnecessary; there were simpler, better and more accurate ways of assessing a candidate's suitability for a job. He said, 'if you have worked for me, say for six months, I can tell how [suitable] you are [for a given job]. This is how it has been done generally and how it ought to be'. He had some friends in senior positions in both the places that he had applied to. However, they were helpful only to the extent of sharing some insider knowledge of what to expect in the interviews – a favour that they would have discreetly extended to other candidates as well. Peter was shortlisted for both vacancies but was not selected for either of them.

When the Enhanced Programme was in full swing and the HIV sector was awash with money, according to Peter, a number of his junior people could get 'better, stable and well paid jobs' in the UN agencies and international NGOs only because he had recommended them for those jobs. But he had not realised what was in store for himself. The ACP was now an organisation that had 'neither money nor future', in Peter's own words, and finding a job elsewhere in the time of recession in donor funding was proving too difficult. Disappointed with the outcome, he requested Maya to speak to someone in a very high position, whom they both avoided to name in my presence; 'please tell *him* to do something to accommodate me. Tell him, Peter is a person who has worked in the government and has good experience to cover that side too'. For Maya, it was time to payback for the 'investment' that Peter had made in her over several years of the Enhanced Programme. It was perhaps an opportune moment for her to reverse the flow of investment in their mutual entrepreneurial relationship.

Conclusions

In the World Bank-financed Enhanced Programme, formal rules, regulations and procedures were engulfed, if not replaced, by 'informal networks and emphasis on individual creativity and deal-making' (du Gay, 1994, p. 671). The 'subjectivation' of the

ACP in this way gave rise to forms of patronage and struggle for personal power, which have been viewed as characteristic of entrepreneurial conduct. Like in Egypt, where the objective of 'planting seeds for future and growing economic enterprise' through microfinance was inverted when a 'successful businessperson remodelled himself as a micro-entrepreneur to gain access to funds' (Elyachar, 2002, p. 505). In Pakistan too, the stated objective of institutional strengthening under the Enhanced Programme was turned on its head by moulding public servants into 'entrepreneurs of the self'. Although I have presented the argument of this paper through an extended case study of a single employee at the ACP, the entrepreneurial relations and job-related insecurities and anxieties that I have outlined here were widespread in the HIV sector in Pakistan, as I observed while working with federal and provincial HIV bureaucrats and the HIV staff of NGOs and donor agencies (Qureshi, 2013a). Private accumulation by public servants' 'moon-lighting' in the private sector to supplement their salaries has been observed in other sections of the bureaucracy, too (Anders, 2005; Pfeiffer & Chapman, 2010, pp. 154–156). However, this paper has highlighted the moral embeddedness of these practices in the flexible work cultures of the external aid and neoliberal modalities working on public servants at a subjective level.

The landscape of power that emerged as a result of conditioning the 'scaling-up' of the HIV response with neoliberal policies of contractualisation and partnership with private sector afforded new opportunities to forge creative alliances and occupy new spaces. The officials at the ACP turned their offices into personal enterprises, as I have shown through the extended case study of Peter. Nevertheless, the uncertainty following the withdrawal of Bank's funding left their jobs precarious – pointing to the vulnerability of the HIV sector to 'scaling-down' as well as 'scaling-up', due to the reliance on donor funding. A number of market-based contractual employees were laid off whereas others left the organisation to work in NGOs and donor agencies where they were valued for their insider knowledge of the government departments. The ones left behind engaged in unhealthy competition with each other, keeping their job hunts secret and spreading false rumours about each other.

This paper has taken a different path from other evaluations of the HIV response in Pakistan. Rather than pointing to the inadequacies of the government bureaucracy and its need for 'capacity building', I have offered an ethnographic critique of the work cultures pervading the transnational HIV apparatus. The dependence on external aid enticed government employees into a politics of upscaled expectations, but also left them precariously exposed to job insecurity, and undermined the continuity of HIV prevention and treatment services in the country. I suggest that this Pakistan-derived analysis is more widely relevant for the post scale-up decade. Globally, the HIV epidemic has now entered a post-scale-up era. However, this has not translated into scaled-down expectations at the receiving end, or indeed, a decrease in the need for interventions in many places. This paper has argued for investigating this mismatch between declining scale of global HIV response and the up-scaled expectations of bureaucrats in the sector for a better understanding of the challenges ahead.

Acknowledgements

I wish to thank the staff of the ACP for allowing me to carry out this fieldwork and welcoming me among them. I am grateful for their generosity. Thanks also to Caroline Osella, Kaveri Qureshi and the two anonymous reviewers from Global Public Health for their valuable inputs. The doctoral research on which this paper is based was made possible by the generous funding from the

Commonwealth Scholarship Commission. Ethical approval was granted by the School of Oriental and African Studies.

References

Anders, G. (2005). *Civil servants in Malawi: Moonlighting, kinship and corruption in the shadow of good governance* (PhD thesis). Erasmus University, Rotterdam.

Biehl, J. (2007). *Will to live: AIDS therapies and the politics of survival*. Princeton, NJ: Princeton University Press.

Burawoy, M. (1998). The extended case method. *Sociological Theory, 16*(1), 4–33. doi:10.1111/0735-2751.00040

Crozier, M. (1964). *The bureaucratic phenomenon*. Chicago, IL: University of Chicago Press.

du Gay, P. (1994). Making up managers: Bureaucracy, enterprise and the liberal art of separation. *The British Journal of Sociology, 45*, 655–674. doi:10.2307/591888

Elyachar, J. (2002). Empowerment money: The World Bank, non-governmental organizations, and the value of culture in Egypt. *Public Culture, 14*, 493–513. doi:10.1215/08992363-14-3-493

Feher, M. (2009). Self-appreciation; or, the aspirations of human capital. *Public Culture, 21*(1), 21–41. doi:10.1215/08992363-2008-019

Fink, B. (1997). *The Lacanian subject: Between language and jouissance*. Princeton, NJ: Princeton University Press.

Gumpertz, J. (1982). *Discourse strategies*. Cambridge: Cambridge University Press.

Harper, I. (2011). World health and Nepal: Producing internationals, health citizenship and the compolitan. In D. Mosse (Ed.), *Adventures in aidland: The anthropology of professionals in international development* (pp. 123–138). Oxford: Berghahn Books.

HASP. (2011). *HIV second generation surveillance in Pakistan, national report round IV*. Islamabad: HIV and AIDS Surveillance Project, National AIDS Control Programme.

Hastings, J. G. (2013). 50,000 frequent flier miles: Thoughts on a multi-sited organizational ethnography. *Practicing Anthropology, 35*(2), 33–37. Retrieved from http://www.sfaa.metapress.com/content/A474132344627J64

Hawkes, S., Zaheer, H. A., Tawil, O., O'Dwyer, M., & Buse, K. (2012). Managing research evidence to inform action: Influencing HIV policy to protect marginalised populations in Pakistan. *Global Public Health, 7*, 482–494. doi:10.1080/17441692.2012.663778

Homer, S. (2005). *Jacques Lacan*. London: Routledge.

Hull, M. S. (2012). *Government of paper: The materiality of bureaucracy in urban Pakistan*. Berkeley: University of California Press.

Hussain, S., Kadir, M., & Fatmi, Z. (2007). Resource allocation within the National AIDS Control Programme: A qualitative assessment of the decision-makers's opinion. *BMC Health Services Research, 7*(11), 1–8. doi:10.1186/1472-6963-7-11

Karim, M., & Zaidi, S. (1999). Poor performance of health and population welfare services in Sindh – Case studies in governance failure. *Pakistan Development Review, 38*, 661–668. Retrieved from http://www.popline.org/node/528391

Kelly, P. (2006). The entrepreneurial self and 'youth at-risk': Exploring the horizons of identity in the twenty-first century. *Journal of Youth Studies, 9*(1), 17–32. doi:10.1080/13676260500523606

Khanna, A. (2009). Meyeli Chhele becomes MSM – Transformation of idioms of sexualness into epidemiological forms in India. In A. Cornwall, J. Edström, & A. Greig (Eds.), *Politicising masculinity* (pp. 47–57). London: Zed Books.

Li, T. M. (2010). To make live or let die? Rural dispossession and the protection of surplus populations. *Antipode, 41*, 66–93. doi:10.1111/j.1467-8330.2009.00717.x

Mayhew, S., Collumbien, M., Qureshi, A., Platt, L., Rafiq, N., Faisel, A., … Hawkes, S. (2009). Protecting the unprotected: Mixed-method research on drug use, sex work and rights in Pakistan's fight against HIV/AIDS. *Sexually Transmitted Infections, 85*, ii31–ii36. doi:10.1136/sti.2008.033670

Mosse, D. (2005). *Cultivating development: An ethnography of aid policy and practice*. London: Pluto Press.

Mosse, D., & Lewis, D. (Eds.). (2006). *Development brokers and translators of aid policy and practice*. London and Ann Arbor, MI: Pluto Press.

NACP. (2010). *UNGASS Pakistan report: Progress report on the declaration of commitment on HIV/AIDS for United Nations General Assembly special session on HIV/AIDS*. Islamabad: National AIDS Control Programme.

NACP. (2012). *UNGASS Pakistan report: Global AIDS response progress report 2012*. Islamabad: National AIDS Control Programme.

Nadesan, M. H., & Trethewey, A. (2000). Performing the enterprising subject: Gendered strategies for success (?). *Text and Performance Quarterly*, *20*, 223–250. doi:10.1080/10462930009366299

Nguyen, V. K. (2010). *The republic of therapy: Triage and sovereignty in West Africa's time of AIDS*. Durham, NC: Duke University Press.

Pfeiffer, J., & Chapman, R. (2010). Anthropological perspectives on structural adjustment and public health. *Annual Review of Anthropology*, *39*, 149–165. doi:10.1146/annurev.anthro.012809. 105101

Pigg, S. (2002). Expecting the epidemic: A social history of the representation of sexual risk in Nepal. *Feminist Media Studies*, *2*(1), 97–125. doi:10.1080/14680770220122891

Pisani, E. (2008). *The wisdom of whores: Bureaucrats, brothels and the business of AIDS*. London: Granta.

Qureshi, A. (2013a). *Bureaucrats, business and the (bio)politics of HIV in Pakistan* (Unpublished doctoral dissertation). SOAS, University of London, London.

Qureshi, A. (2013b). Structural violence and the state: HIV and labour migration from Pakistan to the Persian Gulf. *Anthropology & Medicine*, *20*(3), 209–220. doi:10.1080/13648470.2013. 828274

Qureshi, A. (2014). The marketization of HIV/AIDS governance: Vertical health programming, public private partnerships and bureaucratic culture in Pakistan. In L. Bear & N. Mathur (Eds.), *The new public good: Affects and techniques of flexible bureaucracies*. Oxford: Berghahn Books.

Robins, S. (2004). 'Long live Zackie, long live': AIDS activism, science and citizenship after apartheid. *Journal of Southern African Studies*, *30*, 651–672. doi:10.1080/03057070420002 54146

Rose, N. (1996). *Inventing our selves: Psychology, power, and personhood*. Cambridge: Cambridge University Press.

Rowden, R. (2009). *The deadly ideas of neoliberalism: How the IMF has undermined public health and the fight against AIDS*. London: Zed Books.

Sennett, R. (2006). *The culture of the new capitalism*. New Haven, CT: Yale University Press.

Shore, C., & Wright, S. (1997). *Anthropology of policy: Critical perspectives on governance and power*. London: Routledge.

Stirrat, R. L. (2000). Cultures of consultancy. *Critique of Anthropology*, *20*(1), 31–46. doi:10.1177/ 0308275X0002000103

UNAIDS. (2013). HIV and AIDS estimates (2012). Retrieved from http://www.unaids.org/en/ regionscountries/countries/pakistan/

UNODC. (2013). *The drug use in Pakistan 2013 – Technical summary report (2013)*. Retrieved from http://www.unodc.org/unodc/en/frontpage/2013/March/Key-findings-of-the-drug-use-in-pak istan-2013-technical-summary-report.html?ref=fs2

Zaidi, S. (2008). *A policy analysis of contracting NGOs in Pakistan: NGO-government eng- agement, HIV prevention and the dynamics of policy and political factors* (Unpublished PhD dissertation). London School of Hygiene and Tropical Medicine, London.

Zaidi, S., Mayhew, S. H., & Palmer, N. (2011). Bureaucrats as purchasers of health services: Limitations of the public sector for contracting. *Public Administration and Development*, *31*(3), 135–148. doi:10.1002/pad.581

Žižek, S. (1992). *Looking awry: An introduction to Jacques Lacan through popular culture*. Cambridge: The MIT Press.

HIV testing as prevention among MSM in China: The business of scaling-up

Elsa L. Fan

Department of Behavioral and Social Sciences, Webster University, St. Louis, MO, USA

In this paper, I examine the emergence of *goumai fuwu*, or contracting with social organisations to provide social services, in the HIV/AIDS sector in China. In particular, I interrogate the outsourcing of HIV testing to community-based organisations (CBOs) serving men who have sex with men (MSM) as a means of scaling-up testing in this population, and how the commodification of testing enables new forms of surveillance and citizenship to emerge. In turn, I tie the scaling-up of testing and its commodification to the sustainability of CBOs as they struggle to survive. In recent years, the HIV/AIDS response in China has shifted to expanding testing among MSM in order to reduce new infections. This response has been catalysed by the transition to sexual contact as the primary transmission route for HIV and the rising rates of infection among MSM, leading government institutions and international donors to mobilise CBOs to expand testing. These efforts to scale-up are as much about testing as they are about making visible this hidden population. CBOs, in facilitating testing, come to rely on outsourcing as a long-term funding base and in doing so, unintentionally extend the reach of the state into the everyday lives of MSM.

Introduction

In 2002, the United Nations Theme Group on HIV/AIDS in China released a report entitled 'HIV/AIDS: China's Titanic Peril' which underscored a potential crisis around the epidemic, reiterating concerns that up to 10 million people could be infected with HIV by 2010. By the end of 2011, however, the Joint United Nations Programme on HIV/AIDS (UNAIDS, 2013), estimated that 780,000 people were living with HIV, with 48,000 new infections reported in the same year. Although the numbers were less dramatic than imagined, the report foregrounded an emerging trend in the epidemic landscape: an increasing number of infections from sexual transmission. At the end of 2011, this mode accounted for 63.9% of all existing infections and 81.6% of all new infections (UNAIDS, 2013). Sexual contact had become the leading route of transmission for HIV in China, and a new crisis had appeared, reshaping in crucial ways the response to the epidemic.

In recent years, the national response has converged around HIV testing as a form of prevention, focusing specifically on men who have sex with men (MSM). Interventions have increasingly turned to scaling-up testing in this population in order to reduce new infections, and have mobilised MSM-focused community-based organisations (hereafter

CBOs) to do so. The shift to these groups is due, in part, to the presumed hidden nature of MSM that makes them difficult to access. One report suggests that the emergence of these groups stems from the government's reluctance (or inability) to address certain health topics directly; as a result, these organisations have become instrumental in reaching and providing services to high-risk populations (Xu, Zeng, & Anderson, 2005). CBOs, I suggest, composed of and serving this population, are able to reach MSM in ways that elude government institutions such as the Chinese Center for Disease Control (CCDC). To this end, new models have emerged in order to scale-up testing, reconfiguring this technology as a commodity and enabling the elicitation of new kinds of knowledge and solicitation of new kinds of citizens.

One particular model, called *goumai fuwu*, has come to the fore in this effort, mobilised largely by international donors.[1] It refers to contracting with social organisations to provide social services and has emerged in tandem with the focus on testing MSM.[2] For instance, in a joint project between one donor and the Chinese Ministry of Health (MOH), the Changsha CDC in Hunan Province contracted with a local CBO to conduct HIV prevention services. The arrangement included remuneration to the CBO for the delivery of set outputs in 1 year: (1) train 20 peer educators; (2) provide interventions for 1200 MSM engaging in high-risk behaviour; and (3) refer 200 MSM to the Changsha CDC for testing.[3] At the end of the contract period, the CBO had exceeded the outputs, referring twice as many MSM for testing, thus illustrating their ostensible success in reaching this population [National Center for AIDS/STD Control & Prevention (NCAIDS), 2011].

In this paper, I interrogate the unintended consequences that emerge from the mobilisation of *goumai fuwu* as a means to scale-up testing among MSM in China. This model is intended to address some of the challenges faced by the CCDC in reaching MSM, while offering a long-term funding source for CBOs. Although not new in China, this practice is still nascent in the HIV/AIDS sector, and its emergence signals a wider shift in the preference for market-driven models, in contrast to traditional public health paradigms. This paper draws from 21 months of field research in China carried out between 2008 and 2011 among CBOs, activists, donors and government institutions working on HIV/AIDS programmes. While *goumai fuwu* refers to the outsourcing of service provision, I focus on one component of this, the commodification of testing, or payment in return for HIV tests.

I begin by examining the HIV/AIDS discourse that focuses on the need to expand testing among MSM, predicated on the assumption that they are 'almost always already infected'. This representation is what instantiates the need for this intervention and what makes possible the commodification of testing. I then illustrate how commodification through *goumai fuwu* renders hidden MSM populations visible. What concerns me is how power and politics can be found in unexpected spaces, such as in a testing intervention intended to save lives. Finally, I tie the scaling-up of testing to the sustainability of CBOs. In foregrounding these groups, I illustrate how the expansion and commodification of testing configures new forms of biological citizenship.

The crisis of MSM bodies

Over dinner one night in Beijing, a colleague working for a local CCDC in Yunnan Province noted that their agency was anxious to find more HIV infections among MSM, and had begun stepping up efforts to do so. I commented that it seemed counterintuitive to *want* to find more infections; would not that mean the epidemic was out of control? On the contrary, she replied, it is because there is such limited knowledge about MSM that the detection of more infections indicates the epidemic is under control. She clarified:

> There is a fear and assumption that there are many more infections *out there* [my emphasis] especially among MSM, so we are pushing [testing] and hoping to find more HIV-positives because this means that the more people you find, the more you can control the epidemic. There is a real fear that [infections in] the MSM population will explode.

I considered her point. 'But why all this fear around MSM', I asked, 'if the leading transmission route is from heterosexual contact?' After all, by the end of 2011, heterosexual transmission accounted for 46.5% of all existing HIV infections and 52.2% of all new infections in China (UNAIDS, 2013). My colleague replied, 'Because MSM are married to women'. In other words, 'even though the numbers point to heterosexuals', she explained, 'they are really just MSM who don't admit to their identification'. Her point was that most of the men who came into the CCDC for testing represented themselves as heterosexual; thus, it was their deception of identification, she implied, that accounted for the deception of data.

Her assumption that MSM occlude their sexual identification underscores not only the need to detect more HIV infections in this population, but also the need to know precisely *who* is infected. In public health literature, MSM are often considered to be a bridge group that 'as long as they continue to engage in sex with both males and females, they can spread the epidemic' (He & Detels, 2005, p. 828). This caution is echoed in another study that found a 'high level of potential bridging from MSM to the general population through regular and casual female partners' (He et al., 2006, p. S22). In such representations, MSM are configured as a high-risk group separate from the general population, an important distinction that articulates the need to contain HIV *in* MSM bodies and protect it *from* other bodies. The visibility of their heterosexual lives juxtaposed against the invisibility of their engagement in sex with men reproduces their exclusion from the general population and reinforces the need to protect the general population from them (Choi, Gibson, Han, & Guo, 2004; Choi, Zhen, Gregorich, & Pan, 2007; He et al., 2006; Zhang & Chu, 2005).

The notion of infected MSM bodies 'out there' conjures up images of what Ann Anagnost (1995) calls a 'surfeit of bodies' in China, an excess population of rural farmers marked only by their backwardness who are in need of transforming from bodies that consume *suzhi*, or quality, into bodies that produce it. In the public (health) imagination, MSM exhibit a similar kind of excess, a surfeit of potentially infected (and infecting) bodies that need to be culled through testing and cultivated into responsible, productive bodies. It is the perception that there are more bodies 'out there' yet rendered invisible that underscores the urgency with which the project of testing and scaling-up is mobilised.

This imagined surfeit underscored a meeting I once attended in Henan Province. I had travelled there in 2011 with some colleagues from a US-based foundation to monitor their project that funded CBOs to provide testing to MSM. On the train ride there, Harold, the director of the foundation, prepped me about our upcoming meeting with Ms Li from the local CCDC.[4] Ms Li had heard about the project from another CBO and was interested in participating. 'It's a strange place to want to do a testing project for MSM', Harold remarked. I agreed, since this area was one of the main sites of the commercial plasma donors epidemic, in which thousands of rural farmers in central China were infected with HIV through blood and plasma donations (see Asia Catalyst, 2007).[5] Nonetheless, Ms

Li's insistence that this project was needed intrigued Harold, prompting him to meet with her.

Ms Li and her colleague, a local entrepreneur planning to start his own CBO, met us at the train station and took us to a teahouse for the meeting. Harold asked, 'Are there even MSM here?' expressing what had clearly been on all our minds. Our colleague echoed this concern, saying, 'Is there enough of a population to do a testing project here?' Ms Li replied, 'For now, there are probably about 50 men, but the project could help more of them come out and get tested'. She suggested that there could be more, but that they were just not 'out' or 'visible'. MSM had just begun emerging in the area, she clarified, and noted that, 'I didn't even know there were any here until I first met one in 2010'.

Her concerns echo the presumption that there could be a surplus of potentially infected (and infecting) MSM bodies 'out there' that need to be tested and detected but are not yet 'out'. Her rhetoric aligns with the public health discourse that characterises MSM as a hidden population, embedded in but separate from the general population, thus requiring them to be excised from it. But it is an excision that can only be done through testing, as implied in Ms Li's suggestion that such a project could help more men come out, predicated on the assumption that there are more of them *to* come out. Testing, then, is envisioned as a kind of coming out, an especially acute point considering the infected population in this area consists primarily of former blood and plasma donors (FPDs), *not* MSM. In articulating the need for this project, Ms Li does not reference the FPD population, but rather turns her attention to testing MSM. In doing so, she reproduces testing as a specifically MSM endeavour, while imagining this population to be an excess in need of culling. Implicit in her insistence is the potential for only MSM to infect, and not for FPDs to do the same.

The turn to testing intersected with two notable changes in the HIV/AIDS landscape in China. The first was an emerging discourse coalescing around the need to expand testing among MSM due to their rising rates of infection (Choi, Diehl, Guo, Qu, & Mandel, 2002; Choi, Lui, Guo, Han, & Mandel, 2006; Chow, Wilson, & Zhang, 2012; Fan et al., 2012; Tucker, Wong, Nehl, & Zhang, 2012). The reported percentage of infections resulting from homosexual contact increased from 2.5% in 2006 to 13.7% in 2011; of the 780,000 people estimated to be living with HIV at the end of 2011, 17.4% were infected through homosexual transmission (Ministry of Health of the People's Republic of China, 2012). For 2011, the Ministry of Health (2012) reported a 6.3% HIV prevalence rate among MSM populations. These trends underscored fears that the epidemic could transition from high-risk populations into the general public.

The second change was the rise in the number of MSM-focused groups that had become inseparable from the epidemic itself. This link became clear during a trip to Hainan Island when I met with a number of CBOs that had, in fact, been created by the local CCDC to conduct testing among MSM. I had accompanied some colleagues from a donor-funded project to meet with their local CCDC counterparts. This project focused on scaling-up testing among MSM through outreach by CBOs. In one of our meetings, CCDC staff reminded us that prior to this project, there were no MSM organisations in that area. The few that had been established were done so through the CCDC, specifically to expand testing among MSM.

The creation of these organisations by government institutions is not an unfamiliar practice in China. Much like the CBOs I encountered in Hainan, it is not uncommon for government agencies to establish similar groups as a conduit for international funding. In Hainan, for instance, most of the CBOs formed through the CCDC were specific to a particular project and were established to absorb grants from The Global Fund to Fight AIDS, Tuberculosis and Malaria (GFATM), among other donors. This ambivalent relationship with the government is especially pronounced in government-organised nongovernmental organisations, reflecting the quasi-autonomous nature of these groups and their intimate, if not dependent, relationship to the state. In part, the registration process restricts the formation of CBOs by requiring them to find a government sponsor in order to officially register with the Ministry of Civil Affairs. Many groups, unable (or unwilling) to do so, tend to operate at the margins of legality, functioning in a perpetual state of insecurity. That these CBOs are formed for the specific purpose of channelling HIV/AIDS funding both tethers them to the epidemic and forestalls their identity outside of it. As one activist pointed out in Hainan, such CBOs cannot exist outside of the epidemic.

This inseparability is reflected in the increase of MSM groups in recent years. In the 2006/2007 *China HIV/AIDS Directory*, of the more than 300 organisations listed, fewer than 100 were focused on MSM (China AIDS Info, 2007). In the 2010 follow-up directory, the number of MSM groups had increased to more than 180 (NCAIDS & China HIV/AIDS Information Network, 2010). One report found that out of 337 unregistered groups surveyed in the HIV/AIDS sector, 36% focused on MSM, compared to 27% focused on people living with HIV/AIDS (PLHIV), 9% on sex workers (SWs) and 7% on injecting drug users (IDUs) (Li et al., 2010). This trend both reflects and reinforces the significance of MSM to the HIV/AIDS response.

The attention to MSM is part and parcel of the evolution of China's epidemic (see Sun et al., 2007; Wu, Rou, & Cui, 2004). Historically, HIV infections have concentrated around IDUs and SWs along the drug-trafficking routes in southern China; in the mid-1990s, there was an outbreak among FPDs in central China due to unsafe donation practices. These shifts informed the national response to HIV/AIDS, which initially focused on prevention through public health education and condom promotion, then on scaling-up treatment and care (see Cui, Liau, & Wu, 2009; Wu, Sullivan, Wang, Rotheram-Borus, & Detels, 2007). The latter crystallised in the 2003 'Four Frees and One Care' policy, which provides free testing and treatment to PLHIV, and more recently the 'Five Expands, Six Strengthens' supplement.[6]

The current focus on testing MSM perhaps defines the next stage of China's response. The concerns around MSM are elicited not only from what little is known about them but also from presumptions about their sexual practices. It is in this context that the scaling-up of testing among MSM and the turn to *goumai fuwu* becomes salient. What makes this intervention unique, I contend, is not just the test but what it enables. It is a technology that gains traction only in so far as it extends to MSM. If a crisis is articulated around an imagined surfeit of potentially infected (and infecting) MSM bodies 'out there', then the aversion of that crisis lies in their detection. Thus, testing is not only about containing the virus *in* MSM bodies but also about extracting knowledge *from* them in order to produce particular kinds of citizens.

The mobilisation of *goumai fuwu*

One night, as part of a monitoring trip with a donor to assess their testing projects, I attended a training workshop intended to educate MSM about HIV prevention. The training was organised by a local CBO in Henan Province, and recruited men using MSM websites, online chat rooms, and personal and social networks. Also present, I noticed, were staff from the local CCDC office.

The training consisted of various exercises informing participants how to protect themselves against HIV and other sexually transmitted infections. At the end of the training, the facilitator invited the CCDC doctor to the front of the room, telling the participants that he was here to administer testing to those who wanted to get tested. He encouraged them to do so, and handed out questionnaires to complete. The doctor began spreading out his supplies on the conference table: the needles to draw the blood, the test tubes to collect it and the gauze to cover the wound. The men began rolling up their sleeves and one by one, lined up to get tested.

This scenario raised two questions for me: why was testing being offered at a CBO training and why were men voluntarily lining up to get tested? I found one of the organisers, who explained to me that:

> The CCDC came to us asking if we could help them organise a training workshop for MSM. They had gotten funding from GFATM to do outreach but had no means of reaching MSM, so they turned to us. It is quite common for the CCDC to use funding from international sources to outsource testing.

Indeed, many other CBOs I encountered practised similar forms of *goumai fuwu* to conduct testing, and it had become a model par excellence to expand testing among MSM. In this particular incarnation, the CCDC contracted with the CBO using GFATM funding because, as the organiser clarified, the CCDC could not access this population. The challenge of reaching MSM became a common motif among the staff I met. In Hainan, for instance, one person noted the difficulties for the CCDC in scaling-up testing because of the institution's inability to reach MSM; hence, the turn to creating CBOs for this purpose. One study notes that 'as a socially marginalized and hidden population, government-initiated interventions often have limited impacts on MSM', thus the need for CBOs to play a greater role in HIV prevention (Chow, Wilson, & Zhang, 2010, p. e33). Donors are especially eager to push forward *goumai fuwu* in the HIV/AIDS sector but funded directly from government budgets rather than international sources.

This model is exemplified by one CBO I met in Hunan Province and is consistently highlighted as a best practice by one of their donors. The organisation was paid 25,000 RMB per 6 months (approximately US$4000) directly from government budgets by their local CCDC in return for organising one training workshop a month, to reach a total of 2000 MSM, and testing 400 MSM in the same period. A volunteer from this CBO noted that the local CCDC had recently begun accepting results from another testing project that allowed the CBO to administer rapid HIV tests for MSM. He explained that 'instead of the CCDC going to intervention sites to administer testing, we can now use our rapid tests directly at the sites and submit the results to the CCDC'.

His comment underscores two important points that help to elaborate my earlier questions about testing at the training. The first is the reconfiguration of health as defined in terms of a return on investment, based on the cost of testing one MSM and the test's potential yield for containing the epidemic. As explained by one CBO volunteer:

> The CCDC approached us to help with collecting HIV tests from MSM. It cost them 1000 RMB [approximately US$163] each time to go out to bars and collect HIV tests from the men, but they only ever succeeded in getting a few. Their method wasn't cost-effective. It was cheaper to go through us to collect the tests, and we could reach many more men.

Thus, administering rapid HIV tests directly to MSM and submitting them to the CCDC is both cost-effective and efficient. Similarly, outsourcing this intervention to CBOs and then collecting the tests directly at the site, as in the case of the training, fulfils the same objective. This logic undergirds the decision of one donor to reallocate funding exclusively to testing MSM, rather than other high-risk populations:

> Initially our project targeted three populations: SWs, IDUs and MSM. In most of the program cities, however, there were minimal to no new infections found among SWs and IDUs. Among MSM, though, we were finding a lot of new infections; we had spent a lot of money for these two groups [SWs and IDUs] with no results to show for it, while we spent less money on MSM and yielded more results. So we decided to reallocate the funding to MSM because it was much more financially efficient.

The second point highlights the comparative advantage of CBOs in reaching MSM, and thus the reason for outsourcing. The model of *goumai fuwu* brings into sharp relief the presumed failure of the CCDC to test MSM, against the ostensible success of CBOs to do so. Outsourcing ensures not only that more MSM are reached, but also that more lives can (presumably) be saved; the assumption behind testing, after all, is that prevention (testing) will necessarily lead to behavioural change and treatment. Thus far, initial reports from testing projects demonstrate some success among CBOs in testing men and retaining them through the treatment process. Retention is especially important since an ongoing challenge for the CCDC is that men do not return for their test results or are unreachable having provided false contact information. In China, all HIV tests must be confirmed by a second test performed by the CCDC in order for the tested individual to be eligible for antiretroviral therapy (ART). Once confirmed, the person's data are uploaded into a centralised database to monitor his or her status. One testing project I encountered reported significantly higher detection rates from CBOs in comparison to hospitals, by as much as 10%. The follow-up rate for a confirmation test among men tested by CBOs was also higher than those tested by hospitals.

These findings gesture to two points: CBOs are more effective at reaching MSM and MSM are more likely to go to CBOs for testing. This preference is related, in part, to fears of confidentiality breaches and stigma against MSM more broadly (Choi et al., 2006; Feng, Wu, & Detels, 2010; Li et al., 2012). In fact, many MSM I met expressed similar concerns, and one man I encountered lost his job when the CCDC informed his employer.[7] In a meeting of MSM groups participating in a testing project I once attended in Beijing, a participant remarked that their beneficiaries often refuse to go to the CCDC for testing for fear of registering their identity. Another echoed that some men do not return to the CCDC for a confirmation test for the same reason. On the other hand, participants noted that men feel more comfortable getting tested at a CBO because there is less judgement, and some prefer getting tested by another MSM. Furthermore, men getting tested at a CBO may be more likely to follow through with the treatment process. In one testing project, for instance, almost all CBOs had a 100% rate of confirmation testing from the CCDC, meaning that all of the men who received an HIV test from one of the CBOs also had a confirmation test at the CCDC, thus enabling them to receive ART if needed.

Testing through *goumai fuwu*, in this regard, does something crucial; it elicits certain kinds of knowledge not possible through other means and makes demands of MSM while simultaneously enabling their surveillance. That men resist getting tested at the CCDC yet choose to get tested at CBOs, which ultimately results in a confirmation test at the CCDC – and, in the case of a least one group, also results in the original tests being submitted directly to the CCDC – illustrates the salience of and tension emerging from *goumai fuwu* that expands testing in an otherwise invisible population while securing the future of CBOs through the commodification of testing. It is testing, I suggest, that evokes a new form of biological citizenship that compels men in a training to line up to get tested as people who are 'almost always already infected'.

Cultivating biological citizens through HIV testing

Nikolas Rose and Carlos Novas (2005) refer to biological citizenship as projects that reshape how individuals are thought about and acted upon as citizens, converging around their biological existence. These projects, they contend, become instantiated through such things as public education campaigns and the push towards scientific literacy, a process of 'making up' biological citizens. In other words:

> By 'making up citizens', we mean, in part, the reshaping of the way in which persons are understood by authorities…in terms of categories such as the chronically sick, the disabled, the blind, the deaf, the child abuser, or the psychopath. …It [classification] delimits the boundaries of those who get treated in a certain way – in punishment, therapy, employment, security, benefit, or reward …By making up biological citizens, we also mean the creation of persons with a certain kind of relation to themselves. (Rose & Novas, 2005, p. 445)

The category of MSM presupposes them to be chronically at risk for HIV, necessitating not only an obligation to get tested but also the scaling-up of testing in this population. That Ms Li envisioned testing as a means to draw out MSM who potentially could be infected (and infecting), to the exclusion of FPDs, illustrates the obligation for these men not only to get tested but to be responsible for regulating their health. In getting tested, MSM come to inhabit a particular subject-position that embodies risk, one that shapes their conduct such that they need to be tested. The identification of risk is what compelled one man I met in Hunan Province to get tested. During a meeting of PLHIV, he and other men participating in a local CBO support group described their experiences of being HIV-positive. He explained:

> You know, up until 2006 or 2007, no one knew anything about AIDS, especially in our circle (*quanzi*). We always thought about AIDS as something far away, that it could never happen to us. It was something that happened in big cities like Beijing or Shanghai, not in smaller places like Changsha.

This particular man noted that it had only been in the last few years that information about HIV/AIDS began circulating among them. He had not identified himself as at risk for HIV until he *learned* that he was at risk through these public health campaigns. He himself had only been tested 2 years ago although he had been having sex with men for years. What is crucial here is how testing modulates behaviour and cultivates biological citizens who identify themselves in biological terms – at risk for HIV – and make judgments on how they should act.

This distinction became especially pronounced later in the same meeting, when the men began admonishing other MSM for marrying women and potentially spreading the infection in order to maintain confidentiality about their HIV status and their MSM lives. One man criticised such men for 'spreading the infection because they don't want to tell their wives they are infected'. At that moment, an HIV-positive heterosexual man entered the room, and the men began joking that he too was searching for a wife, much like other MSM. However, they teased, no one wanted to marry him because he was too ugly; *not,*

I noticed, because he was infected. Implicit in this conversation was a glaring disjuncture between the admonishments directed at MSM for their desire to marry women in spite of their infection and the absence of such criticisms for the heterosexual man. The cultivation of biological citizens, in this regard, becomes a project specific to MSM, and not to others.

The role of CBOs is crucial to this process through *goumai fuwu*. In their facilitation of testing, CBOs become critical interlocutors that act both on behalf of and at the expense of MSM, making visible this population to the state while simultaneously ensuring their own survival. These organisations function similarly to what Kristin Peterson (2001) calls 'bioprospecting NGOs', referring to groups involved with the procurement and commodification of biological, chemical and genetic materials used for pharmaceutical products. Bioprospecting NGOs become important brokers in safe-guarding the rights of and compensation for communities from which these materials are extracted, while also expediting the expropriation of these resources for private industries.

There are two important points to highlight in her argument: first is the turn to market-driven approaches, in contrast to traditional development paradigms and second is the role of NGOs in mediating these transactions. What bioprospecting NGOs do is not dissimilar to the practice of *goumai fuwu* in facilitating the extraction of blood from MSM bodies in return for remuneration. The success of this intervention lies not only in the ability of CBOs to reach this population but also in the commodification of this technology, which enables CBOs to scale-up testing. What is commoditised is not the biological material, or blood, but rather the HIV test that necessitates its extraction. Inasmuch as the blood holds value, it is testing that configures this value only once it is extracted from the MSM body, in terms of eliciting an HIV status for the MSM and knowledge of *who* is infected for the state. Similar to bioprospecting NGOs, CBOs mediate the transformation of biological materials into a valuable product because of what these materials can proffer once outside the body. In so far as CBOs act on behalf of MSM in getting them tested, they also act at their expense in making them visible to the state.

It is in this context that the scaling-up of testing becomes especially productive. Testing is a technology that reinscribes MSM as biological citizens, making certain demands of their conduct. Not only do men come to regard themselves in a particular way – as MSM at risk for HIV – but they are also obligated to get tested. In the same vein, it is this practice that enables their detection, mapping and monitoring, a feat long eluding the CCDC but now made possible in ways that allow for even greater surveillance.

What becomes particularly valuable in this process of testing, commoditising and scaling-up testing is what this knowledge can do not only for MSM and the state but also for other bodies writ large. Health, in other words, is configured *for* others; that is, MSM health is reconfigured *for* the general population. It is a transformation that Anagnost (2006) articulates as the potential for 'some bodies ... as having more "value" than others, or that some bodies *have* "value" *for* others, but only when they are disassembled into their several parts and grafted onto other bodies' (p. 523). The metaphorical grafting is elicited from the blood of MSM that, once found to be infected, is transferred onto noninfected bodies. The scaling-up of testing makes it possible for the virus to be contained in MSM bodies and forestalled in others. The culling of an imagined surfeit of potentially infected (and infecting) MSM bodies 'out there' through testing translates into the saving of MSM lives and of those precluded from being infected.

Failure and success, in this context, can be redefined in terms of return on investment. Failure of development projects, argues James Ferguson (1994), tends to be the norm, while success lies in the cultivation of their broader interests. In his interrogation of World Bank practices in Lesotho, he illustrates how the failure of specific projects enables the expansion of state bureaucratic power. Similarly in China, success is not found in the ability of CBOs to scale-up testing among MSM, but rather in the failure of the CCDC that enables *goumai fuwu* and the commodification of testing, which in turn extends surveillance in ways even greater than had previously been possible. Perhaps the most telling moment was watching the men roll up their sleeves and extend their arms to get tested; it was an ironic twist that men who came *to* the CBO to elude the CCDC were now being made visible to that very institution. What makes this practice unique, I contend, is the scaling-up of bodies and biological citizens that make themselves visible for surveillance.

Scaling-up and the politics of sustainability

During my research, I often posed a question to the CBOs I encountered, 'What happens when there are no more MSM to test?' The question was rhetorical, but it indexed the temporality of funding related to the current HIV/AIDS focus on testing MSM. In the past decade, the HIV/AIDS landscape in China has shifted dramatically in terms of funding. In the early 2000s, donors flooded the sector, buttressing and at times surpassing government support. This funding accounted for almost one-third of HIV/AIDS programmes in China since 1988; from 1988 to 2009, international partners contributed more than US$526 million for these programmes (Sun et al., 2010).

In the mid- to late 2000s, donors began shifting their priorities elsewhere. CBOs were especially impacted by this financial drain, since many had been nurtured into maturity through this support. Perhaps the biggest blow to the sector was the suspension and eventual withdrawal of GFATM from China. As one of the largest funders for HIV/AIDS programmes, GFATM was more than a grant for CBOs, it was a lifeline. Their departure, along with other donors, left a critical gap in the HIV/AIDS funding structure, especially for CBOs that needed to find a new role for themselves. In light of the funding recession, a more crucial question came to the fore: If the lifeline for CBOs disappeared, what would that mean for the organisations? What role did they have in China, if any? This gap did not just underscore the insecurity of funding but called into question the pertinence of CBOs to the HIV/AIDS response more broadly.

It was against this backdrop that the mobilisation of *goumai fuwu* emerged, acting as a safeguard for the sustainability of CBOs when confronting risky futures. The focus on testing MSM enabled CBOs to parlay their comparative advantage in reaching this population into a marketable asset, thus ensuring their continued participation in the epidemic response. More than that, it legitimised their indispensability to containing the epidemic, making it possible for CBOs to reclaim a place in the HIV/AIDS landscape. Commoditising testing, especially in partnership with the CCDC, secures for the time being CBOs' very existence.

To that end, the sustainability of CBOs is inextricable from the scaling-up of testing. In so far as the success of this intervention is to mobilise MSM as biological citizens to get tested, CBO preservation is contingent upon the expansion of this practice. In other words, the more MSM tested, the more funding in return. As a donor once said to me, CBOs now use testing as a mode of survival. Thus, inasmuch as CBOs aim to forestall the spread of the infection, they are also profiting from it in ways that are crucial to their survival. The scaling-up of testing is also the securitisation of risky futures.

Conclusion

The turn to *goumai fuwu* highlights the tensions emerging from the scaling-up of testing intended to save lives and the unintentional expansion of state surveillance into the everyday lives of MSM. These tensions, I suggest, gesture to broader issues in the global health landscape that index the temporality and insecurity of funding that often requires CBOs to continually redefine themselves in order to exist, but in ways that come to bear on their beneficiaries. Undoubtedly, the push towards testing is a critical one, particularly in getting ART to those who need it. During my research, I continually met men who credited testing with saving their lives. One man in particular had a CD4 count of 20 when he was first tested by a local CBO, and had since started ART and had increased his CD4 up to 160. What needs further interrogation is not testing itself, but rather its commoditisation, which reproduces the social and political marginalisation of MSM. Inasmuch as *goumai fuwu* intends to be apolitical, CBOs are nonetheless entangled in wider transactions of power, politics and money. In examining what these interventions do ethnographically, perhaps we can gain insight into the broader politics that enmesh and shape global health priorities. In his interrogation of global health strategies, João Biehl (2008) argues that one of the unintended consequences of scaling-up treatment has been the cultivation of therapeutic markets that reconfigure patienthood and civic participation.[8] What he draws attention to, and what I argue here, are the limits to market-driven models that have come to permeate the global health landscape, and the need to decouple HIV/AIDS as an epidemic from the industry that so often has come to define it.

Acknowledgements

The author wishes to thank Britt Halvorson, Denielle Elliott and David Strohl for reviewing earlier drafts of this article. Additional thanks are extended to the anonymous reviewers for their careful reading and constructive feedback.

Notes

1. All references made to donors in this paper refer to international donors.
2. For more on outsourcing in China, see Irish, Salamon, and Simon (2009), Jing (2008), Jing and Bin (2012), and Teets (2012).
3. Funding came from a special AIDS fund administered by the Changsha Finance Department.
4. All names are pseudonyms.
5. For more on the commodification of blood in this context, see Erwin (2006) and Shao (2006).
6. The 'Four Frees and One Care' policy provides free ART to rural residents or those with financial hardship in urban areas, free voluntary counselling and testing services, free drugs to HIV-infected pregnant women and free testing for newborns, and free schooling for AIDS orphans. In 2010, the Chinese government added the 'Five Expands, Six Strengthens' policy for more extensive coverage and regulation of the epidemic.
7. In 2010, a case was publicised involving a man who was fired from his job due to his HIV status (Jacobs, 2010).
8. The more recent campaigns advocated by international health organisations promote treatment as prevention for people found to be seropositive. For a critical perspective on these models, see Nguyen, Bajos, Dubois-Arber, O'Malley, and Pirkle (2011) and Patton (2011).

References

Anagnost, A. (1995). A surfeit of bodies: Population and the rationality of the state in post-Mao China. In F. D. Ginsburg & R. Rapp (Eds.), *Conceiving the new world order: The global politics of reproduction* (pp. 22–41). Berkeley: University of California Press.

Anagnost, A. (2006). Strange circulations: The blood economy in rural China. *Economy and Society, 35,* 509–529. doi:10.1080/03085140600960781

Asia Catalyst. (2007). *AIDS blood scandals: What China can learn from the world's mistakes* (Research Report). New York, NY: Author. Retrieved from http://www.asiacatalyst.org/news/ AIDS_blood_scandals_rpt_0907.pdf

Biehl, J. (2008). Drugs for all: The future of global AIDS treatment. *Medical Anthropology, 27*(2), 99–105. doi:10.1080/01459740802022777

China AIDS Info. (2007). *2006/2007 China HIV/AIDS directory.* Beijing: Author.

Choi, K.-H., Diehl, E., Guo Y., Qu, S., & Mandel, J. (2002). High HIV risk but inadequate prevention services for men in China who have sex with men: An ethnographic study. *AIDS and Behavior, 6,* 255–266. doi:10.1023/A:1019895909291

Choi, K.-H., Gibson, D. R., Han, L., & Guo, Y. (2004). High levels of unprotected sex with men and women among men who have sex with men: A potential bridge of HIV transmission in Beijing, China. *AIDS Education and Prevention, 16*(1), 19–30. doi:10.1521/aeap.16.1.19.27721

Choi, K.-H., Lui, H., Guo, Y., Han, L., & Mandel, J. S. (2006). Lack of HIV testing and awareness of HIV infection among men who have sex with men, Beijing, China. *AIDS Education and Prevention, 18*(1), 33–43. doi:10.1521/aeap.2006.18.1.33

Choi, K.-H., Zhen, N., Gregorich, S. E., & Pan, Q. (2007). The influence of social and sexual networks in the spread of HIV and syphilis among men who have sex with men in Shanghai, China. *Journal of Acquired Immune Deficiency Syndromes, 45*(1), 77–84. doi:10.1097/QAI.0b013e3180 415dd7

Chow, E. P. F., Wilson, D. P., & Zhang, L. (2010). The next era of HIV in China: Rapidly spreading epidemics among men who have sex with men. *Journal of Acquired Immune Deficiency Syndromes, 55*(4), e32–e34. doi:10.1097/QAI.0b013e3181f3d3c1

Chow, E. P. F., Wilson, D. P., & Zhang, L. (2012). The rate of HIV testing is increasing among men who have sex with men in China. *HIV Medicine, 13,* 255–263. doi:10.1111/j.1468-1293.2011. 00974.x

Cui, Y., Liau, A., & Wu, Z.-Y. (2009). An overview of the history of epidemic of and response to HIV/AIDS in China: Achievements and challenges. *Chinese Medical Journal, 122,* 2251–2257. doi:10.3760/cma.j.issn.0366-6999.2009.19.013

Erwin, K. (2006). The circulatory system: Blood procurement, AIDS, and the social body in China. *Medical Anthropology Quarterly, 20,* 139–159. doi:10.1525/maq.2006.20.2.139

Fan, S., Lu, H., Ma, X., Sun, Y., He, X., Li, C., … Ruan, Y. (2012). Behavioral and serological survey of men who have sex with men in Beijing, China: Implication for HIV intervention. *AIDS Patient Care and STDs, 26,* 148–155. doi:10.1089/apc.2011.0277

Feng, Y., Wu, Z., & Detels, R. (2010). Evolution of men who have sex with men community and experienced stigma among men who have sex with men in Chengdu, China. *Journal of Acquired Immune Deficiency Syndromes, 53*(Suppl 1), S98–S103. doi:10.1097/QAI.0b013e3181c7df71

Ferguson, J. (1994). *The anti-politics machine: "Development," depoliticization, and bureaucratic power in Lesotho.* Minneapolis: University of Minnesota Press.

He, N., & Detels, R. (2005). The HIV epidemic in China: History, response, and challenge. *Cell Research, 15,* 825–832. doi:10.1038/sj.cr.7290354

He, Q., Wang, Y., Lin, P., Liu, Y., Yang, F., Fu, X., … McFarland, W. (2006). Potential bridges for HIV infection to men who have sex with men in Guangzhou, China. *AIDS and Behavior, 10,* S17–S23. doi:10.1007/s10461-006-9125-3

Irish, L. E., Salamon, L. M., & Simon, K. W. (2009). *Outsourcing social services to CSOs: Lessons from abroad* (World Bank Report). Retrieved from http://siteresources.worldbank.org/DEVDIA LOGUE/Resources/OutsourcingtoCSOs.pdf

Jacobs, A. (2010, November 12). Discrimination law fails in Chinese court. *The New York Times.* Retrieved from www.nytimes.com

Jing, Y. (2008). Outsourcing in China: An exploratory assessment. *Public Administration and Development, 28,* 119–128. doi:10.1002/pad.488

Jing, Y., & Bin, C. (2012). Is competitive contracting really competitive? Exploring government–nonprofit collaboration in China. *International Public Management Journal, 15,* 405–428.

Retrieved from http://www.tandfonline.com/doi/abs/10.1080/10967494.2012.761054?journal Code=upmj20#.Utw1KGTnYy4

Li, H., Kuo, N. T., Liu, H., Korhonen, C., Pond, E., Guo, H.., … Sun, J. (2010). From spectators to implementers: Civil society organizations involved in AIDS programmes in China. *International Journal of Epidemiology*, *39*(Suppl 2), ii65–ii71. doi:10.1093/ije/dyq223

Li, X., Lu, H., Ma, X., Sun, Y., He, X., Li, C., … Jia, Y. (2012). HIV/AIDS-related stigmatizing and discriminatory attitudes and recent HIV testing among men who have sex with men in Beijing. *AIDS and Behavior*, *16*, 499–507. doi:10.1007/s10461-012-0161-x

Ministry of Health of the People's Republic of China. (2012). *2012 China AIDS response progress report*. Beijing: Author.

NCAIDS. (2011). *Our stories*. Beijing: Author.

NCAIDS & China HIV/AIDS Information Network. (2010). *2010 China HIV/AIDS CSO/CBO directory*. Beijing: Author.

Nguyen, V.-K., Bajos, N., Dubois-Arber, F., O'Malley, J., & Pirkle, C. M. (2011). Remedicalizing an epidemic: From HIV treatment as prevention to HIV treatment is prevention. *AIDS*, *25*, 291–293. doi:10.1097/QAD.0b013e3283402c3e

Patton, C. (2011). Rights language and HIV treatment: Universal care or population control? *Rhetoric Society Quarterly*, *41*, 250–266. doi:10.1080/02773945.2011.575328

Peterson, K. (2001). Benefit sharing for all? Bioprospecting NGOs, intellectual property rights, new governmentalities. *PoLAR: Political and Legal Anthropology Review*, *24*(1), 78–91. doi:10.1525/pol.2001.24.1.78

Rose, N., & Novas, C. (2005). Biological citizenship. In A. Ong & S. J. Collier (Eds.), *Global assemblages: Technology, politics, and ethics as anthropological problems* (pp. 439–463). Malden, MA: Blackwell.

Shao, J. (2006). Fluid labor and blood money: The economy of HIV/AIDS in rural central China. *Cultural Anthropology*, *21*, 535–569. doi:10.1525/can.2006.21.4.535

Sun, J., Liu, H., Li, H., Wang, L., Guo, H., Shan, D., … Ren, M. (2010). Contributions of international cooperation projects to the HIV/AIDS response in China. *International Journal of Epidemiology*, *39*, ii14–ii20. doi:10.1093/ije/dyq208

Sun, X., Wang, N., Li, D., Zheng, X., Qu, S., Wang, L., … Wang, L. (2007). The development of HIV/AIDS surveillance in China. *AIDS*, *21*(Suppl 8), S33–S38. doi:10.1097/01.aids.0000304694.54884.06

Teets, J. C. (2012). Reforming service delivery in China: The emergence of a social innovation model. *Journal of Chinese Political Science*, *17*(1), 15–32. doi:10.1007/s11366-011-9176-9

Tucker, J. D., Wong, F., Nehl, E. J., & Zhang, F. (2012). HIV testing and care systems focused on sexually transmitted HIV in China. *Sexually Transmitted Infections*, *88*(2), 116–119. doi:10.1136/sextrans-2011-050135

UNAIDS. (2013). HIV in China: Facts and figures [web page]. Retrieved from http://www.unaids.org.cn/en/index/page.asp?id=197&class=2&classname=China+Epidemic+%26+Response

The United Nations Theme Group on HIV/AIDS in China. (2002). *HIV/AIDS: China's titanic peril: 2001 update of the AIDS situation and needs assessment report*. Beijing: Author.

Wu, Z., Rou, K., & Cui, H. (2004). The HIV/AIDS epidemic in China: History, current strategies and future challenges. *AIDS Education and Prevention*, *16*, 7–17. doi:10.1521/aeap.16.3.5.7.35521

Wu, Z., Sullivan, S. G., Wang, Y., Rotheram-Borus, M. J., & Detels, R. (2007). Evolution of China's response to HIV/AIDS. *The Lancet*, *369*, 679–690. doi:10.1016/S0140-6736(07)60315-8

Xu, H., Zeng, Y., & Anderson, A. F. (2005). Chinese NGOs in action against HIV/AIDS. *Cell Research*, *15*, 914–918. doi:10.1038/sj.cr.7290368

Zhang, B., & Chu, Q. (2005). MSM and HIV/AIDS in China. *Cell Research*, *15*, 858–864. doi:10.1038/sj.cr.7290359

Bringing the state back in: Understanding and validating measures of governments' political commitment to HIV

Radhika J. Gore[a], Ashley M. Fox[b], Allison B. Goldberg[a] and Till Bärnighausen[c,d]

[a]Department of Sociomedical Sciences, Mailman School of Public Health, Columbia University, New York, NY, USA; [b]Department of Health Evidence and Policy, Mount Sinai School of Medicine, New York, NY, USA; [c]Department of Global Health and Population, Harvard School of Public Health, Boston, MA, USA; [d]Wellcome Trust Africa Centre for Health and Population Sciences, University of KwaZulu-Natal, Mtubatuba, South Africa

Analysis of the politics of HIV programme scale-up requires critical attention to the role of the state, since the state formulates HIV policies, provides resources for the HIV response and negotiates donor involvement in HIV programmes. However, conceptual and methodological approaches to analysing states' responses to HIV remain underdeveloped. Research suggests that differences in states' successes in HIV programme scale-up reflect their levels of 'political commitment' to responding to HIV. Few empirical measures of political commitment exist, and those that do, notably the AIDS Program Effort Index (API), employ ad hoc scoring approaches to combine information from different variables into an index of commitment. The indices are thus difficult to interpret and may not have empirically useful meaning. In this paper, we apply exploratory factor analysis to examine whether, and how, selected variables that comprise the API score reflect previously theorised dimensions of political commitment. We investigate how variables associated with each of the factors identified in the analyses correspond to these theorised dimensions as well as to API categories. Finally, we discuss potential uses – such as political benchmarking and accountability – and challenges of factor analysis as a means to identify and measure states' political commitment to respond to HIV.

Introduction

The global HIV treatment access movement is considered one of the most successful transnational social movements in recent history (Mbali, 2013). Millions of poor people in poor countries are now receiving life-saving antiretroviral therapy (ART), an outcome that was unthinkable a decade ago. However, the scale-up of HIV programmes has been uneven. Based on a comparison of countries with similar background factors, such as socio-economic conditions and health system infrastructure, some countries have met or exceeded expected performance in terms of overall outcomes, such as Botswana and Rwanda, and other countries have fallen short, such as Swaziland, Zimbabwe and, in the early years of the treatment access movement, South Africa (Desmond, Lieberman, Alban, & Ekstrom, 2008; Nattrass, 2008).

Research suggests that a state's 'political commitment', also referred to as political will or political support, can help explain differences in the adequacy of HIV programme scale-up (Ainsworth, Beyrer, & Soucat, 2003; Bor, 2007; Nattrass, 2008; Nunn, 2009; Stoneburner & Low-Beer, 2004). However, both the analysis of the state's role in responding to HIV and the conceptualisation of political commitment remain under-developed in the literature on HIV programme response. In this literature, the dominance of civil society and donor organisations in ART provision has tended to overshadow attention to the role of the state in shaping responses to HIV, and states have been viewed largely as recipients of donor aid rather than active participants in shaping HIV response. Yet studies show a reciprocal relationship between a state's degree of political commitment to HIV and donor attention (Lieberman, 2009). States that signal that they are committed to responding to the HIV epidemic (e.g., by dedicating their own scarce resources towards HIV) may receive more technical and financial support from donors (Lieberman, 2009). Moreover, despite concerns about the vertical nature of HIV programmes and the potential for donor aid to build parallel health system structures (Fukuyama, 2004, pp. 40–42; Shiffman, 2006), the state remains an important entity in health systems in low- and middle-income countries. In these countries, it is the state, rather than the private or non-governmental sector, which is typically the primary funder of the health system and, in many cases, is the major provider of health services (Kruk & Freedman, 2008). Assessing states' contribution to HIV programme response is therefore important for understanding reasons why countries are excelling, or falling behind, in the fight against this disease. Much as social scientists' calls for "bringing the state back in" argued for greater analytical attention to the state—in balance to a focus on societal actors—as an agent that shapes economic, political, and social processes (Evans, Rueschemeyer, & Skocpol, 1985), a similar imperative applies to the analysis of states' role in HIV programme response.

Studies that have examined states' political commitment towards HIV have largely viewed political commitment as an attribute of individual leaders whose public pronouncements on the subject and policy platforms signal their support for HIV response (Fox, Goldberg, Gore, & Bärnighausen, 2011). This view of political commitment does not account for the common conception of the state as 'the institutions of government providing the administrative, legislative, and judicial vehicles for the actual exercise of public authority and power' (Frenk, 1994, p. 25). As such, a state is not entirely a reflection of its political leadership. Rather, the state apparatus remains in existence even while individuals within it, such as political leaders, change. The state's institutional arrangements enable and constrain the actions of individuals within it, and these arrangements affect whether their commitment towards a particular policy initiative is 'credible' (e.g., a commitment that cannot be easily reneged) (Jan, 2003). As we discuss below, states can display political commitment in multiple ways, encompassing several state institutions and functions.

In previous work, we reviewed existing attempts in the public health literature to measure states' political commitment to respond to HIV and, based on this review, conceptualised three dimensions of political commitment: expressed, institutional and budgetary commitment (Fox et al., 2011; Goldberg, Fox, Gore, & Bärnighausen, 2012). *Expressed commitment* refers to verbal declarations of support for an issue by high-level, influential political leaders. *Institutional commitment* comprises the adoption of specific policies and organisational infrastructure in support of an issue. Finally, *budgetary commitment* consists of earmarked allocations of resources towards a specific issue relative to a particular benchmark. The combination of the three dimensions signals that a state has an explicit intention or policy platform to address this health area. However, we also theorise that these dimensions can be examined separately. For instance, we suggest that expressions of commitment that are unsupported by institutional commitment and budgetary allocations may be viewed as rhetorical commitment – declarations without substance. By contrast, states that adopt compulsory institutions and make budgetary allocations without building widespread attention to the issue may reflect the objective trappings of commitment, without actual buy-in from leadership. Although the dimensions of political commitment are conceptually distinct, in practice they are often linked. For example, budget allocations for a particular HIV programme would typically follow institutional measures established for the programme. Announcements made by political leaders to publicise the HIV programme are likely to precede both institutional and budgetary measures.

Our review of the literature identified that in addition to the three dimensions described above, states' commitment to respond to HIV has been assessed along normative and ideological lines. Normative aspects of commitment refer to the inclusivity of a state's response and its protection of human rights, meaning the extent to which policies realise the rights of people living with HIV and marginalised groups that may be disproportionately affected by the epidemic. Ideological aspects of commitment capture whether responses are grounded in scientific evidence; for example, whether they are guided by prevailing medical and social scientific norms, or instead by cultural or political ideology that may contradict or ignore accepted scientific evidence. We suggest that normative and ideological aspects cut across the three dimensions of political commitment.

Our review also found that where empirical studies have estimated political commitment using quantitative measures, they have largely relied on two major indices developed to capture national programme effort to respond to HIV and to monitor progress in meeting HIV-related outputs and outcomes: the AIDS Program Effort Index (API) (USAID, UNAIDS, WHO, & POLICY Project, 2003) and the United Nations General Assembly Special Session on HIV/AIDS (UNGASS) Declaration of Commitment Indicators (UNAIDS, 2010).

The API is a survey tool designed to improve accountability and benchmark progress in HIV programme scale-up efforts across countries (USAID, UNAIDS, WHO, & POLICY Project, 2003). Similar to the Program Effort Score used in the field of reproductive health (Family Planning Program Effort Score, 2009), the API uses key informant interviews to collect information about countries' policy environment, programmes, organizational and legal structures and budgets related to HIV. The API contains a set of questions pertaining to political commitment, which have been used extensively in academic scholarship on the politics of states' responses to the HIV epidemic (Bor, 2007; Lieberman, 2007, 2009; Patterson, 2006). In addition, the Joint United Nations Programme on HIV/AIDS (UNAIDS) has adapted the API to devise the biannual reports that, beginning in 2003, countries have been required to submit to UNAIDS on their progress towards fulfilling the 2001 UNGASS Declaration of Commitment on HIV/AIDS (Gruskin, Ferguson, Peersman, & Rugg, 2009; UNAIDS, 2010). UNGASS' National Commitments and Policies Instrument (NCPI), which assesses the status of HIV-related policies and legal environment in reporting countries, is adapted from various API modules and incorporates a number of the same questions (UNAIDS, 2010). The NCPI, formerly known as the National Composite Policy Index, was updated in 2011, but the majority of its questions remain unchanged from its previous versions to allow for trend analyses (UNAIDS, 2011a). The API is therefore of foundational importance as a measure of political commitment, and it is the focus of this paper.

Although researchers have used the API, the API is based on an ad hoc scoring approach, in which the weights assigned to the different variables in the computation of the index score are not empirically derived. The API variables are grouped into 10 categories based on a conceptual framework of the relationship between HIV programme effort and desired outcomes (USAID, UNAIDS, WHO & POLICY Project, 2003). In its current version, each category of the API includes *yes–no* questions and questions asking respondents to provide a summary score on a scale of 0–10 (USAID, UNAIDS, WHO, & POLICY Project, 2003). The *yes–no* questions are factual, such as questions that ask about the existence of a particular policy. In addition to *yes-no* factual questions, scored 1 for *yes* and 0 for *no*, the 'programme resources' category of the API includes questions about the adequacy of budgetary resources for a number of HIV programme elements, each scored on a scale of 0–3. The factual item score for each category is the proportion of maximum possible points for that category. The questions asked on a 10-point scale elicit subjective judgements, such as the respondents' ratings of political support for HIV programmes, which are a function of an individual's expectations and norms and thus difficult to compare across individuals and settings. A country's score in each category is an average of its factual item and subjective summary scores, which mixes factual and subjective responses. The final score for each country is an average of its category scores, and it assigns equal weight to each category of programme effort.

The resulting country scores, in which a higher score value is thought to represent stronger HIV policy effort, have raised questions about the validity of the API. Researchers have noted that the API assigns higher than expected scores to certain countries that have a poor international reputation on HIV programme response (Busby, 2007; Lieberman, 2007; Patterson, 2006). For instance, the 2003 API rated South Africa's policy effort towards addressing HIV (with an index value of 75) almost as high as Uganda's (76) at a time when South Africa had an international reputation for having low levels of political commitment while Uganda was commonly thought to have strong commitment to fighting HIV.

The above discussion shows that in the literature on HIV programme response, states' political commitment has been inadequately conceptualised, and the validity of existing measures of political commitment, such as the API, has been questioned. Without conceptual clarity on political commitment, and without validating measures such as the API, health system actors can neither hold states accountable for their programme efforts to respond to HIV, nor draw policy lessons from the efforts of relatively more committed states.

In this paper, we have two aims. The first is to establish whether, and how, constructs derived empirically from selected API variables correspond to our theorised dimensions of political commitment. We select variables from the API based on our previous review of the literature and conceptualisation of political commitment as a multidimensional construct with expressed, institutional and budgetary dimensions (Fox et al., 2011). The second aim is to determine the extent to which constructs derived empirically from selected API variables correspond with the intended content of the API categories. This tests the content validity of the API variables by examining how the selected variables group together against their API-assigned categories. Overall, we expect to find that the selected API variables convey more complex information about political commitment than is suggested by the API-assigned categories.

We proceed in four steps: (1) select API variables that capture states' political commitment to HIV, looking beyond the 'political support' category of the API in order to include the multiple ways in which states can signal political commitment; (2) conduct exploratory factor analysis of the selected API variables in order to identify the latent constructs that undergird the observed responses on the selected API variables; (3) compare these empirically identified constructs to our theorised constructs of political commitment; and (4) compare the latent constructs to the API categories. Finally, we discuss the challenges in measuring and validating political commitment given the data used in the analysis.

Findings from the analysis will help researchers and planners develop more theoretically and empirically informed metrics of political commitment that can better assess states' level of political commitment to respond to HIV and that can be applied to existing national reporting systems such as UNGASS. An improved understanding of states' role in HIV programme response can inform practical efforts to build political commitment where it is weak or lacking.

Methods

Data

The API was developed to measure the amount of 'effort' domestic institutions and international organisations have put into national HIV programmes across 10 different categories of indicators: (1) political support; (2) policy and planning; (3) organisational structure; (4) programme resources; (5) evaluation, monitoring and research; (6) legal and regulatory environment; (7) human rights; (8) prevention programmes; (9) care and treatment services; and (10) mitigation programmes. The full questionnaire is available from the 2003 API report (USAID, UNAIDS, WHO, & POLICY Project, 2003).

Sample

The API indicators were first collected in 40 countries in 2000. The questions were subsequently revised and applied in 54 countries, including the original 40, in 2003 (USAID, UNAIDS, WHO, & POLICY Project, 2003). In the third round, data were collected in 2005 from 47 countries. In this paper, we use API data for 2005, adding 27 countries from the 2003 round that were not available in the 2005 round.[1] Data on all variables included in our analysis were available for 72 countries. Two countries were excluded because of missing data. As described in more detail elsewhere (Goldberg et al., 2012), data to construct the API were derived from expert interviews with 5–15 key informants in each country, holding a variety of positions in the governmental and non-governmental sectors. Data are available upon request.

Variables and data properties

Questions on the API are designed as factual items and subjective summary ratings. As mentioned above, factual items are mostly in the form of *yes–no* questions, while subjective questions are on a 10-point scale and aim to elicit respondents' judgements (USAID, UNAIDS, WHO, & POLICY Project, 2003). Some factual item questions, such as questions on the adequacy of budgetary resources, are a mix of fact and judgement. For instance, questions on budgetary allocations are asked on a four-point scale to assess adequacy of resources available for a variety of HIV programmes and services. Although the adequacy of resources can be externally validated, rating whether resources are adequate also requires a degree of judgement.

To produce the API, the factual item scores and subjective summary scores are averaged and multiplied by 100 to produce a score for each of the 10 categories ranging from 0 to 100, with 100 being the highest possible policy effort and 0 constituting no effort. The scores for the 10 categories are then averaged to produce the single index API score. This scoring technique weights all variables equally. Furthermore, the API 'political support' category, which consists of questions about public pronouncements made by government leaders and public officials, the establishment of a national commission for HIV, and the country's application to the Global Fund to Fight AIDS, Tuberculosis and Malaria, may exclude certain variables that are theoretically related to political commitment and are included under other API categories.

Selection of variables

To conduct the exploratory factor analysis, we selected variables from the API that capture states' intentions, or signals of political commitment, to address HIV, but which are unlikely to be affected by other state characteristics. Exploratory factor analysis is a method used to identify the structure of correlations among measured variables. It is applied when researchers expect there to be latent constructs (here political commitment), known as factors, driving the measured variables (Fabrigar, Wegener, MacCallum, & Strahan, 1999). Inclusion of variables that are not relevant to the domain of interest could result in spurious common factors or obscure true common factors (Fabrigar et al., 1999). Based on our previous characterisation of the expressed, institutional and budgetary aspects of political commitment (Fox et al., 2011), we selected variables that might be theoretically relevant from seven API categories: (1) political support; (2) policy and planning; (3) organisational structure; (4) programme resources; (5) evaluation, monitoring and research; (6) legal and regulatory environment; and (7) human rights. We employed several criteria to select which variables to include in the factor analysis.

First, in order to avoid an inference of political commitment from evidence of *outputs* of political processes, we did not use items in API categories (8), (9) and (10) – 'prevention programmes', 'care and treatment services', and 'mitigation programmes', respectively – which measure programme implementation. Variables in these categories are likely to be affected by political commitment, rather than constitutive of political commitment. For instance, ART coverage is believed to be higher in countries that are politically committed to responding to HIV. Measuring political commitment in terms of the output it is supposed to foster, such as ART coverage, would be tautological (Fox et al., 2011; Youde, 2007). Instead, we include the availability of funds for ART, an input measure, as one signal of political commitment. Another possible signal could be adequate staff to deliver ART. These signals of political commitment are precursors to the output of ART coverage.

To capture efforts that most prominently and distinctly signal political commitment, we required that the selected variables from API categories (1)–(7) meet the following additional criteria:

- *Sufficiently demonstrate an aspect of political commitment, and do not qualify responses to another variable.* For example, the question 'Has the country submitted an application for funding to the Global Fund to Fight AIDS, Tuberculosis and Malaria?' is adequate evidence of political commitment for our purposes, so we excluded the qualifying question on whether the application has been approved by the Global Fund. Similarly, the question of whether a national strategic plan for AIDS includes formal programme goals, multi-sectoral strategies, or a monitoring and evaluation plan is contingent on the existence of such a strategic plan. We, therefore, exclude qualifying follow-up questions.

- *Are neutral to the severity of a country's HIV epidemic.* For example, a negative response to the question 'Has AIDS been declared a national disaster?' could reflect either a mild HIV epidemic or the reluctance of political leaders to express commitment towards responding aggressively to a severe epidemic. On the other hand, low scores on questions about the 'adequacy of resources' for essential HIV programme components, such as voluntary counselling and testing (VCT) and ART, would reflect low political commitment to HIV at any level of severity of the epidemic.

- *Are neutral to a state's capacity to respond to HIV.* State capacity, which is conventionally measured in terms of overall public resources (e.g., GDP per capita, health system infrastructure), affects the ability of countries to respond to HIV. Well-resourced health systems would likely have sufficient funds for functions such as policy development, management, evaluation and implementation. Moreover, state resources can affect the types of programmes that the state supports, such as whether it undertakes effort in behavioural prevention, which requires fewer resources, or treatment, which requires more resources (Parkhurst & Lush, 2004). To separate effort from output, we focused on the adequacy of resources for selected HIV programme components (namely blood safety, behaviour change communication, VCT, ART and prevention of mother-to-child transmission [PMTCT]) that are considered essential to an HIV programme (Centers for Disease Control and Prevention [CDC], 2013) and avoided questions that would likely reflect overall public resources. As noted above, whether the selected programme components are funded largely from the state's own funds or donor funds may be of limited concern since donors have funded HIV programmes in states that have allocated public funds towards the programmes.

- *Are independent of governance structure.* API indicators for 'adequacy of staff and structure' refer to three administrative levels: national, province and district. We focused on the national and district level. Responses to the question about 'adequacy of staff and structure at province level' are contingent on features of public administration, and specific to countries with federal structures. By contrast, adequate staff at the national (high administrative tier) and district (low administrative tier) levels would reasonably indicate a state's political commitment to reach a population irrespective of the form of its political and administrative structure. National staff is typically needed for overall decision-making and oversight functions. Local staff is needed for implementation and programme delivery. Moreover, states with federal structures, in which the province level might play a significant decision-making role, would still require district staff for local implementation and national staff to coordinate regional activities. Brazil's decentralised HIV programme is one such example (Berkman, Garcia, Muñoz-Laboy, Paiva, & Parker, 2005). Likewise, a state's existing administrative arrangements may influence whether evaluation results are used in policy development and planning. On the other hand, the appointment of an evaluation and monitoring officer for HIV could be a minimum requirement upon which the possibility of generating and using evidence rests (Management Sciences for Health & World Health Organization, 2006; UNAIDS, 2009).

- *Are designated as 'factual' questions in the API.* We include only factual questions that can be externally validated and exclude questions that were designed as subjective summaries. Subjective summary questions, such as 'Overall, how would you rate the political support for the HIV/AIDS program', rank responses on a 10-point scale. Whereas factual items in the analysis allow researchers to independently verify answers, subjective questions cannot be directly externally validated and may be more subject to response biases. For example, respondents who have low expectations from the state might rate a level of effort favourably, whereas the same level of effort would receive a lower rating from a respondent who expects high performance from the state (USAID, UNAIDS, WHO, & POLICY Project, 2003). The inclusion of the subjective summary scores would make international comparisons of countries with API data difficult to interpret. Although budget questions assess adequacy on a four-point scale, we do include these because the adequacy of budgetary resources can be externally validated and are primarily of a factual nature. We discuss the implications of the inherently subjective nature of measures of political commitment in the Discussion section.

- *Do not reflect normative evaluations about involvement of marginalised groups or civil society in the HIV response, and do not reflect subjective evaluations of whether the HIV response is 'evidence-based'.* A large portion of the questions on the API can be considered *normative* – capturing the degree to which a state conforms to international best practices on HIV or a 'Geneva Consensus' response (Gauri & Lieberman, 2006), including how rights-based and inclusive policies are of marginalised groups and civil society. For instance, including the question 'Was the national policy developed in a participatory manner with significant involvement of civil society?' denotes a normative and process-related concern for the inclusion of non-governmental actors in a state's response. A state that does not include civil society or address HIV in a participatory manner may nonetheless allocate political attention and organisational and budgetary resources to HIV. Likewise, API questions related to 'policy and planning' and 'programme resources' ask whether human rights, gender and vulnerable populations are addressed in the national plan and whether budgetary allocations are adequate for these groups. These concerns with inclusivity involve normative and process-oriented judgements about the type of approach that *should* be taken to respond to HIV, which we view as separate from a state's degree of commitment. We view the *type* of response taken (e.g., rights-enhancing versus rights-constraining) as conceptually distinct from the *degree* of response taken. In this view, the budgetary question regarding whether there are 'resources allocated according to priority guidelines including considerations of need, cost-effectiveness and available infrastructure' reflects a concern that responses should follow specific global standards, which might exclude innovative or heterodox responses that are not proven. In general, we view normative and evidence-based dimensions of responses as a separate category on which to assess the nature of commitment indicated by different responses. Thus, we exclude a majority of questions relating to concerns about human rights, social inclusion, participation and following internationally prescribed best practices. We do include two measures that represent policies to ensure the confidentiality of HIV-related information, known or reported in the course of employment, and programmes that are designed to change attitudes of discrimination and stigmatisation associated with HIV to understanding and acceptance. Although still normative, we view these as basic policies that might signal the state's commitment to improving the well-being of individuals living with HIV within its borders. We expected that these variables would undergird all aspects of a state's response to HIV and would be distinct from efforts signalling any one dimension of political commitment.

- *Provide adequate variations in responses, which would clearly distinguish degrees of states' expressions of, institutions for, or budget allocations for HIV.* We included only questions for which fewer than 90% of countries answered affirmatively. For example, 94% of countries in the sample reply positively to the question 'Is there a national strategic plan for AIDS?' With nearly all countries adopting national strategic plans, this leaves insufficient variation for judging differences across countries. In contrast, we included the question 'Does a favourable national policy exist?' that receives positive replies in 78% of countries. We have selected 90% as the cut-off so that we do not end up exclusively with measures that are universal signals of commitment – the lowest common denominators by which states can show that they have committed to responding to HIV – as these indicators would not be able to distinguish between states that are substantively or 'genuinely' committed to HIV and states that are only committed in form.

The 14 variables[2] that were ultimately selected for the exploratory factor analysis according to the above criteria are described in Table 1. The variables are either dichotomous or (for the budgetary questions) ordered-categorical. The ordered-categorical budget variables, which were captured on a scale of 0–3, were dichotomised, with 0 representing 'limited or no resources to meet needs' and 1 representing 'substantial or adequate resources to meet needs'.

Analysis

After selecting variables for the analysis, we applied exploratory factor analysis to the correlation matrix of the selected API variables to ascertain whether, and how, the resulting factor structure among the variables reflects distinct dimensions of political commitment and corresponds to our theorised dimensions. Exploratory factor analysis finds the least number of factors that account for the common variance of a set of variables, excluding variable-specific variance, and allows us to identify latent constructs that explain correlations among the selected variables (Gorsuch, 1997).

Beginning with the initial 14 variables, we undertook a stepwise elimination[3] of variables to optimise the factor structure and remove factors that did not appear to contribute substantially to the overall solution (Henson & Roberts, 2006; Costello & Osborne, 2005). To determine the number of factors to retain, we visually inspected the scree plot and also considered the criterion of retaining factors with eigenvalues >1.[4] To facilitate interpretation of factor loadings, we rotated the solution.[5]

Next, we tested the content validity of the selected API variables. *Content validity* refers to the degree to which indicators grouped under a particular API category capture the aspect of political commitment that the category is intended to measure (American Educational Research Association, American Psychological Association, & National Council on Measurement in Education, 1999; Goodwin & Leech, 2003). We examined the extent to which the selected variables correspond with the *intended* content of the API

Table 1. Variables selected for exploratory factor analysis.

AIDS Program Effort Index category	Variables
(1) Political support	1. Does the head of government speak publicly and favourably about AIDS issues at least twice a year? 2. Has the country applied to the Global Fund to Fight AIDS, Tuberculosis and Malaria? 3. Is there a National AIDS Commission outside the Ministry of Health?
(2) Policy and planning	4. Does a favourable national policy exist?
(3) Organisational structure	Is there an adequate administrative structure and staff for HIV/AIDS activities either through the national AIDS programme or through the Ministry of Health: 5. At the national level? 6. At the district level?
(4) Programme resources	Rate the resources available for the following programmes. Use a scale of 0–3 where 0 = no resources, 1 = limited resources, 2 = substantial but insufficient resources and 3 = adequate resources to meet needs. 7. Voluntary counselling and testing. 8. Behaviour change communication. 9. Blood safety. 10. Prevention of mother-to-child transmission. 11. Antiretroviral therapy.
(5) Evaluation, monitoring and research	12. Is there an evaluation officer responsible for monitoring and evaluation activities of the national programme?
(6) Legal and regulatory environment	13. Legislation and policies require that information related to HIV, known or reported through the course of employment, is subject to strict rules of data protection and confidentiality.
(7) Human rights	14. There are programmes that are explicitly designed to change attitudes of discrimination and stigmatisation associated with HIV/AIDS to understanding and acceptance.

Note: All of the variables included in the exploratory factor analysis are originally coded on a 0–1 scale, with 0 representing 'no' and 1 representing 'yes', except for the variable included in category 4. This variable, originally on a 0–3 point scale (0 = no resource; 1 = limited resources; 2 = substantial, but insufficient resources; and 3 = adequate resources to meet needs), was dichotomised as follows: response options 0 and 1 were collapsed into a score of 0, representing 'limited or no resources' and response options 2 and 3 were collapsed into a score of 1, representing 'substantial or adequate resources'.

categories. Below, we provide possible explanations for any divergence between the content of the empirically derived factors and the intended content of the API categories. To examine whether the factors reflect the actual HIV programme response of countries surveyed in the API, we computed countries' factor scores[6] on the three dimensions of political commitment. Factor scores indicate the relative standing of a country on each aspect of political commitment. We illustrate and discuss factor scores for a selection of

Table 2. Factor loadings[a] and communalities for theoretically plausible factors of political commitment after rotation.

Variable	Factor 1: institutional commitment	Factor 2: expressed commitment	Factor 3: budgetary commitment	Communality
Head of government speaks about HIV	.01	**.55**	−.03	0.34
NAC exists outside of Ministry of Health	−.15	**.57**	−.03	0.31
Favourable national policy exists	.07	**.43**	.05	0.23
Adequate administrative structure and staff exist:				
At national level	**.66**	−.06	.04	0.41
At district level	**.60**	.07	.06	0.44
There is an evaluation officer	**.37**	.18	−.07	0.23
Adequacy of resources available for:				
Blood safety	**.53**	−.01	−.14	0.29
Voluntary counselling and testing	.04	**.36**	**.33**	0.31
Antiretroviral therapy	−.02	−.05	**.66**	0.42
Prevention of mother-to-child transmission	.02	.02	**.67**	0.48
Proportion of common variance explained by each factor	.73	.40	.21	

[a]Absolute factor loadings >.3 are shown in bold font.

countries, namely, Brazil, Kenya, Nigeria, South Africa, Thailand and Uganda, which are considered iconic cases in HIV programme response.

Finally, we discuss the challenges in conducting the above analysis given the data that are available, with a view to helping researchers develop more theoretically and empirically informed metrics of political commitment and more comprehensive assessments of states' level of political commitment to respond to HIV. All statistical analyses were conducted using Stata, version 11.2 (StataCorp, 2009).

Results

Exploratory factor analysis

The exploratory factor analysis generated a final solution of three factors based on the scree test.[7] Rotated factor loadings and communalities[8] for the 10 variables used in the final factor analysis are shown in Table 2. Four variables dropped out of the analysis. These items, including, as expected, the normative variables referring to workplace discrimination policies for people living with AIDS and policies to reduce stigma, did not load highly onto the primary three factors and were not retained in the analysis.

Based on the variables that loaded onto the factors, we assigned factor labels to capture the essence of the loadings (see Table 2). Factor 1 had high (>0.3) loadings from variables related to staffing and the appointment of an evaluation officer. These variables, which belong to the 'organisational structure' and 'evaluation, monitoring and research' categories of the API, are substantively related to the adequacy of public sector administration and technical expertise. We thus labelled factor 1 'institutional commitment' in order to capture evidence of political commitment as demonstrated through investment in organisational resources. Factor 2 indicated positive and high loadings for the questions on whether the head of government speaks, an independent National AIDS Commission (NAC) exists, and a favourable national policy exists. These indicators, which belong to the 'political support' and 'policy and planning' categories of the API, are declarations of political commitment, made not only through public statements, but also through the creation of institutions that have a high political profile. Therefore, we labelled factor 2 'expressed commitment'. Factor 3 had high and positive factor loadings for most of the budget-related variables and was thus labelled 'budgetary commitment'. Of the four budget-related variables in the final analysis, only one did not load highly onto factor 3.

The factors indicate our theorised dimensions of expressed, institutional and budgetary aspects of political commitment. Notably, factors labelled as expressed and institutional commitment consist of variables from multiple API categories. Of particular interest is the expressed commitment factor, which includes items that refer not only to the 'political support' API category, but also the items regarding the existence of a favourable national policy for HIV (which belongs to the API category 'policy and planning') and the perceived adequacy of resources for VCT (which belongs to the API category 'programme resources'). The institutional commitment factor comprises variables related to three API categories: 'organisational structure', 'programme resources', and 'evaluation, monitoring and research'.

Content validity analysis

The structure of the factor loadings – namely, variables from multiple API categories loading onto a distinct factor, and one API variable cross-loading onto multiple distinct factors – does not completely conform to the categorisation of variables according to API categories. Table 3 provides a comparison of variables as they load onto the factors and as

Table 3. Content validity of AIDS Program Effort Index variables.

Variable	AIDS Program Effort Index category	Loads onto factor
Head of government speaks about HIV	Political support	Expressed
National AIDS Commission exists outside of Ministry of Health	Political support	Expressed
Favourable national policy exists	Policy and planning	Expressed
Adequate administrative structure and staff exist:		
At national level	Organisational structure	Institutional
At district level	Organisational structure	Institutional
There is an evaluation officer	Evaluation, monitoring and research	Institutional
Adequacy of resources available for:		
Blood safety	Programme resources	Institutional
Voluntary counselling and testing	Programme resources	Budgetary and expressed
Antiretroviral therapy	Programme resources	Budgetary
Prevention of mother-to-child transmission	Programme resources	Budgetary

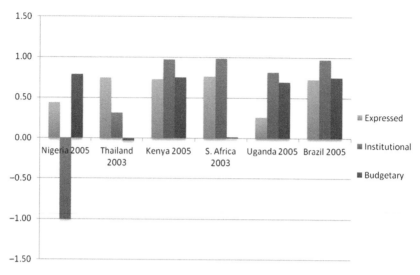

Figure 1. Factor scores along expressed, institutional and budgetary aspects of political commitment.

they are categorised under the API. Notably, variables from the API categories 'political support' and 'policy and planning' load together; variables from 'organisational structure' and 'evaluation, monitoring, and research' load together; and variables from the 'programme resources' category are associated with all three factors. Variables from the API categories 'legal and regulatory environment' and 'human rights' do not load onto the primary factors. Factor scores for selected countries (see Figure 1) show variation across countries on their relative positions on dimensions of political commitment.

Discussion

The results from this exploratory analysis and content validity tests lend support for the three dimensions of political commitment to the HIV response that we previously hypothesised – expressed, institutional and budgetary. Our findings further suggest that the three dimensions of political commitment cannot be read directly from scores on the named API categories. The factor structure that emerged from the exploratory factor analysis shows multiple constructs (expressed, institutional and budgetary) and heterogeneity within those constructs. Rather than being purely expressed, institutional and budgetary indications of political commitment, the constructs comprise variables from more than one API category. Conversely, variables in the API do not all fit under their intended API categories. Variables capturing normative issues did not load onto the primary factors, suggesting that normative issues are conceptually distinct from the theorised dimensions of political commitment. We discuss the content of each of the three factors in turn.

The expressed commitment factor includes variables from API categories outside the 'political support' category, which is the module most directly intended to capture political commitment. (Table 4 provides the full set of the API 'political support' variables and the set of variables selected for and retained in this analysis, which extend beyond the 'political support' category.) The expressed commitment factor confirms that some expressions of political commitment may be offered not only through public

Table 4. Comparison of original AIDS Program Effort Index 'political support' questions and identified political commitment questions meeting inclusion criteria and retained in the exploratory factor analysis.

Original API 'political support' category questions

Does the head of the government, and/or other high officials, speak publicly and favourably about AIDS issues at least twice a year?
  Head of government Y/N[a]
  Other high officials Y/N
Is there a National AIDS Council or Commission outside the Ministry of Health that coordinates the multi-sectoral AIDS programme? Y/N[a]
  If so, is the Head of the Council or Commission chaired by the President, Vice President, Prime Minister or Deputy Prime Minister? Y/N
  Does the Council or Commission include active participation of representatives of civil society? Y/N
Has AIDS been declared a national disaster? Y/N
Has the country submitted an application for funding to the Global Fund to Fight AIDS, Tuberculosis and Malaria? Y/N
  If so, has the application been approved by the Global Fund? Y/N
Overall, how would you rate the political support for the HIV/AIDS programme? 0–10 scale

---

API questions drawn from categories (1)–(7), meeting inclusion criteria and retained in the exploratory factor analysis

---

Questions from API 'political support' category
  Does the head of the government seak publicly and favourably about AIDS issues at least twice a year? Y/N
  Is there a National AIDS Council or Commission outside of the Ministry of Health that coordinates the multi-sectoral AIDS programme? Y/N
Questions from other API categories
  Does a favourable national AIDS policy exist? Y/N
  Is there an adequate administrative structure and staff for HIV/AIDS activities either through the national AIDS programme or through the Ministry of Health?
    a. At the national level? Y/N
    b. At the district level? Y/N
  Is there an evaluation officer responsible for monitoring and evaluation activities of the national programme? Y/N
  How would you rate the resources available for the following programmes? Scale of 0–3
    a. Blood safety
    b. Voluntary counselling and testing
    c. Antiretroviral therapy
    d. Prevention of mother-to-child transmission

---

[a]Questions retained in the analysis in this paper.

statements, but also through the establishment of policies and institutional entities, such as an NAC and the existence of a National AIDS Policy (Putzel, 2004). Although an NAC may be thought of as a quintessential HIV institution, the existence of an NAC and National AIDS Policy may also be largely symbolic or rhetorical expressions of political commitment rather than actualisations of political commitment, signalling countries' commitment to respond to HIV to the international community. By parallel example, researchers have pointed to the diffusion of election monitoring in autocratic countries as a means of signalling a government's purported commitment to democracy (Hyde, 2011). Over time, not having election monitoring has come to be seen as an admission that a country is not democratic, such that even countries that are not genuinely committed to democracy invite election monitors to symbolically show their commitment. The establishment of an independent NAC and the existence of a National AIDS Policy may thereby constitute more symbolic than functional institutions.

By contrast, variables that emerge in the institutional commitment factor are more concrete, substantive institutions that mobilise and enhance a state's administrative and technical capacity and health-care infrastructure. Actions taken to ensure that adequate staff are positioned at the national and sub-national levels to deliver HIV programmes, and to put in place the technical capacity to evaluate programmes, signal greater credibility of political commitment than the notional institutional efforts under expressed commitment. Not only are staffing decisions in the public sector more difficult to reverse once they are executed, but they also typically involve continuity of funds (Management Sciences for Health & World Health Organization, 2006). In comparison, the signing of a policy or formation of a national commission is relatively inexpensive and is 'toothless' without the administrative and technical staff to implement policy prescriptions or commissioned recommendations.

A surprising finding is that the adequacy of resources for ensuring blood safety, an item belonging to the 'programme resources' API category, loads highly onto institutional commitment, while none of the other selected items from the 'programme resources' category correlate with institutional commitment. The correspondence between adequacy of resources for blood safety programmes and adequacy of staffing suggests that some elements of HIV programme response may be closely tied to the existence of sufficient technical staff and organisational structure. Ensuring blood safety represents a core function or first response that all states, regardless of the severity of their epidemic, may make in response to HIV. However, a state's ability to supply safe blood depends upon the availability of trained staff, technical guidelines, administrative procedures, and distribution and logistics systems for blood safety (U.S. President's Emergency Plan for AIDS Relief, 2006; WHO, 2008). Donor aid for blood safety programmes may include technical assistance to develop a nationally regulated system for safe blood supply (U.S. President's Emergency Plan for AIDS Relief, 2006), which would reinforce the link between adequacy of resources for blood safety and the availability of staff and systems. For those HIV programme areas that rely on technical protocols and trained staff, the adequacy of resources for the programme might be a stronger signal of the state's institutional readiness for the programme rather than its budgetary commitment towards HIV.

The variables that comprise the budgetary commitment factor – adequacy of resources for VCT, ART and PMTCT – refer to programme elements that, while also requiring trained staff, additionally involve substantial budgetary allocations for operating physical facilities and supplying drugs (UNAIDS, 2011b; World Bank, 2011). Responses that note adequate resources in these programme areas are likely to capture the country's budgetary commitment to HIV. It is also possible that these measures reflect donor support more so than a state's political commitment, but as we note in the introduction, research has generally found that states that invest more in their HIV response domestically receive more donor assistance (Lieberman, 2009).

The adequacy of resources for VCT, an item from the 'programme resources' category, loads onto both the expressed and budgetary commitment factors and contributes to defining the state's expressed as well as budgetary commitment. In the context of HIV programme scale-up, counselling and testing for HIV has been identified as a critical gateway service for HIV prevention, care and treatment (WHO, 2005). Our findings suggest that resources allocated to VCT programmes constitute not only a signal of budgetary commitment, but also serve as another facet of expressed commitment. The adequacy of resources for VCT might be a bellwether of additional or forthcoming commitment to HIV response, similar to expressions of support such as public pronouncements by heads of government, the establishment of an independent NAC and the existence of a favourable national policy.

Variables that capture a country's normative orientation to address HIV are not associated with any of the factors, suggesting that rights-based aspects of a state's response to HIV are less signals of political commitment to HIV than they are indicators of states' commitment to human rights. State actions to incorporate a rights-based approach to HIV programme response, such as instituting anti-discrimination policies and programmes to reduce stigma, may be more appropriately conceptualised as indicators of the state's normative orientation towards addressing public health threats in a rights-based versus rights-constraining manner. Rights-based measures could inform the nature of a state's actions to responding to HIV, such as the social inclusiveness of its programmes. But rights-based measures may not, in themselves, serve as a substitute for, or supplant, the expressions, institutions and budgetary allocations that constitute political commitment.

In empirical terms, the normative variables do not load onto any factor. However, the fact that the normative variables are not associated with any of the other variables does not mean that normative dimensions are unimportant as a metric of political commitment, but rather suggests that they are conceptually distinct from other measures of commitment. Because many researchers and advocates will likely view the *type* of response as equally or more important than the *degree* of response, we suggest that normative variables be analysed separately to understand how they interrelate with one another. Baldwin (2005), for instance, has examined why some countries responded to HIV in a rights-promoting versus rights-constraining manner. Organisations concerned with government accountability may be more interested in measuring process-related indicators than input-related measures.

The above analysis shows that latent factors derived from the selected API variables can be meaningfully interpreted. The factors reflect our conceptualisation of political commitment as comprising multiple dimensions, encompassing not only political statements and commissions as per the API 'political support' category, but also policies, staffing and notional budget allocations.

Figure 1 illustrates how factor scores for selected states with varying international reputations on HIV programme response perform across the three dimensions of political commitment. For instance, Nigeria performs poorly on institutional commitment and Thailand and South Africa perform poorly on budgetary commitment, suggesting that commitment in these states has been more rhetorical than substantive. Uganda's poor performance on expressed commitment, which comprises items from both the 'political support' and 'policy and planning' categories of the API, reflects how failure to issue an enabling national policy may undermine the credibility of public pronouncements on HIV by political leaders. The variability across the three dimensions also demonstrates the utility of dissecting political commitment into its constituent dimensions in order to assess performance. For example, South Africa receives relatively high scores on expressed and institutional commitment but low scores on budgetary commitment, suggesting where

South Africa's performance falls short. Brazil scores highly in all three dimensions in keeping with expectation.

Challenges and limitations

The findings of this analysis lend insight into the content validity of existing measures of political commitment to respond to HIV and how these measures can be conceptualised to better represent common dimensions of political commitment. However, there are a number of limitations to this analysis that must be discussed. First, the findings are based on variables selected from the API according to our inclusion criteria. A different set of assumptions and choice of variables might have yielded an alternate set of dimensions of political commitment. The methods and interpretation of results are subject to at least three additional challenges, which we describe in more detail below: limitations of sample size of API data, the inherently subjective nature of questions on political commitment, and the possibility of policy reversals.

First, factor analytical techniques require a sufficient sample size relative to the number of included variables to achieve stable solutions, which forced us to be strict in our application of inclusion criteria to limit the number of variables in the analysis. Our results could be substantively affected by the selection of API variables, and by the use of an alternate or larger sample of countries. However, sample size may not be the only, or even the main, concern (MacCallum, Widaman, Preacher, & Hong, 2001; Velicer & Fava, 1998). When the communalities of the variables in the factor analysis are low, the influence of sample size on the quality of the solution becomes particularly important (MacCallum et al., 2001). In our analysis, the communalities of the variables are relatively low, ranging between 0.2 and 0.5, and the design of the data could affect our findings. Due to these methodological constraints, we recommend that a similar analysis also be conducted with data including a wider set of countries, such as from the UNGASS indicators; this would permit the inclusion of more variables.

Second, the inherently subjective nature of the API questions, including to some extent the factual questions, makes it difficult to rank countries with API data. As the API report states:

Some items that appear to be simple statements of fact actually require some judgment, such as 'Senior government officials speak out favourably about HIV/AIDS at least twice a year'. This statement requires an assessment about the number of officials speaking out, their ranking in the government hierarchy, and the content of their statements (USAID, UNAIDS, WHO, & POLICY Project, 2003, p. 7).

We include the factual variables because among the API variables, these are the least prone to respondents' subjective evaluation. Our analysis looks for relationships among the variables, rather than treating the country scores as absolute measures. We recognise that any ranking based on the questions, however combined into a single score, is partly a ranking of the stated perceptions of survey respondents, which may not fully capture how committed or uncommitted states actually are. The perceptions may be inaccurate, and respondents may misrepresent their perceptions for a number of reasons. For instance, key informants from government may have a vested interest in protecting their countries' international reputation, whereas key informants from civil society may have a vested interest in blaming and shaming governments; both interests may bias responses. Furthermore, perceptions are inherently subjective and it is unclear what standards or 'anchors' respondents have in mind when making subjective evaluations, such as on the adequacy of the HIV response. The subjective nature of responses limits cross-individual comparability of answers and calls into question whether variables reflecting such responses can be used in factor analysis. Researchers have suggested ways around this bias, such as devising methods to 'anchor' survey responses to ratings of standardised vignettes (King, Murray, Salomon, & Tandon, 2004).

Finally, our analysis captures states' programme efforts at a point in time, whereas state responses evolve over time. As leadership and representative bodies change, so do policies and platforms. As more global resources have become available, states' degree of commitment and methods of signalling commitment have changed in response. Conversely, if donor resources decrease or shift their emphasis, this too could affect states' HIV programme response. Isolating state commitment from international influences may not be practically possible in the era of HIV programme scale-up and much global attention to the epidemic. Conceptions of the global health system emphasise relations of interdependence between states, private organisations and social movements, among other actors (Frenk & Moon, 2013). Decisions that affect health are influenced by multiple non-state entities, including civil society organisations, multinational corporations, foundations, academic institutions and hybrid entities such as the GAVI Alliance and the Global Fund to Fight AIDS, Tuberculosis and Malaria (Frenk & Moon, 2013). Given these changing influences on policy decisions, states' political commitment should also be viewed in historical context and as an interaction between the priorities of domestic and international actors.

While the API usefully captures a range of HIV programme components, the present analysis is concerned with distinguishing aspects of political commitment based on selected essential and, to the extent possible, objectively measured elements of HIV programme response. Findings from the analysis, taken alone, may not reflect a state's performance on specific HIV programme response categories. For example, although Brazil earns a perfect 100 for the API 'programme resources' category, its relative position on budgetary commitment does not appear much different from that of Kenya, Uganda and Nigeria, countries that have varied API 'programme resource' scores, but which share with Brazil a commitment to core resource investments in testing and treatment. The findings should be read together with a broad set of factual benchmarks and subjective assessments of policy effort.

Global benchmarking surveys repeated on a regular basis, such as UNGASS, provide a monitoring tool that allows for change to be observed over time. UNGASS has collected information from countries every two years since 2003. UNGASS also includes additional information not available on the API, such as objective data on national and international AIDS expenditures. We did not use UNGASS reports for this analysis because it was not available in a readily usable format.

Improving measures and analysis of political commitment

Research suggests that political commitment can shape the scale-up of HIV programmes. The methods and insights from the present study can be used to improve global benchmarking efforts and assess states' political commitment to respond to HIV. Guided by our previously theorised characterisation of the expressed, institutional and budgetary aspects of political commitment, we selected variables from the API and applied factor analysis to identify variables that comprise dimensions of political commitment. As used in this paper, factor analysis is one special, and limited, case of the general class of models called structural equation models (Kaplan, 2000) to explore the latent variables generating the data captured by the API variables and examine how far these latent variables relate to the theorised dimensions of political commitment to respond to the HIV epidemic. A major advance for future efforts to validate the theorised dimensions of political commitment would be to confirm hypothesised relationships between the dimensions and outcomes in structural equation models. Future studies may also employ principal components analysis to generate a summary measure for global benchmarking purposes, bearing in mind the limitations of the survey measures described above.

Contemporary approaches in policy analysis acknowledge the increasing plurality of domestic and international actors involved in policy processes and highlight the importance of subjective assessments captured in indices such as the API. Previous policy analysis frameworks focused largely on the content of policy and the 'politicians, bureaucrats and interest groups' conceived to comprise the policy environment (Walt et al., 2008, p. 309). In contrast, in recent decades, policy research has acknowledged global shifts in the policy environment, such as partnerships between public and private actors, the rise of global civil society actors, market growth in the health sector and decentralisation of health services, which impact the role and capacities of the state (Reich, 2002; Walt et al., 2008). Recent approaches to analysing health policy and health systems emphasise taking a relational view, that is, focusing on how relations among actors as well as actors' values and beliefs shape policy decisions (Sheikh et al., 2011; Walt et al., 2008).

Although the present analysis is based on (as far as possible) objective measures of states' commitment to respond to HIV, its findings underscore the need for systematic study of subjective assessments of states' contribution to HIV programme response. Explaining divergence among the dimensions of political commitment (e.g., low expressed commitment but high budgetary commitment as in Uganda), and gaps between objective and subjective assessments by respondents in the API survey (e.g., Nigeria's API score of a perfect 100 on factual items measuring 'political support' but lower score of 60 on subjective assessment of 'political support') require examining the varied influences, ideas and beliefs that undergird state actions and stakeholders' perceptions. One method to elicit both factual and subjective information, and use alternative sources and types of information to validate measures of country progress in HIV programme response, is illustrated in the NCPI module of the UNGASS. The NCPI explicitly guides countries to gather concrete evidence of policies and laws for HIV programme response; conduct participatory, deliberative events among stakeholders to discuss views and validate assessments of policies and laws; and provide comments on any disagreements or discrepancies (UNAIDS, 2011b, p. 83). Analysis of subjective views would complement analysis of objective measures of states' commitment to HIV programme response.

Conclusion

Early in the response to HIV, a number of countries took the lead, rapidly scaling up HIV treatment and prevention programming, while others did far less. This variation in initiative spurred both global benchmarking efforts to track country responses and academic research to analyse reasons for variations in country responsiveness to the HIV epidemic. Existing research suggests that states' political commitment contributes to HIV programme response. However, attention to the role of the state in HIV programme response and the construct of political commitment remain underdeveloped in the literature, and the validity of existing benchmarking tools to capture states' HIV policy effort has been questioned. This paper calls for greater attention to the state's role in shaping HIV programme response and uses a conceptual framework of political commitment to describe multiple ways in which states can display political commitment. The factor analytical approach employed in this paper identified variables from the API that can be integrated into a theoretically and empirically derived metric of political commitment. Although this approach cannot overcome underlying limitations from the data collection process, it offers a more principled method to generate valid measures of political commitment than those constructed in the past. Improved measures of political commitment can be used for global benchmarking and accountability purposes, as well as academic research into the politics of HIV programme scale-up.

Notes

1. In the data that we obtained from the 2005 round, the survey questions were the same as in the 2003 round. The difference in the two rounds was in the countries that were sampled. Data from the two years were pooled in order to get the maximum number of countries for analysis.
2. A potential constraint under exploratory factor analysis is that sample size can affect the precision and the stability of the solution: factors obtained from a relatively small sample may not be congruent with population factors and may vary in repeated samples (MacCallum, Widaman, Zhang, & Hong, 1999). However, researchers caution against relying solely on sample size in assessing the adequacy of the sample (Bandalos & Boehm-Kaufman, 2008; MacCallum, Widaman, Zhang, & Hong, 1999; Costello & Osborne, 2005). We discuss implications of our sample size in the 'challenges and limitations' section below.
3. In successive iterations of the factor analysis, variables were eliminated one at a time if (1) the variable had a loading of 0.3 or higher only on those factors that we would not consider significant to the analysis based on the scree test or (2) the variable did not have a loading of 0.3 or higher on any factor (Costello & Osborne, 2005). In all cases, we used prior knowledge and theory as a parallel guide to decide whether a variable should be left out (Costello & Osborne 2005). For example, if a variable loaded onto multiple factors, then we considered whether the cross-loadings could be plausibly interpreted based on the substantive content of the variable and the factors.
4. The scree plot graphs eigenvalues in descending order of their magnitude; the eigenvalue of a factor refers to the amount of variance explained by that factor (Preacher & MacCallum 2003). In the scree test, the inflection point of the scree plot indicates the point where further factors do not substantially increase the proportion of common variance explained and it is used as a cut-off for the number of factors. Whereas the scree test tells us where the addition of further factors does not increase the proportion of common variance explained relative to the explanatory power of the other factors, the eigenvalue test (i.e., retaining factors with eigenvalues > 1) assesses the percent of the common variance explained in absolute terms.
5. We applied a standard oblique (oblimin) rotation, allowing for correlation among the factors.
6. Three factor scores were computed for each country, one for each dimension of political commitment, using the regression scoring method.
7. Based on the alternative, arbitrary cut-off criterion of eigenvalues > 1, we would retain two factors, but we defer to the scree test and theoretical plausibility, which suggest three factors.
8. Factor loadings represent the weights or contribution of each variable to a given factor. Communalities refer to the proportion of a variable's total variance that is explained by common factors (Preacher & MacCallum 2003).

References

Ainsworth, M., Beyrer, C., & Soucat, A. (2003). AIDS and public policy: The lessons and challenges of 'success' in Thailand. *Health Policy, 64*(1), 13–37. doi:10.1016/S0168-8510(02) 00079-9

American Educational Research Association, American Psychological Association, & National Council on Measurement in Education. (1999). *Standards for educational and psychological testing*. Washington, DC: Author.

Baldwin, P. (2005). *Disease and democracy: The industrialized world faces AIDS*. Berkeley: University of California Press.

Bandalos, D. L., & Boehm-Kaufman, M. R. (2008). Four common misconceptions in exploratory factor analysis. In C. E. Lance & R. J. Vandenberg (Eds.), *Statistical and methodological myths and urban legends: Doctrine, verity and fable in the organizational and social sciences* (pp. 61–87). New York, NY: Taylor & Francis.

Berkman, A., Garcia, J., Muñoz-Laboy, M., Paiva, V., & Parker, R. (2005). A critical analysis of the Brazilian response to HIV/AIDS: Lessons learned for controlling and mitigating the epidemic in developing countries. *American Journal of Public Health, 95,* 1162–1172. doi:10.2105/AJPH.2004.054593

Bor, J. (2007). The political economy of AIDS leadership in developing countries: An exploratory analysis. *Social Science & Medicine, 64,* 1585–1599. doi:10.1016/j.socscimed.2006.12.005

Busby, J. (2007). Review of Amy Patterson, The politics of AIDS in Africa. *Political Science Quarterly, 122,* 530–532. doi:10.1002/j.1538-165X.2007.tb01677.x

Centers for Disease Control and Prevention (CDC). (2013). *Elements of successful HIV/AIDS prevention programs*. CDC, National Prevention Information Network. Retrieved from http://www.cdcnpin.org/scripts/hiv/programs.asp#eleven

Costello, A., & Osborne, J. (2005). Best practices in exploratory factor analysis: Four recommendations for getting the most from your analysis. *Practical Assessment, Research & Evaluation, 10*(7), 1–9. Retrieved from http://pareonline.net/pdf/v10n7.pdf

Desmond, C., Lieberman, E., Alban, A., & Ekstrom, A. M. (2008). Relative response: Ranking country responses to HIV and AIDS. *Health and Human Rights in Practice, 10,* 105–119. doi:10.2307/20460106

Evans, P., Rueschemeyer, D., & Skocpol, T. (Eds.). (1985). *Bringing the state back in*. Cambridge: Cambridge University Press.

Fabrigar, L. R., Wegener, D. T., MacCallum, R. C., & Strahan, E. J. (1999). Evaluating the use of exploratory factor analysis in psychological research. *Psychological Methods, 4,* 272–299. doi:10.1037/1082-989X.4.3.272

Family Planning Program Effort Score (PES). (2009). *Futures group*. Retrieved from http://futuresgroup.com/projects/family_planning_program_effort_score_pes

Fox, A. M., Goldberg, A. B., Gore, R. J., & Bärnighausen, T. (2011). Conceptual and methodological challenges to measuring political commitment to respond to HIV. *Journal of the International AIDS Society, 14*(Suppl 2), S5. doi:10.1186/1758-2652-14-S2-S5

Frenk, J. (1994). Dimensions of health system reform. *Health Policy, 27*(1), 19–34. doi:10.1016/0168-8510(94)90155-4

Frenk, J., & Moon, S. (2013). Governance challenges in global health. *New England Journal of Medicine, 368,* 936–942. doi:10.1056/NEJMra1109339

Fukuyama, F. (2004). *State building: Governance and world order in the 21st century*. Ithaca, NY: Cornell University Press.

Gauri, V., & Lieberman, E. S. (2006). Boundary institutions and HIV/AIDS policy in Brazil and South Africa. *Studies in Comparative International Development, 41*(3), 47–73. doi:10.1007/BF02686236

Goldberg, A., Fox, A., Gore, R., & Bärnighausen, T. (2012). Indicators of political commitment to respond to HIV. *Sexually Transmitted Infections, 88,* 79–84. doi:10.1136/sextrans-2011-050221

Goodwin, L. D., & Leech, N. L. (2003). The meaning of validity in the new standards for educational and psychological testing: Implications for measurement courses. *Measurement and Evaluation in Counseling and Development, 36,* 181–191.

Gorsuch, R. L. (1997). Exploratory factor analysis: Its role in item analysis. *Journal of Personality Assessment, 68,* 532–560. doi:10.1207/s15327752jpa6803_5

Gruskin, S., Ferguson, L., Peersman, G., & Rugg, D. (2009). Human rights in the global response to HIV: Findings from the 2008 United Nations General Assembly Special Session reports. *Journal of Acquired Immune Deficiency Syndromes, 52*(Suppl 2), S104–S110. doi:10.1097/QAI.0b013e3181baeeac

Henson, R., & Roberts, J. (2006). Use of exploratory factor analysis in published research common errors and some comment on improved practice. *Educational and Psychological Measurement, 66,* 393–416. doi:10.1177/0013164405282485

Hyde, S. D. (2011). Catch us if you can: Election monitoring and international norm diffusion. *American Journal of Political Science, 55,* 356–369. doi:10.1111/j.1540-5907.2011.00508.x

Jan, S. (2003). A perspective on the analysis of credible commitment and myopia in health sector decision making. *Health Policy*, *63*, 269–278. doi:10.1016/S0168-8510(02)00119-7

Kaplan, D. (2000). *Structural equation modeling. Foundations and extensions*. Thousand Oaks, CA: Sage.

King, G., Murray, C. J. L., Salomon, J. A., & Tandon, A. (2004). Enhancing the validity and cross-cultural comparability of measurement in survey research. *American Political Science Review*, *98*, 191–207. doi:10.1017/S000305540400108X

Kruk, M. E., & Freedman, L. P. (2008). Assessing health system performance in developing countries: A review of the literature. *Health Policy*, *85*, 263–276. doi:10.1016/j.healthpol.2007.09.003

Lieberman, E. (2007). Ethnic politics, risk, and policy-making. A cross-national statistical analysis of government responses to HIV/AIDS. *Comparative Political Studies*, *40*, 1407–1432. doi:10.1177/0010414007306862

Lieberman, E. (2009). *Boundaries of contagion: How ethnic politics have shaped government responses to AIDS*. Princeton, NJ: Princeton University Press.

MacCallum, R., Widaman, K. F., Preacher, K. J., & Hong, S. (2001). Sample size in factor analysis: The role of model error. *Multivariate Behavioral Research*, *36*, 611–637. doi:10.1207/S15327906MBR3604_06

MacCallum, R. C., Widaman, K. F., Zhang, S., & Hong, S. (1999). Sample size in factor analysis. *Psychological Methods*, *4*(1), 84–99. doi:10.1037/1082-989X.4.1.84

Management Sciences for Health & World Health Organization. (2006). *Tools for planning and developing human resources for HIV/AIDS and other health services*. Cambridge, MA: Management Sciences for Health. Retrieved from http://www.who.int/hrh/tools/tools_planning_hr_hiv-aids.pdf

Mbali, M. S. (2013). *South African AIDS activism and global health politics*. New York, NY: Palgrave McMillan.

Nattrass, N. (2008). Are country reputations for good and bad leadership on AIDS deserved? An exploratory quantitative analysis. *Journal of Public Health*, *30*, 398–406. doi:10.1093/pubmed/fdn075

Nunn, A. (2009). *The politics and history of AIDS treatment in Brazil*. New York, NY: Springer.

Parkhurst, J. O., & Lush, L. (2004). The political environment of HIV: Lessons from a comparison of Uganda and South Africa. *Social Science & Medicine*, *59*, 1913–1924. doi:10.1016/j.socscimed.2004.02.026

Patterson, A. (2006). *The politics of AIDS in Africa*. Boulder, CO: Lynne Reinner.

Preacher, K. J., & MacCallum, R. C. (2003). Repairing Tom Swift's electric factor analysis machine. *Understanding Statistics*, *2*(1), 13–43. doi:10.1207/S15328031US0201_02

Putzel, J. (2004). The global fight against AIDS: How adequate are the national commissions? *Journal of International Development*, *16*, 1129–1140. doi:10.1002/jid.1167

Reich, M. (2002). Reshaping the state from above, from within, from below: Implications for public health. *Social Science & Medicine*, *54*, 1669–1675. doi:10.1016/S0277-9536(01)00334-3

Sheikh, K., Gilson, L., Agyepong, I. A., Hanson, K., Ssengooba, F., & Bennett, S. (2011). Building the field of health policy and systems research: Framing the questions. *PLoS Medicine*, *8*(8), e1001073. doi:10.1371/journal.pmed.1001073

Shiffman, J. (2006). HIV/AIDS and the rest of the global health agenda. *Bulletin of the World Health Organization*, *84*, 923. doi:10.2471/BLT.06.036681

StataCorp. (2009). *Stata Statistical Software: Release 11 [computer program]*. College Station, TX: StataCorp LP.

Stoneburner, R. L., & Low-Beer, D. (2004). Population-level HIV declines and behavioral risk avoidance in Uganda. *Science*, *304*, 714–718. doi:10.1126/science.1093166

UNAIDS. (2009). *12 components monitoring & evaluation system assessment tool: Guidelines to support preparation, implementation and follow-up activities*. Geneva: UNAIDS.

UNAIDS. (2010). *Monitoring the Declaration of Commitment on HIV/AIDS: Guidelines on construction of core indicators, 2010 reporting*. Geneva: UNAIDS. Retrieved from http://www.unaids.org/en/resources/presscentre/featurestories/2009/march/20090331ungass2010/

UNAIDS. (2011a). *Global AIDS response progress reporting: Monitoring the 2011 political declaration on HIV/AIDS: Guidelines on construction of core indicators: 2012 reporting*. Geneva: UNAIDS.

UNAIDS. (2011b). *Manual for costing HIV facilities and services*. Geneva: UNAIDS Programmatic Branch, UNAIDS. Retrieved from http://www.unaids.org/en/media/unaids/contentassets/documents/document/2011/20110523_manual_costing_HIV_facilities_en.pdf

USAID, UNAIDS, WHO, & POLICY Project. (2003). *The level of effort in the national response to HIV/AIDS: The AIDS Programme Effort Index (API), 2003 round*. Geneva: UNAIDS. Retrieved from http://www.policyproject.com/abstract.fm/1677

U.S. President's Emergency Plan for AIDS Relief. (2006). *Report on blood safety and HIV/AIDS*. Retrieved from http://www.state.gov/documents/organization/74125.pdf

Velicer, W. F., & Fava, J. L. (1998). The effects of variable and subject sampling on factor pattern recovery. *Psychological Methods*, *3*, 231–251. doi:10.1037/1082-989X.3.2.231

Walt, G., Shiffman, J., Schneider, H, Murray, S., Brugha, R., & Gilson, L. (2008). 'Doing' health policy analysis: Methodological and conceptual reflections and challenges. *Health Policy & Planning*, *23*, 308–317. doi:10.1093/heapol/czn024

World Bank. (2011). *The fiscal dimension of HIV/AIDS in Botswana, South Africa, Swaziland, and Uganda*. Washington, DC: Author.

World Health Organization (WHO). (2005). *Scaling-up HIV testing and counselling services: A toolkit for programme managers*. Geneva: Author.

World Health Organization (WHO). (2008). *Universal access to safe blood transfusion: Report of the global consultation on universal access to safe blood transfusion*, 9–11 June 2007, Ottawa, Canada. Geneva: Author.

Youde, J. (2007). Ideology's role in AIDS policies in Uganda and South Africa. *Global Health Governance*, *1*(1), 1–16.

'Low-hanging fruit': Counting and accounting for children in PEPFAR-funded HIV/AIDS programmes in South Africa

Lindsey J. Reynolds

Department of Sociology and Social Anthropology, Stellenbosch University, Matieland, South Africa

The article traces the social life of a policy that aimed to define and circumscribe the ambiguous and contested category of 'orphaned and vulnerable children' (or OVC) in South Africa at the height of the 'emergency response' to HIV/AIDS. Drawing on several months of institutional ethnographic research conducted over the course of five years with South African organisations receiving funding from the US President's Emergency Plan for AIDS Relief to provide services to 'OVC', the project interrogates the influence of governmental forms of counting and accounting on health policy and practice in South Africa. Focusing on the experiences of one organisation, the article describes a process of policy 'translation' typified by a series of disconnects between the intentions of a policy and the exigencies of implementation, structured by the ambiguous and flexible nature of the 'OVC' category. In this context, the article argues that the uncertainty produced by the implementation of the guidelines was not simply an artefact of a poorly designed policy, but rather signals an underlying epistemological tension in the practice of 'global health', in which quantitative metrics designed for monitoring and evaluation are often incapable of approximating the complexities of everyday life.

Introduction

In 2008, five years after the passage of legislation authorising the President's Emergency Plan for AIDS Relief (PEPFAR), President George W. Bush hosted an event at the Smithsonian National Museum of African Art to highlight the important effects of the initiative. 'This work of health and redemption', he proclaimed in his introductory speech, 'is both a matter of conscience and a wise exercise of American influence' (Wolfe, 2008). In a film produced for the occasion, President Bush narrated, 'This is really a story of the human spirit, one of the great untold stories of our time' (United States President's Emergency Plan for AIDS Relief, 2008a). In the film, impact numbers were set to dramatic music and combined with images of African children, poor neighbourhoods, and US-funded HIV clinics (United States President's Emergency Plan for AIDS Relief, 2008).

Such outcome statistics were celebrated as a sign of PEPFAR's significance and success. With other impact numbers for treatment, prevention and care, the statistics became important tools for policy-makers and advocates in debates around the reauthorisation of the legislation, and were cited as a justification for increased funding for PEPFAR in its second five years. In introducing the legislation, the chairman of the House Committee on Foreign Affairs commented, 'Every dollar saves lives. I don't know of any other legislation that is this direct' (House Committee on Foreign Affairs, 2007). 'PEPFAR has succeeded', a *Wall Street Journal* editorial claimed, 'precisely because it is the one foreign-aid program that channels money toward specific targets. The statistics are astounding: since 2004, the program has provided counseling and testing for more than 33 million people, and administered care to nearly 7 million, including more than 2.7 million children and orphans' (Editorial Staff, 2008, p. A10).

Nearly five years later, on 1 December 2012, World AIDS Day, the US Secretary of State Hillary Clinton officially released a new report entitled *PEPFAR Blueprint: Creating an AIDS-Free Generation*. The report opens with the following description:

> What a difference a decade makes. Ten years ago, AIDS was wiping out a generation of individuals and reversing important health and development gains being made in Africa. [...] AIDS threatened the very foundations of societies. It took people in the prime of their lives when they should have been caring for their families. It created millions of orphans, unable to attend school without the support provided by their parents. (US Department of State, 2012, p. 2).

By 2012, the report contrasts, citing 2012 programme outcome statistics, AIDS was no longer a certain death sentence and important steps had been made in prevention and control. 'These results are not just numbers', the report went on:

> They represent lives saved and infections averted—and that is the true test of success. For PEPFAR, it is all about results. By adopting a targeted approach to address one of the most complex global health issues in modern history, and by then taking it to scale with urgency and commitment, the U.S. has helped demonstrate what is possible with focus, resources and science. (United States Department of State, 2012, p. 2)

On the occasion of the 10th anniversary of PEPFAR, this article explores the multiple impacts of the programme through an in-depth examination of the effects of the implementation of one set of PEPFAR guidelines in South Africa. While the majority of research and media attention on PEPFAR, and on 'HIV scale-up' more broadly, has focused on prevention and treatment programmes, my research has centred on programmes for 'OVC' – the smallest and, in many respects, least controversial of PEPFAR's programmatic initiatives. By tracing the effects of OVC policies and programmes, the aim of the project has been to highlight how frameworks and models of intervention drawn from the world of public health have increasingly been inscribed onto what would generally be considered 'social' concerns – the raising of children, the functioning of families and the structure of social relations.

Rather than interrogating the effects of these technologies on young people and families, a concern I take up elsewhere, I take the entry of PEPFAR guidelines as a site for examining how the creation and implementation of such categories is shaped by negotiations between forms of knowledge, expert discourses, and local, national, and international politics. More specifically, the article is concerned with the production and management of epistemological uncertainty surrounding the deployment of enumerative technologies required to produce metrics of PEPFAR programme 'success'. Focusing on the experiences of staff at one PEPFAR-funded organisation in South Africa, I describe a process of policy 'translation' typified by a series of disconnects between the intentions of a policy, designed to satisfy the requirements of a system of assistance dependent on the production of evidence and accountability, and the exigencies of implementation, structured by the complex dynamics of local relations and lived experience and which come together in the ambiguous and flexible nature of the category of the 'OVC'.

Through this analysis, I show how the uncertainty produced by PEPFAR OVC guidelines was not simply an artefact of a poorly designed policy, but rather signalled an underlying epistemological tension in the practice of 'global health', in which quantitative metrics designed for monitoring and evaluation are often incapable of approximating the complexities of everyday life. This challenge was readily acknowledged by policy-makers, who highlighted the need to maintain a clear distinction between so-called 'operational' and 'programmatic' definitions and encouraged programme implementers to 'be flexible' or 'use their common sense' to deal with the incommensurability of such categories. Nonetheless, the contradictions between the sedimented notions of such categories spelled out in policy and the flexibility encouraged by programme officers created powerful uncertainties and fears for those who were dependent on the beneficence of strangers to secure their own livelihoods and provide care for children in need. In this context, measures of programme 'success' did not in fact stand simply for effective programming, but rather signalled the ability of actors to negotiate deeply contradictory mandates and fraught relationships across multiple levels of authority.

PEPFAR and technologies of global health

In 2003, one week before the declaration of war against Iraq, President George W. Bush made a pledge in his State of the Union address to commit US$15 billion over five years to the US President's Emergency Plan for AIDS Relief (PEPFAR), a new initiative in the global fight against HIV/AIDS (Bush, 2003). Further, he pledged that by the end of 2008, PEPFAR-funded programmes would have supported treatment for two million people living with HIV/AIDS; prevented seven million new HIV infections and supported care for 10 million people infected with and affected by the disease, including two million 'OVC'. On 27 May 2003, the US Congress passed the US Leadership against HIV/AIDS, Tuberculosis and Malaria Act of 2003 with strong bipartisan support, authorising the requested $15 billion for global AIDS programmes and establishing the new Office of the Global AIDS Coordinator (OGAC) to oversee the plan. In 2005, Congress passed an additional law, the Assistance for Orphans and Other Vulnerable Children in Developing Countries Act, which called for increased attention and funding for programmes for 'OVC affected by HIV/AIDS', mandating that at least 10% of PEPFAR funds be disbursed to OVC programmes, and created an additional set of oversight and reporting requirements for these programmes.

As the flagship programme of President George W. Bush's 'compassionate conservat-ism' agenda,[1] PEPFAR was significant not only for its immense monetary commitment but also for its targeted and strictly regulated approach. The PEPFAR legislation mandated specific funding and outcome targets for different elements of the programme, enshrining President Bush's pledge into law, and required the submission of annual reports to Congress to document progress towards these goals. To reach these goals and document impacts across programmes implemented by thousands of partners and sub-partners across many countries, strict monitoring and evaluation became a central component of the PEPFAR approach. By mandating quantitative funding and outcome targets for specific categories of individuals perceived to be in need of intervention, the legislation mobilised a series of estimations and assumptions regarding the number of individuals in specific target groups in need of intervention and necessitated the production of definitions of each of these categories, a point I take up below.

Because of its regulated approach and focus on results, as the second director of the programme recalled in a 2009 article entitled 'How to Save Lives by Breaking all the Rules', PEPFAR was seen as a fundamentally different kind of development initiative. 'The idea', he described, 'was to favour personal and national responsibility, rethinking the traditional roles of "donor" and "recipient"' (Dybul, 2009). To this end, he went on:

> Bush called for local problems to be solved by local governments and people; for good governance and an end to corruption; for accountability that focused on results rather than how much money was committed; for people from every sector of society—government and nongovernment alike—to contribute to the effort; and for an emphasis on trade and economic best practices as the ultimate engine of sustainable growth. (Dybul, 2009)

Through its massive financial investment – the 'largest commitment ever by any nation for an international health initiative dedicated to a single disease' (White House Press Office, 2007) – and its strictly regulated approach, PEPFAR has played a major role in shaping an expanding form of development and philanthropic aid structured around global public health initiatives (Oomman, Bernstein, & Rosenzweig, 2007). In the new approach to 'global health', health programmes and development funds have shifted towards the free market, and into the control of donor nations and private industries, thus creating a series of 'vertical', technical interventions framed by, as Brown describes, 'the new international political economy structured around neoliberal approaches to economics, trade, and politics' (Brown, Cueto, & Fee, 2006, p. 68).

In this new approach, as many have argued, forms of surveillance and control have shifted from the state's regulation of individual bodies and populations to globalised forms of sovereignty mediated through biomedical technologies (Biehl, 2004; King, 2002; Nguyen, 2005; Redfield, 2012). Funding agencies, donors and public–private partnerships declare a need to intervene and set strict conditions for their assistance and support, compelling recipients to comply in order to access support. Citizenship is thus reconfigured in biological terms, and distributed through complex relations between donors, states and non-governmental organisations (NGOs).

Through their particular focus on children impacted by one disease, PEPFAR OVC policies and programmes can be seen to represent the apex of this expanding biopolitical imaginary. This discursive terrain can be framed in reference to the work of medical anthropologists who have espoused ideas about health, biological or therapeutic citizenship to understand the increasing medicalisation of individuals' lives and the ways in which they adapt (Biehl, 2004, 2007; Lakoff, 2005; Nguyen, 2005; Petryna, 2002; Robins, 2004; Rose, 2005). Like the radiation exposure in Adriana Petryna's work, the OVC category cannot easily be defined by, nor reduced to, a definitive biomedical dichotomy but is still placed in a biomedically oriented classificatory system framed around a single disease. Because of this ambiguity, individuals (policy-makers, NGO officers and families) negotiate their own uses of the category. For the child affected by HIV/AIDS, however, it is hard to imagine that the market-based modes of biological citizenship described in the work of others could operate. Children, when they are discussed at all in this literature, are seen as something other than a patient-citizen or an advocate. They are painted as the victim, the recipient of support or the surrogate for someone else's claims to biological citizenship. Thus, to complicate the biological citizenship literature, the larger project from which this paper is drawn has attempted to explore the dynamics of citizenship for young people classified as 'OVC' and to explore more seriously other forms of belonging that hold great importance in the lives of these children. This article, however, is not focused on interrogating the effects of these technologies on programme recipients. Instead, the article examines their effects on the 'middle figures', to use Nancy Hunt's term (1999), who are forced to negotiate divergent forms of knowledge; local, national and international politics; and complex everyday encounters in the implementation of public health policies and programmes.

Documenting the 'local' lives of a policy

The research was initially organised around the implementation of the 2006 US PEPFAR guidelines for programmes for 'OVC' in South Africa. The project has taken the entry of the guidelines as a site for examining the effects of policy and programmatic definitions of vulnerable children on governmental techniques, NGO practices and the experiences of children and families in rural South Africa. Drawing from this frame, I structured my project around two guiding questions. The first sought to comprehend how definitions of the OVC category and understandings of child vulnerability move through donor and policy domains and through implementing organisations to service provision in local communities, and then how they penetrate individuals' lives. The second has explored forms of vulnerability and structures of care for children in rural KwaZulu-Natal in order to identify points of divergence between programmatic approaches and paradigms of policy-makers and programme implementers and the experiences of children and families.

Following these guiding questions, the project was framed around two distinct, though overlapping, methodological approaches or phases: a multi-site, institutional ethnography of PEPFAR-funded care programmes in South Africa and an in-depth study of the experiences of 20 young people and families in one area of northern KwaZulu-Natal, chosen based on their reported membership in this category of vulnerability. The research did not simply proceed from one phase to the other, however, but rather moved back and forth between them. To study such processes of power and governance, Michel Foucault suggests, we must not begin at the centre looking for homogeneous domination, but rather look towards power's extremities, its capillaries (Foucault, 1975, p. 30). Thus, while the temporal unfolding of the project necessarily proceeded from policy-makers to children, I attempted to complicate this temporality by moving back and forth between spaces in each phase. In the end, the looping and folding between these 'sites' become in itself a central focus of the research. This paper draws primarily on material from the first of these methodological approaches.

The institutional research drew primarily on techniques of archival research, discourse analysis, participant observation and key informant interviews. First, to understand the formation of categories of vulnerability and eligibility in global health programmes oriented around children affected by HIV, I reviewed US government documents, including transcripts of congressional hearings and PEPFAR programme documents, and tracked media representations of PEPFAR and of OVC programmes over several years. Second, to explore the ways in which PEPFAR policies were translated, adapted and co-opted in South Africa, I conducted several months of institutional ethnographic research between 2006 and 2010 with PEPFAR-funded OVC programmes in South Africa, the country with the highest number of HIV-infected individuals and 'AIDS orphans' in the world (Joint United Nations Programme on HIV/AIDS [UNAIDS], 2011; United Nations Children's Fund [UNICEF], 2010) and the largest recipient of PEPFAR funds (PEPFAR,

2012). I conducted interviews with staff members at all levels of the PEPFAR structure of implementation within South Africa (policy-makers, programme directors and local implementers) and extensive documentary record of e-mail communications, meeting minutes, and inter-organisational memos involved in the development and dissemination of PEPFAR guidelines.

One South African NGO providing services for children affected by HIV/AIDS, whom I call Orphan Care, served as the focal point of this institutional research. I interviewed staff at head offices in Durban and Johannesburg, pored over the organisation's records and informational materials, travelled with area managers to visit project sites in rural KwaZulu-Natal, and spent time with project staff at local programme sites. In all of these settings, I was given free access to talk to staff, attend meetings, sit in on daily activities, and study reports, correspondence, child monitoring forms, and data collected for reporting purposes. Through these diverse sources, I have been able to piece together a detailed account of the organisation's experience with PEPFAR.

When I began the research, Orphan Care was generally considered one of PEPFAR's 'poster child NGOs', as one staff member put it. By the end of 2007, however, the organisation appeared to have fallen entirely out of the favour of PEPFAR programme officers and seemed to be at risk of losing their PEPFAR funding. Staff at the organisation traced this shift to the vocal concerns they had raised about the new PEPFAR guidelines and their active role in the debates that ensued. Thus, the organisation offers an interesting study of the complex effects of policy for organisations charged with implementing programmes in South Africa and of the sometimes fraught relationships between global health policy-makers and programme officers and those who must implement programmes and policies in locality.

Categorising the 'children of AIDS'

Despite the focus on numerical targets, neither the Leadership Act nor the Assistance for OVC Act defined the term 'OVC' or set specific programming requirements for OVC programmes. The 2006 *Orphans and Other Vulnerable Children Programming Guidance* represented the programme's first attempt to formalise its use of the 'OVC' term. The new guidelines explicitly restricted the use of the term in programmes supported by PEPFAR funds, defining an 'OVC' as 'a child, 0–17 years old, who is either orphaned or made more vulnerable *because of* HIV/AIDS' (United States President's Emergency Plan for AIDS Relief, 2006, p. 2). The language of the *Guidance* thus excluded as beneficiaries other children living in high HIV prevalence areas, stating in several places that funds could not be given to any programme 'not directly supporting HIV/AIDS-affected OVCs' or to any child who did not fit the definition (United States President's Emergency Plan for AIDS Relief, 2006, p. 19).

The restrictive focus was in direct contradiction with dominant international opinion and research on the subject at the time. The 2004 *Framework for the Protection, Care and Support of Orphans and Vulnerable Children Living in a World with HIV and AIDS*, a document authored by UNICEF, UNAIDS and the United States Agency for International Development (USAID), stated clearly that 'programmes should not single out children orphaned by HIV/AIDS' as 'targeting specific categories of children can lead to increased stigmatization, discrimination and harm to those children while, at the same, denying support to other children in the community whose needs may be profound' (United Nations Children's Fund, Joint United Nations Commission on HIV/AIDS, and United States Agency for International Development [UNICEF, UNAIDS, & USAID],

2004, p. 28). Further, a large body of quantitative and qualitative evidence published before the release of the guidelines offered contradictory results as to whether this category of children constituted a high-risk population that should be targeted for particular interventions.[2]

Despite its bounded definition of the OVC category, the *Guidance* itself also openly acknowledged the limitations of the definition it used, providing the following clarification:

> The above operational definition identifies those who are potentially eligible for PEPFAR supported services, but does not identify those most in need of services. For programmatic decisions, each community will need to prioritize those children most vulnerable and in need of further care. (United States President's Emergency Plan for AIDS Relief, 2006, p. 4)

The tension between the need for a clearly quantifiable indicator to measure the number of children served with PEPFAR funds and the practicalities of effective programme implementation was clearly of major concern from the early years of PEPFAR. A 2004 USAID report, for example, described how the terms 'orphan' and 'vulnerable children' could take on different meanings when developed for the purpose of gathering and presenting quantitative data (an 'operational' definition) or for the purpose of designing and implementing policies and programmes (a 'programmatic' definition). It was essential, the report suggested, establishing a 'firewall' between these two kinds of definitions:

> Problems occur in the field when definitions established for quantitative purposes are picked up and used for program targeting or eligibility criteria in policy and program implementation. The quantitative process must have clear boundaries and allow for absolute distinctions. In contrast, developing and implementing policies have to take into account local variations in what factors cause or constitute vulnerability. In the latter case, no one prescriptive notion will suffice for every occasion. (Williamson, Cox, & Johnston, 2004, p. 1)

The ambiguity introduced by the distinction between operational definitions and the necessities of programmatic decision-making became a central component in the debates and disagreements the guidelines inspired as they were disseminated to local organisations in South Africa. Further, the tension between these concepts underscores exactly the epistemological challenge the paper attempts to elucidate. By establishing a 'firewall' between these two fundamentally different kinds of definitions but expecting individuals in the field to be able to negotiate both of them in their everyday experiences, policymakers forced NGO staff to find ways of reconciling these seemingly irreconcilable imperatives.

Resistance and accommodation: the implementation of PEPFAR OVC policy in South Africa

As I walked off the plane in Durban, South Africa in 2006 and entered the international arrivals terminal, I was greeted by an enormous lighted sign advertising the services of a South African company specialising in the creation of data management systems for HIV/ AIDS programmes. The sign highlighted in bold, red letters that the company's software was designed to generate reports specifically tailored to PEPFAR reporting requirements. The presence of this lighted billboard was an immediate and powerful signal of the expanding importance of HIV/AIDS programmes, international donors and the 'audit cultures' (Strathern, 2000) they bring with them in this landscape. Since the early 2000s, when I began to conduct research on HIV/AIDS in South Africa, the humanitarian concern, media attention and donor funding the epidemic generated had increased by several orders of magnitude. As a result of this expanding concern, from the early 2000s, many existing South African organisations began to shift their programming to focus on HIV/AIDS and numerous new organisations were formed, particularly after the arrival of funds from PEPFAR in 2004. From a list of a few hundred organisations when it was founded in 2003, by 2012, the Centre for HIV/AIDS Networking's directory of HIV/AIDS organisations in South Africa listed more than 12,000 organisations that provided HIV-related health and social welfare services.

Orphan Care was one of these vast numbers of new organisations founded in the early 2000s to address the effects of the rapidly expanding epidemic. The goal of Orphan Care was to 'franchise', as the organisation's advertising materials termed it, a community-based model of care for orphans that could be implemented sustainably throughout the country. Since it began offering services to children in early 2003, the organisation had garnered increasing support and had started to expand, growing from 12 centres in 2003 to more than 100 sites across KwaZulu-Natal and Gauteng by 2006. Staff members at other organisations labelled Orphan Care 'PEPFAR's darling' because its business-based model of programming was highly respected by PEPFAR programme officers. By the time the guidelines were rolled out, Orphan Care was one of the largest recipients of PEPFAR OVC funding and had a strong track record of success.

Shortly after the release of the *Guidance* in South Africa, however, Orphan Care staff were informed that their funding for certain services would be cut because they could not identify which children in the services fit within the new PEPFAR definition. Despite the necessary reallocations and programmatic changes, it was repeatedly emphasised that Orphan Care's reported target numbers could not 'under any circumstances' go down. Senior Orphan Care staff resisted these new requirements, insisting that it was both unethical and unfeasible to track HIV status of children or parents and that their inclusive approach was appropriate in a context where the overwhelming majority of children were affected by HIV/AIDS.

Orphan Care staff members were not alone in their objections to the new guidelines. In interviews conducted in December and January 2006, NGO officers at several of the major PEPFAR-funded organisations in South Africa expressed profound frustration about the problematic nature of the OVC definition as well as other restrictions on services, arguing that the guidelines were misguided, potentially stigmatising and impossible to implement in many communities. Further, as several individuals high-lighted, the guidelines were in direct contradiction with South African government policy, which emphasised that the definition of orphanhood and vulnerability should make 'no reference to the causes of orphanhood' (South African Government, 2005, p. 4), making the situation even more difficult for South African organisations.

For Orphan Care, their insistence that their existing eligibility criteria and service models were effective, and that they were not willing to change them in the face of PEPFAR demands, became a constant source of tension in discussions with PEPFAR programme officers. Rather than accepting what they saw as an unethical and impossible policy, Orphan Care staff began to work with their counterparts at 11 other major PEPFAR-funded organisations affected by the *Guidance* to put together a formal complaint and advocate for a change in the *Guidance* itself.

Outside of this process, prominent Orphan Care board members decided to pursue their concerns regarding the *Guidance* through political and diplomatic avenues, expressing their frustrations to colleagues in high-level positions in government and industry. Further, at the international level, Orphan Care joined a larger collective effort to develop a report advocating for change in the policy. In the report, organisations highlighted a series of concerns regarding the restricted OVC definition, concluding, 'We see the restriction of the term OVC as a dangerous step in the wrong direction, which seemingly overwrites years of research illustrating that NGOs should not limit themselves to serving only those children affected by HIV/AIDS.' In addition to specific concerns about the content of the *Guidance*, the report also raised a general issue with the frequent changes in OVC indicators and guidelines and the significant challenges this had created for organisations.

In response to the pressure being put on them, in early 2007, USAID staff called all of the organisations receiving PEPFAR OVC funds to a meeting to clarify their expectations regarding the new *Guidance*. In the meeting, according to the official minutes, programme officers stated explicitly that PEPFAR would not be requiring verification of the HIV status of individual children or parents to justify 'the provision of OVC support or the selection of sites', but that PEPFAR did expect that organisations could confirm the eligibility of supported OVC 'through viable monitoring and evaluation systems and processes' and that these 'should provide an adequate audit trail that can sufficiently answer the question of "why" any particular OVC was enrolled into the program' (United States Agency for International Development, 2007). While the explanation was intended to clarify matters, it amplified the existing ambiguity and tension between flexible selection criteria and strict audit requirements.

Shortly thereafter, at a meeting held in Washington, DC to discuss concerns regarding the *Guidance*, the Senior Technical Officer for OVC Programs acknowledged the challenges presented by implementing the new OVC definition in explicit terms. 'We do *not* want to have a situation that requires people to exclude orphans that are not vulnerable because of AIDS', he stated strongly, 'but we don't want to lose our focus on HIV/AIDS. This requirement is a part of the legislation that governs PEPFAR' (Global Action for Children, 2007, p. 10). To address this tension, he suggested, 'We need to rely on common sense and find a balance that provides guidance without being so restrictive that we undermine or constrain creative programming in the field' (Global Action for Children, 2007, p. 3). Implementing organisations need not show proof but 'only a possibility' that children are directly affected by HIV/AIDS, such as 'a parent who is chronically ill'. Organisations should 'be flexible' and use their 'common sense', he reiterated several times, in order to do the best they could in applying the *Guidance*.

While they had not managed to incite any real change in the OVC *Guidance*, Orphan Care and other PEPFAR-funded organisations had succeeded, it seemed, in swaying how the *Guidance* would affect their programmes. They had largely avoided having to implement major programmatic changes and had maintained their PEPFAR funding. However, the institutional effects of the contestations over the *Guidance* were more difficult to gauge. As these conversations came to an end, the new CEO of Orphan Care was called to another meeting with PEPFAR programme officers, where she was told in no uncertain terms that there was a need to move on from the debates about the *Guidance* now that it had become clear that organisations were largely going to be able to adapt the *Guidance* to suit their own programme directives. 'They would like to see us being more positive', she reported to staff, 'about a situation that was a directive out of Washington'. There was a possibility of new funds in the near future, she was told, and Orphan Care would be recommended. However, she reported, 'it was noted that [Orphan Care] was a very vocal antagonist about American funding and it was hoped that [Orphan Care] would understand that an aggressive public approach would give us negative press'

(Internal communication, 2007). Speaking to senior staff after the meeting, she explained what she had taken away from the conversation:

> Personally, I think we will get more money and politically I think we need to deliver as best as we can under their new guidelines to ensure this … If we raise money in the future that can replace PEPFAR then we would rethink our approach but at present we need them and so we walk cautiously. (Internal communication, 2007)

Because of the inherent ambiguity of the category and the clearly articulated 'flexibility' given to programmes in terms of implementation, organisations had a great deal of space in the end to adapt the provisions of PEPFAR policy to suit their needs. However, because they were dependent on donors, organisations like Orphan Care were still forced to 'walk cautiously' to satisfy the ambiguous and shifting expectations of PEPFAR and to try to implement the forms of monitoring and reporting they required. In the next section, I take this account further to examine how the OVC definition and the bureaucratic requirements of PEPFAR programming were interpreted by mid-level managers responsible for programme oversight and reporting.

Documenting the child and implementing 'common sense'

In 2007 and 2008, in the midst of the debates regarding the OVC *Guidance*, I spent time working with the coordinator of one of Orphan Care's areas of service on the north coast of KwaZulu-Natal. Prudence was in charge of managing the operations of a number of local care sites spread across northern KwaZulu-Natal. Travelling each day between far-flung projects, she visited local programme offices to check on the status of operations, help resolve issues and provide advice. The central element of her work seemed to be the supervision and oversight of the data collection process. On numerous occasions, I sat with her in cramped project offices as she went about the task of checking the forms and attendance registers filled out by local staff to confirm that they were conducting their programmes appropriately and to verify the numbers being reported to her. 'We must be in a position to explain every number', Prudence told me on several occasions.

In early 2007, in response to a concern expressed by senior staff about eligibility of children in programmes, Prudence began to review every child registration form collected by staff at project sites. 'We've got to be very careful', Prudence asserted, 'because once the donors hear that [there is a concern regarding whether children are eligible], they can come down to the sites and check the forms. So if I am not making sure, if the manager is not making sure, then we are in for it!' Reviewing each line of the form, she pressed local staff to justify the eligibility of each child they were enrolling, asking for more details about illness status, employment, resident relatives, social grants and other forms of support. For more than half of the registration forms she reviewed, Prudence returned the form to the site manager, telling them that they should not enrol the child until they had more information. Interestingly, while the concern had been motivated by fears about the consequences of not following the PEPFAR OVC definition, the decisions being made by Prudence and her staff in reviewing the enrolment forms were not based strictly on the definition of OVC formalised by the PEPFAR *Guidance*. Instead, Prudence had clearly adapted her own definition of what orphanhood and vulnerability meant in her community. When I asked her to define the term, she explained:

An OVC is a child between the ages of 0 and 18. It's the child that doesn't have both parents or one parent. But the condition is that child must be vulnerable, that the child is not having a primary caregiver. But there are also children who don't have both parents who are not vulnerable. Like if my sister and her husband died and I am available to look after their children, they aren't vulnerable as long as I am playing the role of being a parent and doing everything that the parents would have done … But if the primary caregiver has no money— they don't have money to go to school, for food—then the child is vulnerable. He or she gets in.

In a later conversation, I asked Prudence if she had been told about the new PEPFAR guidelines and the focus on children directly affected by HIV. 'Yes, I've heard all about it', she responded, 'but it really is not easy to identify if a person has died of AIDS, and that would stigmatise the child'.

Prudence's definition clearly referenced important notions of kinship and family amongst isiZulu-speaking individuals in the region, where children are generally understood to belong not only to a nuclear family but to a broader extended kin structure, in which care for children is often more distributed.[3] In this context, to call a child an *intandane*, the term most frequently employed to describe an orphan, carries with it a sense of neglect, of lack of care, not simply of loss of a biological parent. As one of the volunteers working for Orphan Care explained to me, a child who had lost their mother and father would no longer be referred to as an *intandane* if a family member took them in, as was most often the case after parental death. 'This name no longer works well', she explained, 'if she is looked after because now she would be getting full support'.

In a small survey, I conducted in 2007 of a random sample of 200 child registration forms from 10 randomly selected Orphan Care programme sites, only one form referenced HIV/AIDS as a cause of parental death or child vulnerability, while 24 referenced deaths due to 'natural causes'. Further, 142 of the 200 registration forms left the location or status of one or both parents (primarily fathers) blank or listed the parental status as 'unknown'. In reality, these forms rarely contained sufficient infor-mation to be able to assess whether children fit within the PEPFAR OVC definition – or even enough information to categorise the children within the kinds of alternate definitions put forward by Prudence and other programme staff. While these forms were religiously stored, counted and photocopied and their information entered in Orphan Care's databases, many of the forms had more questions left blank than completed. In practice, decisions about which children to enrol drew on much more personal, emotional registers, a point I take up in detail elsewhere.

While registration forms may have said little about whether each child was 'an OVC', government identification numbers for the children and their caregivers were almost always included, and many care centres required copies of children's birth certificates and death certificates for their parents. In addition, programme staff were expected to take attendance each day at care sites to document children's participation in different activities and to complete forms for each home visit or other service offered. Despite the large numbers of forms collected by staff to record services received by enrolled children and document their on-going needs and submitted each month to Orphan Care, copies of these forms were generally not included in children's records at the programme sites, making it impossible for staff and volunteers to refer back to them to follow-up on concerns and monitor young people's progress and needs over time. Rather the aim of these extensive record-keeping systems was clearly to document the number of services provided, and to create the requisite paper-based 'audit trail' to back up service counts reported to PEPFAR each month. Further, because enrolment figures were used to make budget allocations, it was very important to centres to report as many children as possible.

To track and collect these figures, Orphan Care area coordinators like Prudence called together the local project managers once each month to collect data for the monthly reports required by PEPFAR. Early in the morning, local programme managers, nearly all women, would converge on a hotel in the largest town of the region, each bearing carefully sorted stacks of forms to be reviewed, including attendance registers for daycare, aftercare and nutrition programmes; committee staff, and volunteer meeting minutes; clinic referral forms and forms documenting bereavement counselling; registration and deregistration forms; and tally sheets of children served for the month. At each meeting, programme staff carefully distilled the many forms and tick marks on daily attendance registers into overall service counts in a spreadsheet on the area coordinator's laptop. As one staff member entered the data, another would double-check the counts to ensure that the numbers were accurate. While the numbers were entered for one project, the other project managers sat sorting and resorting their stacks of forms into plastic sleeves and folders and checking the counts on their attendance forms. Even if a child was listed as having received a service only once during the month (e.g. attended after-school care one out of 31 days), the child would be counted as a full recipient of PEPFAR services. Thus, service counts were based on the number of children visited, not on the depth or quality of engagements. Staff members at Orphan Care and other PEPFAR-funded organisations frequently expressed concern that the over-focus on counting and on formal bureaucratic procedures undermined the quality of services being offered. 'It doesn't matter how well you reach 64 children', one programme officer stated bluntly, 'if you didn't reach your target of 600'.

At most monthly meetings, there was also one or more new forms distributed to be completed for the next month's meeting, accompanied by a long explanation as to how they were to be used. The constant stream of forms and changes in reporting systems inspired frequent complaints from project managers. Over the years since the start of PEPFAR funding, organisations had been required to change the way they reported on services to children several times. Reporting demands had shifted from raw counts of children served to a 'service-based model', first based on a rubric of six different kinds of services, then eight, and then expanded to 11 categories. Each of these changes required the development of costly new systems of monitoring and reporting. In 2007, the director of one of the largest international children's organisations operating in South Africa told me that they were spending nearly half of their PEPFAR funding on database development and monitoring and evaluation. A staff member at another organisation described the situation thus: 'The level of detail that we have to report on is so great that it can take 5 months of intensive work to prepare and submit a report on PEPFAR expenditure and impact'.

By the end of 2008, though the PEPFAR *Guidance* still stood as the official policy document governing practices of PEPFAR-funded OVC organisations, most organisations I worked with reported that they were 'getting used to the *Guidance*'. Most had found ways to work around its strictures, to be 'flexible', as they had been advised, but there had been no official change in the language of the guidelines. 'There's been all of this talk of "being reasonable"', one staff member complained, 'and they are not going to penalise you for being reasonable, but they're also not going to change the policy to make it reasonable'.

In this context, organisations continued to struggle with the tension between the flexibility advocated by PEPFAR officials and the oftentimes more literal interpretations of PEPFAR 'prime partners', who were tasked with disbursing and overseeing funds, and external auditors, who could arrive without warning to review programme documentation, looking for reporting errors and omissions. These audits inspired such levels of fear, a former PEPFAR auditor told me, that it was not uncommon for NGO staff to break into tears during the audit process. PEPFAR reporting requirements had created a management style governed through fear, staff members at several organisations told me – fear that the numbers were not right, that indicators were wrong, that funding would be lost. 'The stress and fear is created at the top and moves all the way down', an Orphan Care staff member explained, 'and the competition with the organisation next to you makes sure you keep it going'.

A central element of the tension inherent in these processes derived from a basic fact about the structure of PEPFAR programmes in South Africa and elsewhere. The companies charged with monitoring and evaluation were generally large, international corporations with strong ties to the US government, while programmes were implemented by local organisations with predominantly local staff. One of the major critiques of PEPFAR and other US bilateral programmes has been the large percentage of funds spent on overhead, travel, equipment, and salary and benefit packages for expatriate staff tasked with evaluation activities (see, for example, Epstein, 2005; Redfield, 2012). As a result, there were often powerful barriers of socio-economic status, education, experience, and race between local programme staff who implemented programmes on the ground and those charged with the oversight of many PEPFAR-funded projects, a point that was articulated in quite powerful terms by the director of Orphan Care:

> As with all USG-funded initiatives, the expenditure of the funding is reported against a set of indicators that are rational, measurable and generally make sense, especially to those that set the indicators. The recipients of funding often find the indicators rather confusing, as they are the poor, the mostly illiterate, the vulnerable, the marginalised and the desperate people of the developing world.

In reality, many local organisations in South Africa relied quite heavily on voluntary labour for the implementation of programmes. At one Orphan Care local site where I spent a good deal of time in 2009 and 2010, PEPFAR reporting forms were completed almost entirely by local volunteers. In many senses, the local volunteers I came to know experienced similar challenges to those whom they 'served.' Often without any other source of income, volunteers relied on small contributions from individual donors and the occasional 'transport money' offered by Orphan Care to attend trainings to get by. In this context, despite the distancing practices of form filling, service provision was shaped by complex interpersonal relationships defined by the complexities of dependence and historical inequalities, a concern I take up more fully elsewhere.

The production of PEPFAR 'success'

While PEPFAR programme officers emphasised the importance of tracking systems for children to ensure quality service provision, the end point of these complex networks of data collection and reporting was in fact the production of raw counts of individuals given assistance for reports to the US Congress. To reach global targets and collapse complex data into digestible statistics for public dissemination, PEPFAR officials were compelled to implement generic guidelines and reporting requirements that allowed for the comparison of standardised data across diverse countries. Despite the ambiguities of the

OVC category and the clearly divergent understandings of eligibility criteria, numbers continued to be counted and services summed in quarterly reports for PEPFAR. The questions raised about which children were to be included and what services they received faded as reports were collected, collated and entered into national data banks. As Andrew Lakoff suggests in his study of pharmaceutical systems in Latin America, the need for 'liquidity' or 'universality' often trumps individual complexities and needs and requires the standardisation of knowledge and forms of practice across institutions, cities and countries (Lakoff, 2005).

Because of concerns regarding audits and accountability, however, numbers of children reported as enrolled in PEPFAR-funded OVC programmes dropped drastically in the first reporting periods after the dissemination of the *Guidance*. The problem of low numbers was a concern from the level of the local service providers, whose annual funding was directly related to the number of children they could report, to that of the Office of the Global AIDS Coordinator, which was responsible for ensuring that PEPFAR programmes were making satisfactory progress towards global prevention, treatment and care targets set by the US Congress. The resultant push for numbers created even greater pressure and competition within and between organisations for children to count.

In addition to the pressure on partner organisations to produce higher service counts, the need for high service numbers was also addressed at the aggregate level through changes in counting and reporting practices. Along with its revised OVC definition and restrictions on services, the OVC *Guidance* had also shifted how organisations were intended to measure the number of OVC served through their programmes. Previously, to count a child as 'directly served', an organisation had to document that they had provided the child with at least three services from a list of 'essential' categories of support. Under the new rules, the category of children 'directly served' was divided into two subcategories: (1) 'primary direct', defined as children receiving three or more services and (2) 'supplementary direct', children who received only one or two services (United States President's Emergency Plan for AIDS Relief, 2006). When the numbers were reported to Congress in the 2007 annual report, however, the subcategories 'primary direct' and 'supplementary direct' were added together and reported as a total number of children 'served' through PEPFAR programmes. Thus, through the change in counting practices, which effectively reduced the depth of support programmes had to provide to children, PEPFAR programmes were not only able to meet their 2007 targets but were able to report significant increases in the number of 'OVC' served, despite the important challenges faced on the ground.

By 2008, numbers of children served, summed and summed again over the preceding four years, resulted in the impressive statistic of 2.7 million children 'supported' by US government funds, as stated in PEPFAR's annual report to Congress (United States President's Emergency Plan for AIDS Relief, 2008b). The number was well above the target of two million OVC set by President Bush and the US Congress for PEPFAR's five-year plan. According to the PEPFAR annual report, all of the numerical targets – treat two million HIV-positive individuals, prevent seven million infections and provide care for 10 million individuals affected by AIDS, including two million OVC – had been met and surpassed.

These outcome statistics were celebrated as a sign of PEPFAR's significance and success. As Mark Dybul wrote in a piece reflecting on the success of PEPFAR's programmes, 'Over time, people came together, and as a result, lives were literally saved... PEPFAR met its ambitious goals early and on budget' (Dybul, 2009, p. 2). With other impact numbers for treatment, prevention and care, the figure of 2.7 million 'OVCs served' became an important tool for policy-makers and advocates and was cited as a justification for increased funding for PEPFAR. When the PEPFAR legislation was reauthorised in 2008 for another five years with a budget of $50 billion, the final legislation included a specific new target for OVC programming the next 5 years of PEPFAR funding: five million OVCs served (Tom Lantos and Henry J. Hyde United States Global Leadership Against HIV/AIDS, Tuberculosis, and Malaria Reauthorization Act, 2008).

'From emergency to sustainability': The new era of PEPFAR programming

The entry of PEPFAR II (as the second five years of PEPFAR programming has been called) in 2009 coincided with a political transition in the USA and with major shifts in the global economic climate. After flattening in 2009, donor government funding for HIV/AIDS fell by 10% between 2009 and 2010, the first decline in more than a decade (Kates, Wexler, Lief, Avila, & Gobet, 2011). Similarly, growth in global health funding overall fell to 4% in 2010, and in 2011 and 2012 appeared to have stopped completely (Garrett, 2012). In this new climate of fiscal austerity, a series of reforms were implemented with the aim of shifting PEPFAR programming and other initiatives away from 'emergency' response and towards a more 'sustainable' model framed around collaboration with recipient governments and evidence-based programming.

A central element of the new PEPFAR approach was a renewed focus on monitoring and evaluation and on research, structured by a new framework of 'implementation science' (United States President's Emergency Plan for AIDS Relief, 2009; Padian et al., 2011a). In an article intended to explain and advocate for the new approach, PEPFAR leadership conceded that monitoring and evaluation activities in the first 'emergency' phase of PEPFAR had functioned solely to 'monitor progress and report to Congress', rather than to improve quality of services (Padian et al., 2011b, p. 200). In a later article, OGAC programme officers openly acknowledged the problems with these initial emphases: 'High targets provided some motivation to offer the most affordable and feasible services rather than the most needed', to reach for the 'low-hanging fruit' (Nyberg et al., 2012, p. S129). Because of this overemphasis on numerical targets, an external review of PEPFAR-funded programmes concluded that the majority of PEPFAR-funded interventions seemed to have had no measurable effect on the young people they were intended to serve (Bryant et al., 2012, p. 1513). To address these concerns, emphasis began to shift from a focus on efficient, inexpensive forms of service provision to an interest in interventions that could be shown to have *measurable* impacts. As PEPFAR leadership argued, 'programs must demonstrate value and impact to be prioritized within complex and resource-constrained environments. In this context, there is a greater demand to causally attribute outcomes to programs' (Padian et al., 2011a, p. 199). To realise these objectives, though the next phase of PEPFAR was framed around a new era of country ownership and a discourse of development, programmes could in fact be subject to more techniques of measurement.

Such shifts in programmatic imperatives could be seen to be part of a broader bureaucratic process of circumscription, framed around appeals to science, truth and bureaucratic efficiency. In a recent analysis of the shifting discourses of global HIV/AIDS funding over the last decade, Alan Ingram describes what he sees as a shift from a 'rationality of salvation (premised upon exception from the neoliberal norm of scarcity)', which defined the early years of global HIV/AIDS intervention, to 'one of administration (premised upon the subsumption of HIV/AIDS back within a discourse of scarcity)'. In these circumstances, he suggests, 'the need for greater visibility, calculability and attributability of all aspects of the response is intensified by a discourse of scarcity (often rendered as "sustainability")' (Ingram, 2013, p. 3).

In August 2012, Secretary Hillary Clinton announced that South Africa was to become the first country to 'nationalise' its PEPFAR programme, as funds would be scaled back and 'responsibility' handed over to the South African government (Govender, 2012). One of the first programmes to lose funding under the new, scaled-back PEPFAR mandate was Orphan Care, which had continued to struggle to keep up with the changing requirements of PEPFAR reporting and the need to demonstrate programme impact. In early September 2012, Orphan Care officially announced that they would be closing down 67 of their 90 centres across the country as a result of their loss of PEPFAR funding (Nkosi, 2012). These closures represented, according to an Orphan Care staff member, 'nearly 11,000 AIDS orphans left out in the cold and over 300 jobs retrenched' (Nkosi, 2012). 'Though [Orphan Care] has been viewed as a model partner of PEPFAR', the organisation's CEO was quoted as stating in a news article, 'the current service offering does not fit the eligibility criteria of this new Partnership Framework' (Nkosi, 2012).

Conclusion

The article has described the ways in which the category of the 'OVC' was circumscribed through particular political and bureaucratic procedures in the USA and in South Africa, and how this bureaucratisation of the category was translated into an overwhelming imperative to produce counts of children served and 'lives saved'. In the emphasis on a restricted definition of the ambiguous category of the OVC, the *Guidance* aimed to bound notions of risk, create certainty and limit the scope of intervention by identifying a circumscribed, apolitical group of 'vulnerable' young people for whom bounded services could be offered and 'results' measured. However, in the context of programme implementation in locality, it quickly became evident that the circumscribed definition was of little use, particularly in the context of programmes designed to provide 'care' for children, and programme officers began to encourage a certain amount of negotiation and adaptation to suit the needs of service providers.

This flexibility was productive in some senses, allowing programme officers and policy-makers to satisfy political agendas and show programme 'success', while still enabling negotiations and adaptations to suit the needs of programme implementers. In the background, however, the production of this coherent narrative of programme 'success' required a great deal of material, intellectual and emotional labour on the part of programme staff and diluted the effectiveness of interventions as resources were expended on negotiating the requirements of an unimplementable policy and program-ming decisions were made in order to facilitate a numerical imperative. In this context, measures of programme 'success' did not necessarily stand for effective programming but, rather, signalled the ability of actors to negotiate deeply contradictory mandates and fraught relationships across multiple levels of authority.

More broadly, by channelling its resources through 'civil society', setting strict conditions for its assistance and support, deploying new biomedical technologies, and requiring complex forms of accounting, PEPFAR has reconfigured forms of governance in the areas where it has intervened beyond the reach or impact of actual funding dollars. As the prominent sign in the Durban airport advertising data management services suggested, the bureaucratic procedures required by PEPFAR and other donors in the HIV/ AIDS 'industry' have reshaped the practices of powerful organisations across South Africa, who have implemented new technologies of counting and accounting in order to satisfy PEPFAR requirements, and of the South African National Government, which has begun to take over these programmes and practices in the new era of PEPFAR and HIV/AIDS programming in South Africa.

This phenomenon is not isolated to PEPFAR in South Africa, but rather represents a broader trend in global health and development programmes in which a renewed concern with cost, impact and efficiency is driving global health and development policy and practice more generally towards an ever-greater focus on counting and accounting, on metrics and quantitative forms of evidence, and on the categorisation and circumscription of forms of suffering and of everyday life. Faced with this expanding emphasis on evidence and accountability, policy-makers and programme officers intending to make a difference in the lives of young people and families must continue to struggle to define and delimit a target population for their interventions. Through these processes, epistemological tensions are produced that create powerful uncertainties in the everyday practice of public health. There is a need for greater attention to the long-term effects of such uncertainties on the experiences of both the individuals tasked with delivering services and their intended beneficiaries.

Acknowledgements

Having studied the impacts of HIV in South Africa for more than a decade, the list of individuals who have helped to shape this project is long and diverse. For the material contained within this article, thanks must go to the many staff members at the organisation I dub Orphan Care and other key interlocutors in the OVC field in South Africa, who gave their time and trust to share their experiences with me. The article is based primarily on research conducted for my doctoral dissertation at Johns Hopkins University. Lori Leonard, Jane Guyer and Randy Packard all served as incredibly generous mentors throughout the process, and their insights have shaped my work in powerful ways. In addition, many friends and teachers in the Departments of Anthropology and Health, Behavior, and Society have offered support and feedback at various stages in the process, most notably Thomas Cousins, who offered important feedback on the paper as it developed. Early versions of this paper were presented at the Isaac Schapera Conference and at the African Studies Seminar at Johns Hopkins, where I received generous feedback. Preliminary and follow-up research for this project was supported by the following awards: the US Department of Education Fulbright-Hays Doctoral Dissertation Research Abroad Award (2008), the Social Science Research Council International Dissertation Research Fellowship (2008–2009) and the US National Institutes of Health Ruth L. Kirschstein National Research Service Award (2009–2012, award number 1F31MH084714-01), as well as several internal awards from Johns Hopkins University (including the Bloomberg School of Public Health Doctoral Distinguished Research Award, the Institute for Global Studies Summer Research Fellowship and the Centre for Africana Studies Summer Research Fellowship). The writing of the article was completed with support from a South African National Research Foundation Innovation Postdoctoral Fellowship in the Department of Sociology and Social Anthropology at Stellenbosch University.

Notes

1. 'Despite charges of simplistic militarism', *Washington Post* columnist Mike Gerson wrote in 2008, 'the Bush Doctrine actually includes three elements: the pre-emption of emerging threats, the encouragement of responsible self-government, and the promotion of development and health as alternatives to despair and bitterness' (Gerson, 2008). 'Government cannot solve every problem', President Bush explained in a 2002 speech, 'but it can encourage people and communities to help themselves and to help one another. It is compassionate to actively help our fellow citizens in need. It is conservative to insist on responsibility and on results' (Bush, 2002). The same principles of compassion and conservatism applied, he stated, when the US offered assistance to developing nations.
2. Studies had not been able to clearly show whether orphans in fact suffered higher rates of morbidity and mortality than non-orphaned children living in the same communities. Similarly,

studies published before the release of the *Guidance* that attempted to assess the effects of orphanhood on factors such as relative socio-economic situation or educational outcomes (e.g. Ainsworth & Filmer, 2002; Case, 2004; Foster & Williamson, 2000; Monasch, 2007) had not shown conclusive results. The most conclusive evidence of increased vulnerability of orphaned children could be drawn from psychological studies, in which orphans have been shown to have higher levels of psychosocial distress than non-orphans (Atwine, Cantor-Graae, & Bajunirwe, 2005; Cluver & Gardner, 2007; Cluver, Gardner, & Operario, 2007). Similarly, much work in the social sciences has questioned the assumptions made about the special vulnerability of orphans of AIDS and those made vulnerable because of the illness of their parents and has identified a vast overlap between the difficult experiences of orphans and the large numbers of other poor children in communities affected by HIV (e.g. Bray, 2004; Henderson, 2006; Meintjes & Bray, 2005; Meintjes & Giese, 2006).

3. This is admittedly a reductive description of a complex field of experience and understanding. I explore the dynamics of kinship and care amongst isiZulu-speaking individuals in post-apartheid South Africa in much more depth elsewhere.

References

Ainsworth, M., & Filmer, D. (2002). *Poverty, AIDS, and children's schooling: A targeting dilemma.* Policy Research Working Paper 2885. Washington, DC: World Bank.

Atwine, B., Cantor-Graae, E., & Bajunirwe, F. (2005). Psychological distress among AIDS orphans in rural Uganda. *Social Science & Medicine, 61*, 555–564.

Biehl, J. (2004). The activist state: Global pharmaceuticals, AIDS, and citizenship in Brazil. *Social Text, 22*(3), 105–132.

Biehl, J. (2007). *Will to live: AIDS therapies and the politics of survival.* Princeton, NJ: Princeton University Press.

Bray, R. (2004). 'AIDS orphans' and the future: A second look at our predictions. *AIDS Bulletin, 13*(2): 124–125.

Brown, T., Cueto, M., & Fee, E. (2006). The World Health Organization and the transition from 'international' to 'global' public health. *American Journal of Public Health, 96*(1), 62–72.

Bryant, M., Beard, J., Sabin, L., Brooks, M. I., Scott, N., Larson, B. A., ... Simon, J. (2012). PEPFAR's support for orphans and vulnerable children: Some beneficial effects, but too little data, and programs spread thin. *Health Affairs, 31*, 1508–1518.

Bush, G. (2002). *President promotes compassionate conservatism.* Retrieved from http://georgewbush-whitehouse.archives.gov/news/releases/2002/04/print/20020430-5.html

Bush, G. W. (2003, 28 January). *Address before a joint session of the congress on the state of the union.* Washington, DC.

Case, A. (2004). Orphans in Africa: Parental death, poverty and school enrollment. *Demography, 41*, 483–508.

Cluver, L., & Gardner, F. (2007). The mental health of children orphaned by AIDS: A review of international and southern African research. *Journal of Child and Adolescent Mental Health, 19*(1), 1–17.

Cluver, L., Gardner, F., & Operario, D. (2007). Psychological distress amongst AIDS-orphaned children in urban South Africa. *Journal of Child Psychology and Psychiatry, 48*, 755–763.

Dybul, M. (2009, September). How to save lives by breaking all the rules. *Foreign Policy.* Retrieved from http://www.foreignpolicy.com/articles/2009/09/22/to_fight_poverty_fight_bureaucracy#sthash.ppgMNr5Z.dpbs

Editorial Staff. (2008, June 28). Coburn of Africa. *The Wall Street Journal.* Retrieved from http://online.wsj.com/article/SB121460665479612081.html?mod=googlenews_wsj

Epstein, H. (2005, November 3). The lost children of AIDS. *The New York review of books.* Retrieved from http://www.nybooks.com/articles/archives/2005/nov/03/the-lost-children-of-aids/

Foster, G., & Williamson, J. (2000). A review of the current literature on the impact of HIV/AIDS on children in sub-Saharan Africa. *AIDS, 14* (Supplement 3), S275–S284.

Foucault, M. (1975). *"Society must be defended": Lectures at the Collège de France, 1975–1976.* (D. Macey, Trans.). New York: Picador.

Garrett, L. (2012, 6 March). Money or die. *Foreign Affairs.* Retrieved from http://www.foreignaffairs.com/articles/137312/laurie-garrett/money-or-die

Gerson, M. (2008, 30 July). An AIDS victory up close. *Washington Post*, p. A15.

Global Action for Children. (2007, 24 May). *Orphans and vulnerable children (OVC) USG guidance and policy meeting notes*. Washington, DC.

Govender, P. (2012, 7 August). US hands more control to South Africa in its AIDS fight. *Reuters*. Retrieved from http://www.reuters.com/article/2012/08/07/us-clinton-safrica-aids-idUSBRE8760ZU20120807

Henderson, P. C. (2006). South African AIDS orphans: Examining assumptions around vulnerability from the perspective of rural youth and children. *Childhood, 13*, 303–327.

House Committee on Foreign Affairs. (2007). *PEPFAR reauthorization: From emergency to sustainability*. Washington, DC: US Government Printing Office.

Hunt, N. R. (1999). *A colonial lexicon: Of birth ritual, medicalization, and mobility in the Congo*. Durham: Duke University Press.

Ingram, A. (2013). After the exception: HIV/AIDS beyond salvation and scarcity. *Antipode, 45*, 436–454.

Joint United Nations Commission on HIV/AIDS. (UNAIDS). (2011). *How to get to zero: Faster, Smarter, Better*. Geneva: Joint United Nations Commission on HIV/AIDS.

Kates, J., Wexler, A., Lief, E., Avila, C., & Gobet, B. (2011). *Financing the response to AIDS in low- and middle- income countries: International assistance from donor governments in 2010*. Washington, DC: Kaiser Family Foundation and Joint United Nations Program on HIV/AIDS.

King, N. B. (2002). Security, disease, commerce: Ideologies of postcolonial global health. *Social Studies of Science, 32*, 763–789.

Lakoff, A. (2005). *Pharmaceutical reason: Knowledge and value in global psychiatry*. Cambridge: Cambridge University Press.

Meintjes, H., & Bray, R. (2005). 'But where are our moral heroes?' An analysis of South African press reporting on children affected by HIV/AIDS. *African Journal of AIDS Research, 4*(3), 147–159.

Meintjes, H., & Giese, S. (2006). Spinning the epidemic: The making of mythologies of orphanhood in the context of AIDS. *Childhood, 13*, 407–430.

Monasch, R. (2007). National response to orphans and other vulnerable children in sub-Saharan Africa: The OVC policy and planning effort index, 2004. *Vulnerable Children and Youth Studies, 2*(1), 40–59.

Nguyen, V-K. (2005). Antiretroviral globalism, biopolitics, and therapeutic citizenship. In A. Ong & S. Collier (Eds.), *Global assemblages: Technology, politics, and ethics as anthropological problems* (pp. 124–144). Malden, MA: Blackwell Publishing.

Nkosi, N. (2012, 3 September). [Orphan Care] forced to cut back support for orphans. *Sowetan*. Retrieved from http://www.sowetanlive.co.za/news/2012/09/03/noah-forced-to-cut-back-support-for-orphans

Nyberg, B. J., Yates, D. D., Lovich, R., Coulibaly-Traore, D., Sherr, L., Thurman, T. R., ... Howard, B. (2012). Saving lives for a lifetime: Supporting orphans and vulnerable children impacted by HIV/AIDS. *Journal of Acquired Immune Deficiency Syndromes, 60* (Supplement 3), S127–S135.

Oomman, N., Bernstein, M., & Rosenzweig, S. (2007). *Following the funding for HIV/AIDS: A comparative analysis of PEPFAR, the Global Fund and World Bank MAP*. Washington, DC: Center for Global Development.

Padian, N. S., Holmes, C. B., McCoy, S. I., Lyerla, R., Bouey, P. D., & Goosby, E. P. (2011a). Implementation science for the US President's Emergency Plan for AIDS Relief (PEPFAR). *Journal of Acquired Immune Deficiency Syndromes, 56*(3), 199–203.

Padian, N. S., McCoy, S. I., Karim, S. S. A., Hasen, N., Kim, J., Bartos, M., ... Cohen, M. S. (2011b). HIV prevention transformed: the new prevention research agenda. *The Lancet, 378*, 269–278.

Petryna, A. (2002). *Life exposed: Biological citizens after Chernobyl*. Princeton, NJ: Princeton University Press.

Redfield, P. (2012). Bioexpectations: life technologies as humanitarian goods. *Public Culture, 24*(1 66), 157–184.

Robins, S. (2004). Long live Zackie, long live: AIDS activism, science and citizenship after apartheid. *Journal of Southern African Studies, 30*, 651–672.

Rose, N. (2005). *The politics of life itself: Biomedicine, power, and subjectivity in the twenty-first century*. Princeton, NJ: Princeton University Press.

South African Government. (2005). *Policy framework for orphans and other children made vulnerable by HIV and AIDS, South Africa: Building a caring society together*. Pretoria, South Africa.

Strathern, M. (Ed.). (2000). *Audit cultures: Anthropological studies in accountability, ethics and the academy*. London: Routledge.

Tom Lantos and Henry J Hyde United States Global Leadership Against HIV/AIDS, Tuberculosis, and Malaria Reauthorization Act of 2008 §22 U.S.C. §7601 (2008).

United Nations Children's Fund (UNICEF). (2010). *Children and AIDS: Fifth stocktaking report*. New York: United Nations Children's Fund.

United Nations Children's Fund, Joint United Nations Commission on HIV/AIDS, and United States Agency for International Development (UNICEF, UNAIDS, & USAID). (2004). *The framework for the protection, care and support of orphans and vulnerable children living in a world with HIV and AIDS*. New York: United Nations Children's Fund.

United States Agency for International Development. (2007, 22 January). *USAID-PEPFAR South Africa OVC Partners Meeting Minutes*. Pretoria, South Africa.

United States Department of State. (2012). *PEPFAR blueprint: Creating an AIDS-free generation*. Washington, DC: US Government Printing Office.

United States President's Emergency Plan for AIDS Relief (PEPFAR). (2006). *Orphans and other vulnerable children. Programming guidance for United States in-country staff and implementing partners*. Washington, DC: President's Emergency Plan for AIDS Relief, Office of the US Global AIDS Coordinator.

United States President's Emergency Plan for AIDS Relief (PEPFAR). (2008a). *Saving lives, creating hope* [Documentary]. United States: Still Life Projects.

United States President's Emergency Plan for AIDS Relief (PEPFAR). (2008b). *The power of partnerships: The US President's Emergency Plan for AIDS Relief 2008 annual report to Congress*. Washington, DC: President's Emergency Plan for AIDS Relief.

United States President's Emergency Plan for AIDS Relief (PEPFAR). (2009). *Next generation indicators reference guide*. Washington, DC: President's Emergency Plan for AIDS Relief.

United States President's Emergency Plan for AIDS Relief (PEPFAR). (2012). *Partnership to fight HIV/AIDS in South Africa*. Retrieved from http://www.pepfar.gov/countries/southafrica/index.htm

White House Press Office. (2007). *Fact Sheet: President Bush Announces Five-Year, $30 Billion HIV/AIDS Plan*. Vol. 2007. Washington, DC: The White House.

Williamson, J., Cox, A., & Johnston, B. (2004). *Conducting a situation analysis of orphans and vulnerable children affected by HIV/AIDS*. Washington, DC: Africa Bureau Information Center, United States Agency for International Development.

Wolfe, R. (2008, 15 February). Bush agenda for next week is Africa. *USA Today*. Retrieved from http://usatoday30.usatoday.com/news/washington/2008-02-14-africa_N.htm

Towards the embodiment of biosocial resistance? How to account for the unexpected effects of antiretroviral scale-up in the Central African Republic

Pierre-Marie David

Department of Medication and Population Health, Faculty of Pharmacy, Université de Montréal, Montreal, Canada

At the fringes of the unprecedented medication scale-up in the treatment of HIV, many African countries have experienced dramatic antiretroviral drug stock-outs. Usually considered the result of irrational decisions on behalf of local politicians, programme managers and even patients (who are stigmatised as immoral), these problems seem not to be so exceptional. However, ethnographic attention to the social consequences of the presence and absence of antiretroviral drugs in the Central African Republic (CAR) suggests that these stock-outs entail far more than logistical failures. In 2010 and 2011 in the CAR, major antiretroviral treatment (ARV) stock-outs resulted in the renewal of 'therapeutic' social ties and also significant social resistance and defiance. While this paper explores reasons for the shortage, its focus is on subsequent popular reactions to it, particularly among people who are HIV-positive and dependent on ARVs. The exceptional and ambiguous consequences of these drug stock-outs raise new concerns relevant to the politics of global public health.

Introduction

In 2012, more than 8 million people had access to antiretroviral (ARV) drugs and associated services (UNAIDS, 2012). The scale-up of these life-saving medicines was an unprecedented international health intervention both in terms of financial and social mobilisation (Hirsch, Parker, & Aggleton, 2007). New institutions were the direct product of this international will and social mobilisation, including the Global Fund to Fight AIDS, Tuberculosis and Malaria (Sidibé, Tanaka, & Buse, 2010) and the President's Emergency Plan For Aids Relief, both of which have committed exceptional funds. New public/private partnerships specifically committed to HIV scale-up policies, such as the Bill and Melinda Gates Foundation, have redesigned the health agenda at the international level (Birn, 2005; Lee, Buse, & Fustukian, 2002). These partnerships have contributed to a reconfiguration of international health interventions in such a way that 'global health' has become a matter of scale with regard to addressing widely disseminated diseases but also in terms of normalised transnational interventions (Adams, Novotny, & Leslie, 2008; Brown, Cueto, & Fee, 2006). 'Health' has returned, through

HIV treatment and its scale-up, as a real issue for international development policies (Boidin, 2007; David, 2011b), and 'global health' appears now as a new laboratory for these policies (Atlani-Duault & Vidal, 2013), as well as for public policy (Eboko, 2013).

The Central African Republic (CAR) is no exception and has benefited from HIV scale-up treatment programmes. CAR's National Council for the Fight Against AIDS (CNLS) was created in 2001 as a multi-sectorial institution with funding from the World Bank. Following international recommendations on national and political leadership, the CNLS was controlled directly by the President of the Republic, who served as its General Assembly President, and the Prime Minister, who served as the institution's second president. In 2002, a programme funded by the Global Fund transformed individual access to treatment, which was previously based on the ability to pay, into a more comprehensive and coherent national programme. In the context of this programme, the United Nations Development Programme became the country's Principal Recipient (PR) and aimed to follow 5000 people undergoing treatment for five years. In late 2007, the Global Fund committed another US$43 million to the country, with the CNLS serving as the PR and the Ministry of Health serving as a sub-recipient. This round of funding aimed to support antiretroviral treatment for 15,000 people by 2013 (GFATM, 2008). In 2011, US$62 million had been disbursed for the fight against AIDS in CAR, thanks to the Global Fund. The same year, foreign aid accounted for more than two-thirds of government expenditure on health (World Health Organization [WHO], 2013).

The 'pharmaceuticalisation' of public health and its local effects

Beyond an international policy achievement, these programmes also created a 'politics of life' (Nguyen, 2010) based on therapeutic power (Fassin, 1996). The pharmaceuticalisation of public health has emerged as a fruitful area of research in anthropology, particularly with regard to various experiences of HIV scale-up (Biehl, 2007; Petryna, 2011). New rights and services have accompanied HIV treatment, including nutritional support, discussion groups and therapeutic education workshops. ARVs are not simply a biomedical treatment that save lives – they encompass a complex network of medications, techniques, guidelines, resources and ideas (Hardon & Dilger, 2011). New forms of subjectivity have also resulted, in some cases, from this heterogeneous assembly, such as 'therapeutic citizenship' (Nguyen, 2005). In this paradigm, citizenship is transformed into 'therapeutic citizenship', legitimated by a state of exception, involving a change of sovereignty beyond national borders (Nguyen, 2009; Rottenburg, 2009).

This seminal global perspective must be considered from the local perspective by integrating the specifics of the field, such as postcolonial dominations, and also the specific negotiations that translate the global HIV scale-up into local moral worlds (Mattes, 2012) and into everyday lived experience (Le Marcis & Ebrahim-Vally, 2005). Indeed, I am careful not to mechanically apply a disciplinary perspective of public health here, which has, at the fringes and especially in Africa, little empirical relevance (Ferguson, 2011; Geissler, Rottenburg, & Zenker, 2012). Alongside new forms of social inclusion based on medication access (David, 2011a; Ecks, 2005; Sanabria, 2010), the discontinuities of global access programmes provide a double opportunity to query and specify the material and temporal importance of treatment in local biosocialisation processes and with regard to the wider deployment of the new politics of global health.

Facing the unexpected: discontinuity, failures, and abandonment

Along with the unprecedented drug scale-up in HIV treatment, many African countries have experienced dramatic antiretroviral drug stock-outs. Usually considered the result of irrational decisions made by local politicians, local programme managers, and even patients (who are stigmatised as immoral), these problems are typically read as unexceptional, and have led to few publications by social scientists or others (Park, 2012). Although not part of AIDS accountability frameworks, international research on AIDS needs to examine these situations for clear operational and ethical purposes.

When I returned to CAR in January 2010, after having worked on ARV access programmes in CAR from 2005 to 2008, it was ultimately the social effects of ARV absence that drew my attention. The Global Fund's freeze on programme funding after only 8 months of national management led to a national ARV shortage, which lasted for 3 months. The social aspects of treatment discontinuity were striking.

Paradoxically, the stock-outs of life-saving medications raised the possibility of a form of 'killing' within a biopolitics of 'making live'. As I will argue, the drug stock-outs I observed produced resistances, both biological and social, that would result in symbolic and material forms of killing. Examining these stock-outs as 'economies of abandonment' (Povinelli, 2011) may enlighten global initiatives' rationality, and their anthropological, as well as biopolitical, consequences. The CAR, its distant state (Bierschenk & de Sardan, 1997) and local micro-sovereignties (Lombard, 2012) constitute a remarkable context in which to track the networks of governance associated with the presence and absence of ARVs.

This article explores the biopolitical consequences of national ARV stock-outs in CAR. Following a short description of my ethnographic methods, I describe the context in which treatment ruptures have appeared. I then describe the subjective embodiment and the social tactics resulting from this crisis. In the final section of the article, I analyse the ambiguous biopolitical consequences the stock-outs have brought about.

Methodology

To highlight the differences between AIDS programmes' claims and the practices through which ARV treatment is socially translated, for this paper and for a related broader study[1] I have relied on observant participation (Favret-Saada, 1990; Soulé, 2007). I make this distinction from participant observation, because in my experience, participation in the field was essential. My experience in various health centres and in supporting various associations in CAR enabled me to take part in an extraordinary diversity of situations and this ethnographical work has been essential to account for the politics of HIV drug scale-up.

Between 2005 and 2007, the first wave of observant participation in CAR included participation in national writing teams for grants from institutions such as the Global Fund, among other activities. This paper is drawn principally from a second wave of research conducted when I returned to CAR in 2010 and joined (as both a socio-anthropologist and a practicing pharmacist) teams that were making about 200 drug deliveries per day. Working three days a week in three different health centres for a period of three months provided me with a rich insight into the diversity of experiences of a range of health professionals and patient practices, as well as the opportunity to identify some similarities across them. Moreover, I carried out *in situ* observations in AIDS clinics in Bangui (the country's capital and largest city), conducted ethnographic interviews with institution representatives, patients and health personnel, and led focus groups with members of community associations. The everyday practices that produce and reproduce the social world surrounding access to ARVs were my main theoretical objects (de Certeau, 1980/1990).

ARVs stock-outs and the local context of drug access

From exceptional funds to national drug stock-outs

Leaving the capital city of Bangui in December 2007 after my first wave of research, I shared an optimistic feeling with regard to the future of antiretroviral therapy in CAR with the people I had worked with. An application to the Global Fund had been accepted and would provide care for 15,000 people for five years with US$43 million. On my return to Bangui in January 2010, the social effects of the lack of treatment took me by surprise. The Global Fund's freezing of programme funding after only eight months of national management led to massive ARV shortages, which had already lasted more than two months in some centres. Availability of all first-line regimens were affected by the freeze, including nucleosidic (AZT/3TC or d4T/3TC) and non-nucleosidic inhibitors (nevirapine or efavirenz).

As explained to me by the national expert for drugs procurement, the CNLS, as PR, could not pay the 'sub-recipient', the National Drugs Distribution Unit's (Unité de Cession du Medicament) bills. Then, generic drug suppliers in India did not want to ship drugs without prepayment. These prepayments were against Global Fund accountability rules, and the ARV supply chain was cut.

From free access to accusations

ARVs had been issued for free since 2008 with the Global Fund's (Round 7) support.[2] This free circulation in a previously fee-based system led to the abandonment of alternative ARV procurement strategies (private and public). Patients therefore became entirely dependent on a unique system financed by the Global Fund. This national supply monopoly contrasted with fragmentation at distribution sites. At the beginning of 2010, all public facilities experienced an average of three months of ARV stock-out, with some variations. International non-governmental organisations (NGOs) could afford exceptional procurements to keep their patients under treatment. Other faith-based local NGOs had managed stocks very cautiously and could overcome a three-month stock-out.

The reasons provided for this fund freezing varied. Officially, the reason was a lack of performance with regard to the programme's key indicators. Unofficially, corruption was the major reason. Some claimed hundreds of thousands of dollars had disappeared, while others suggested the official amount was US$25,000 for which the Ministry of Health, as Sub-Recipient, could not justify to the PR, the CNLS. The Global Fund has never officially reported corruption in this context and has never asked for money back as was done in Mali during the same period.

A joint emergency team of international experts from the private and the public sector, the JURTA Mission (Joint UN Regional Team on AIDS), assembled in Bangui from 14 to 21 January 2010, to account for this situation and to produce recommendations to improve performance and the financial tracking system. The rupture in ARV accessibility was legitimately treated as a crisis that required a technical fix and the mission acknowledged that the Global Fund had frozen its funding as a condition for technical improvements. However, the stories of people affected by ARV stock-outs, which I provide below, illustrate this crisis went beyond a technical problem.

From hope to uncertainty

ARV access through the Global Fund programme had produced great hopes among those living with HIV and AIDS. People receiving treatment could better engage with health facilities. The time between receiving a positive test to being cared for and followed by a doctor was reduced. People could access ARVs or cotrimoxazole chimioprophylaxia. The access to ARVs had made HIV infection 'an infection like any other', as many of my interlocutors stated, and also lowered the stigmatisation experienced by some.

Psychosocial counselling accompanied various types of nutritional support, as well as training for income-generating activities and home care visits, giving credence to the expression 'living positively'. Acting on this hope, people in Bangui increasingly chose HIV testing, as conditions improved to better enable confidentiality and the possibility of treatment. For example, the number of pregnant women tested for HIV rose from less than 20,000 in 2008 to more than 40,000 in 2009 (UNAIDS, 2010).

However, when I returned in 2010, hope had turned into major uncertainty. After meeting my former colleagues, I learned that a fierce battle was raging between the national programme management institutions. The CNLS and the Ministry of Health mutually accused each other of mismanagement, and they were both in turn accused by experts of the international community and by patients. To illustrate this tension around AIDS funding, the Ministry of Health (*Ministère de la Santé Publique et de la Population*) was renamed, following the receipt of US$43 million dollars in Global Fund funding, becoming the MSPPLS: *Ministère de la Santé Publique, de la Population et de la Lutte contre le Sida* (Ministry of Public Health, Population and the Fight against AIDS). Suspicion was widespread with regard to the moral integrity of the different players involved in HIV programmes: national leaders, doctors and even patients, who were accused of enrolling at several sites. AIDS programme civil servants were seen as receiving four-wheel drive vehicles, building houses and hiring family members, while patients were left without drugs. Various social moral worlds would emerge in community-based organisations due to these stock-outs. Some local organisation leaders would try to fight and resist the situation, as I will describe further, but others would tell me that the problem was not that HIV treatment had become a business, but that it should be *theirs*.

Betrayal and outrage: identities in flux

'*It's almost already over for her because of drugs stock-outs*'

In 2010, the secretary of the local management office of the Global Fund (the Country Coordinating Mechanism), with whom I had worked, invited me to participate in the office's next meeting, which brought together national referents, partners (United Nations and international NGOs) and representatives of relevant ministries, as well as two representatives of people living with HIV.

Representatives of those infected had urged leaders to deal with the stock-out situation. 'It is now the resistance that will kill us', said the president of the Central African Conference of people living with HIV/AIDS (COCAPEV), vehemently. 'The vice president is now between life and death, in the hospital. It's almost already over for her because of drug stock-outs'. This person, Francine, who I had met a few years before, was a prominent figure in the fight against HIV and AIDS.

A few weeks later, having learned of Francine's hospital discharge, I called her to find out how she was doing. She invited me to visit her at her home. When I arrived, Francine recognised me: 'You are the white man working at the Community Hospital'. She seemed very thin and still very weak. She had great difficulty walking. Her face was drawn and emaciated, amplified by differences in pigmentation in the folds of the face, hands and feet.

It was the dry season, so we stayed on the terrace to enjoy the breeze, although hot. The house was built of cement and a wood frame supported the roof. Wooden furniture, including a wardrobe, coffee table, sofa and chairs, occupied the visible part of the house and gave an impression of relative comfort. 'You see this house, I paid for it after a mission in Kenya in 2004', she commented. She had represented the Central African women living with HIV and had probably benefited from the *per diem* provided by the international institution that financed the trip. Since the mid-1990s, when she met with representatives of WAB (Women with HIV/AIDS without borders) in South Africa, she became the representative of the association in the CAR on a voluntary basis. She was also vice president of COCAPEV, which was the first association of people living with HIV, and later became a network of associations.

Uncertain rights and the remains of past promises

I asked Francine about her experience with antiretroviral therapy and she told me what had happened to her. She was employed as a psychosocial assistant in an AIDS clinic in the central downtown district, recruited in early 2009, thanks to funding from the Global Fund to provide psychosocial counselling with HIV screening. She earned about 40,000 FCFA per month (roughly US$80), which allowed her to support a family of four children. In autumn 2009, the Global Fund had frozen its funding. Francine explained to me the difficulty of continuing to live normally and especially of obtaining food and medicines. Unable to support herself, she became vulnerable to many common infections (including malaria and intestinal infections). She was subsequently hospitalised in early 2010, when ARVs were not yet out of stock in her health facility.

As she could not pay the hospital costs, she sent her daughter to the CNLS, which adjoined her hospital and was in the same administrative neighbourhood as the Ministry of Health. 'The coordinator asked the minister to sign a waiver for my hospitalisation', she explained. 'He accepted'. At this point in her story, Francine diverged, delving into a vehement speech against the AIDS bureaucracy of her country. 'They live off our backs'. Francine had expressed her dismay, her disappointment, and a sense of betrayal. 'Look, they made us testify openly. We did it for our brothers and sisters. Now what do we have? Nothing. While they have their houses and ride in big cars'. The same system that 'makes live' infected persons also contributes to 'making eat' many government officials who have access to material resources such as 'large vehicles, drivers and villas' as noticed by the infected people.

From Francine's perspective, this was a terrible misallocation of benefits. Francine was indeed one of the first people to give the epidemic a face in the CAR in the 1990s. She emphasised the sacrifices made to engage, train and testify as a person living with HIV, when the '*azo ti SIDA*', the local name for infected people in the CAR, was a social curse. They were called '*kanga na pelle*' – pick and shovel – referring to the 'hole' that awaited them, and that they helped to dig with a thoughtless life. According to Francine, speaking out for those infected had to come along with rights, including being first to have access to resources, paid training workshops, awareness sessions, open testimonies, and later of having drugs and even, as was the case with Francine, getting paid for their work. With the disappearance of ARVs and associated services came the scars of past promises.

Variable geometry of the body and the identity

'The CNLS paid for drugs, but I told my daughter if I die, I do not want the honours of the CNLS'. 'Now nobody gives us anything and they await my death to make a quest, pay for flowers, casket and a big parade with honours'. Francine seemed no longer to want to be the engaged and committed person she once was. The identity of 'PLWHA' she had built was crumbling along with her body. Recurrent financial difficulties and the inability to feed her family all revealed her extreme vulnerability. 'What will I leave my children? At least there will be this house', she added.

I remained silent. She smiled and called her daughter, who came a little later with a photo album. We looked together at pictures of her with other community members in Bangui or on missions outside the country. I was struck by the differences between the two bodies: the one shown in the photos of a young woman rather strong and plump, and the one in front of me, that of a woman so thin and with lines so drawn that I had forgotten that she was only 45-year old.

At the end of our conversation, she asked me to drop by taxi into *ville* (administrative downtown area) to see another community member, the representative of the National Union of girls with HIV. This association was founded in 2001, supported by various international NGOs, and its members benefited from training abroad, as well as support for attending international AIDS conferences. The President had just returned from a mission to Casablanca, where the Francophone AIDS Conference was held. She could probably 'do something' to help, Francine told me. The symbolic passing of the baton between these two iconic leaders symbolised well the ambivalence that treatment involved: one coming back from an international conference with enthusiasm and *per diem*, and the other one feeling betrayed and helpless.

Francine's story revealed the powerful link between treatment materiality and the changing relationship to one's self and the world through her body's experience. Even though the therapeutic citizenship Francine experienced had been powerful, treatment rupture recalls its fragility. Out of necessity, patients like Francine tried to pull through, employing tactics that drew on their social relations. Some also seemed to hope that I could be a resource. This was evident during several encounters I had with patients who were willing to tell me their story, because they wanted something from me in exchange.

Tactics 'from below' and the production of biosocial resistance

This rupture in treatment access paradoxically reinforced other social formations, as revealed by other patients' tactics to navigate the challenges of everyday life. My presence in various support centres provided insight into the concrete practices of solidarity that reflect what Jean-François Bayart has called a 'politics from below' (Bayart, Mbembe, & Toulabor, 2008). The discontinuation of resources inspired multiple forms of social resistance and also displays of creativity.

In treatment centres, uncertainty became widespread among patients and healthcare personnel. 'When will drugs arrive?' they asked. The patients, two-thirds women, explained the very real problems they faced: the difficulty in paying for transport, the difficulty in walking long distances (especially with the long-term side effects of some treatments), the need to leave the city for the countryside to stock up on food or do a 'little business' often necessary for the survival of the household.

Feelings of insecurity were also noticeable in the health centres observed. These feelings translated into multiple ways. When many patients who had tested positive and knew they were eligible for antiretrovirals received the news of the unavailability of drugs, they accused the doctors of keeping the drugs and selling them for their own gains (which many had done at the beginning of the Global Fund programme when they had to provide consultations to HIV patients for free). These exchanges often ended in verbal violence, sometimes physical violence. This violence revealed patients' dismay, as well as confusion and anger towards the people both representing a failing system and suspected of taking advantage of the situation.

Daily tactics vis-à-vis drugs

Access to ARVs during the national programme break cannot be reduced to an economic problem or the whims of an informal private market, in which only those with money would gain access to drugs. Finding ARV, especially one's particular ARV, usually required cunning tactics that drew on both social and economic resources. The health centre and association frameworks described below help to illustrate the different tactics relied upon to obtain treatment. In reality, these frameworks overlap.

In health centres

Half of the patients were able to overcome the stock-out (ranging from 1 to 4 months, depending on the centre) through personally accumulating drug reserves by regularly returning well before their monthly stock was exhausted. Those most concerned with the management of their medication were rewarded. In addition, they could sell part of their reserves to other patients, which frequently occurred. Long queues at health centres played a key role in the exchange of information and created a new supply and demand for drugs. If this situation did not necessarily result in a 'transaction', it still allowed the flow of information with regard to how to provide drugs informally.

In treatment centres, many had access to medicine through people they knew or relatives who were health personnel. Indeed, during daily dispensation of drugs, health staff went to the pharmacy with family members' prescriptions and asked their colleagues to 'do something'.

Despite being free of cost, stock-outs lent an increasing value to ARVs. Centres where I worked were generally integrated, that is, the staff was paid by the Ministry of Health. In drug sale units in hospitals, staff was paid on programme funds, frozen since September 2009. It was therefore ultimately not very surprising to find the drugs were being sold in the black market. You could procure at *Cinq kilo* market, in a popular neighbourhood, antiretrovirals for 1000 or 2000 FCFA from February to March 2010. These facts justified for some international experts the freezing of the programme, while they were actually the consequences.

In associations

Associations offered another pathway to access treatment through the ties of solidarity. In interviewing members of the UNG + (Union of National Girls with HIV), people explained to me how they had faced medication disruptions. First, they exchanged information about treatments and their remaining stocks. Second, if they wished, people with available stocks could exchange them with people undergoing the same therapy line. Third, supervision missions in the province by the headquarters of the association also served as a way to build reserves for members based in Bangui. This latter tactic raised questions about real consumption and management of ARVs in the province (the countryside). These ways to obtain one's drugs in a time of shortage also painted an interesting picture of Bangui's dependency on its province.[3]

All these successful strategies, however, did not reflect stories of those who sought to obtain drugs during the stock-out. Many people did not benefit from the associations' social network and did not know how to find drugs. Patients who did not take their treatment regularly were reminded daily that they were not only sick, but also that they were further damaging their health, as repeated by the COCAPEV President and instilled in them during therapeutic education workshops. Out of fear of running out of drugs, some adopted the tactic of taking their pills every two days, thus promoting the development of biological resistance.

Such 'irrational' tactics from a biomedical perspective seem rather rational, given the context of programmatic failure. Social relations appear to facilitate obtaining treatment. These were thus forms of social resistance and resilience. However, the effects of these tactics were not only symbolic, as they also left traces of biological resistance in the body. These biological traces would vary with the forms of social solidarity that eventually gave access to treatment.

Biosocial resistances

The first figures on virologic failures published in 2011 showed rates of about 30% in a leading health centre supported by an inter-hospital bilateral initiative with a hospital in Paris (Péré et al., 2012) in a study from 2009 to 2011. Much higher rates can hence be expected in the more peripheral centres of the city and the countryside. What will happen to the spread of these resistant viruses that, as shown in the cited study, are already resistant to recent (and unaffordable) second-generation molecules such as etravirine? In 2006, the rate of primary resistance in ARV-naive patients (pregnant women) was still less than 5% (Marechal et al., 2006). This low rate of primary resistance to ARVs is challenged by critical situations as those described above. These biological resistances moreover show how a social event such as ARV rupture can be incorporated into the body, both individually and socially, and can delineate future humanitarian emergencies.

Meanwhile, social resistance became increasingly common in Bangui. Discourses and experiences such as those of Francine showed an early effect of this drug stock-out that was critical vis-à-vis the biomedical discourse. Indeed, it is through the establishment of large-scale therapeutic education counselling or recurring reminders by professionals that biomedical discourse affirmed the need of a *continuous treatment for life*. The same biomedical speech that distinguished the sacred from the profane became incoherent and almost absurd.

How could the same discourse be deployed after these major stock-outs? Health personnel with whom I discussed posed two questions: first, loudly, what would be the future reception of their discourse with regard to education and adherence by patients after this episode? And secondly, in a lower voice, how could they themselves continue to make statements that legitimised them as health professionals and would now delegitimise them in everyday life. The consistency of biomedical discourse and the trust between patients and health professionals was put to the test. Beyond moral dilemmas, the absence of ARVs reveals and updates the very material and difficult relations between health professionals and their own local culture (Fanon, 2011) and between them and the culture of global biomedicine (Lock & Nguyen, 2010).

The ambiguous biopolitical consequences of stock-outs
'They are causing 4000 people to die'

Discourse regarding biological resistance to the virus flourished as a result of the shortages. The discourse was marked by the fact that no study could precisely document the impact of these stock-outs on the production of biological resistance.[4] A doctor from the French cooperation wrote in his reports that biological resistance had increased by 60% after the medication rupture. Even though this doctor's reports do not seem to have been released formally, his remarks circulated widely. In fact, the doctor, who maintained a thriving clinical practice by conducting medical consultations at several sites, had decreed the scale of the emergency to development partners during stock-outs: 'You are causing 4000 people to die'. (This was a sensible choice of phrasing, given that the language that the development partners used highlighted the number of lives saved.) Later, I observed some of these partners repeating his statement with a slight but important modification: '*They* are causing 4000 people to die', pointing at national health authorities.

Other expatriate doctors were more critical towards such discourse and wondered at the fuss over biological resistance as a 'spectrum'. The arguments for such scepticism were generally supported by clinical trials on 'therapeutic vacation' that had not been effective, but also did not show an excessive viral load rebound.[5] This position, however, was not sustained enough to create a public controversy in a politically tense situation. The urgency of the situation was not officially challenged by anyone.

'It is now the resistance that will kill us': these words vehemently expressed by the President of COCAPEV reflected the ownership of a discourse he knew well, since it was the foundation of the entire therapeutic education system in which association members were very involved, including Francine. The discourse on biological resistance also seemed reinforced by the special resonance it had with development partners. After the President of COCAPEV had spoken up at the Global Fund meeting previously described, key individuals in charge of bilateral cooperation gave him their business cards, apparently interested in continuing the discussion.

To practically cope with these biological resistances, the ability to switch to second-line treatment was also mentioned as a solution that caused pharmaceutical Global Fund programme officials to review their orders and integrate new, much more expensive, molecules without real data on the situation. This was a legitimate response and very questionable at the same time in a context where the choice of second-line drugs, if not operationally controlled, could destabilise the programme because of the high price and the greater complexity of their use and follow-up.

Exceptional spending

The practical social and political consequence of the embodiment of these resistances and discourses concerning resistance included the threat that the associations might protest or riot. Below, I will show how the discourses and these local tactics motivated the government to act and hence initiate a state of exception.

The Ministry of Health highly discouraged associations from protesting in the streets of Bangui. The president of the network of patients had a very strong response to these injunctions, showing that patients would not be intimidated: 'We prefer to be killed by bullets than without medication'. A great demonstration was scheduled in February 2010. It would start from the *Place de la Reconciliation*, also called *Place Omar Bongo*. A first phase at the Community Hospital would include the singing of the national anthem, and a second phase in front of the Prime Minister's building would lead to the filing of a memorandum. Then the march would end in front of the Ministry of Health. Association representatives that I met told me that they also wanted to sue the government for breach of human rights, as the government was not providing them with essential drugs.

The Prime Minister finally agreed to accept a meeting with the associations on 22 February 2010. He promised that a government order of EUR 300,000 for antiretroviral medications would arrive in the following days. The government had finally kept its word on this issue, and the expected drugs indeed arrived. They were purchased in a drugs buying group based in Africa, at a much higher price than the international market price. This exceptional intervention represented an unprecedented gesture on behalf of the government. The discourse on resistance, and the power relations involved seemed to have opened new possibilities. This expense returned access to free antiretroviral therapy to part of the population, for a few months at least.

This exception also recalled breaches of the State in carrying out its functions towards the rest of its population (civil servants salaries, poor access to water and sanitation, etc.). This break thus forced the government to choose among its population, and to legitimise *de facto* the special status of people infected with HIV at the expense of others. The consequences of ARV rupture, motivating HIV/AIDS organisations to threaten their government, shed new light on what Nguyen (2009) has called government-by-exception.

This experience enacted the incorporation of a 'therapeutic domination' based on the technologies of making up people and enrolling them into global intervention, and hence forcing the nation-state to continue the effort when the global apparatus withdraws. But at the same time, this exceptional spending resulted from the recognition, by local HIV/ AIDS associations, of a local nation-state that should facilitate their access to resources; arguing for a national political citizenship (although thin) next to a fragile therapeutic citizenship. This very political moment revealed the profound ambiguities embedded within the experience of treatment. In 2011, the ARV access programme was once again threatened by a 'no go' recommendation.

'No go' recommendation and the hypothesis of global 'scriptural economies'

The CAR national drugs stock-outs and their related social effects revealed moving networks of governance (Pandolfi, 2000, 2002). The *accountability* inferred from particular programmatic indicators appeared to be a powerful justification for the continuation or the freeze of such programmes. Preceding the 2010 programme rupture, it was argued (in a letter to national and international partners) that performance on three indicators was not good enough, and was classified as 'C'. The tracking system of both indicators and finances was also insufficient and would necessitate new private partners to lower donors' uncertainty. Although these three indicators[6] did not concern ARV distribution for adults, the entire programme was endangered.

This raises the question of whether low-performing programmes actually require more or less support to improve (not necessarily in the form of increased funding or private consultancies). In 2006, when receiving the Global Fund refusal for the sixth round at a local Global Fund meeting, local and international experts questioned the validity of performance as the major criterion. The problem they acknowledged was that the less capability a country has, the less support it gets. These experts wrote a letter to the Global Fund on this issue. Eventually, the funds were granted with the 7th round application, and an unprepared national institution, the CNLS, had to operate with and account for tens of millions of dollars.

Indicators that feed global goals, such as the Millennium Goals, and the accounting system of success in global health (Birn, 2009) are based on the rise of evidence-based medicine in global health and the audit culture to which it is related (Adams, 2013). Indicators and performance ratings are used at the same time to subcontract activities and expertise. It seems that this treatment device deploys what I call, in reference to Michel de Certeau,[7] global 'scriptural economies' connecting an assemblage of elements such as private and public organisations, antiretrovirals (present or absent), rationalities (operational and research) and practices through the production and circulation of specific knowledge, from body counts to performance and disbursement rates. *Writing*, as a modern practice, takes an important place in these types of interventions (Whyte, Whyte, Meinert, & Twebaze, 2013), transforming values through credited registration forms and debited infected bodies. But practices from below, as I have described, constitute an undisciplined *reading* that leaves traces in the body and the identity. This concept of 'scriptural economies' is heuristic and helpful in the sense that it sheds light not only on writing and calculative technologies but more precisely on the link between them and powerful *inscriptions*, through everyday practices, both with regard to biologies and subjectivities.

Conclusions

ARV ruptures produced paradoxical effects in the CAR. On the one hand, if infected people once believed in a healthy future as 'therapeutic citizens', this perspective changed for many with stock-outs. On the other hand, these ruptures reinforced social ties. Different forms of subjectivities coexisted in Central African society, not depending on the presence of a therapeutic power (ARVs), but according to its discontinuities and the negotiations of various forms of solidarity to cope with them.

Specifically, I have described how abandonment, because of programme freezing, produced biosocial resistances that resulted in a national exceptional intervention. The arguments for this intervention in the context I described reinforced the classical justification of 'lives to be saved', with its corollary: otherwise 'we are causing people to die'. But on the other hand, a less classical justification for this intervention also emerged, one that involved the containment of social and biological resistances through potentially new coercive technologies.

From a global perspective, HIV scale-up programmes should take seriously the effects of local discontinuities in drug access, including effects that fall outside the classic accountability framework. Two avenues for future research are evident: the first would further theorise the embodiment of biosocial resistance, and the second would further explore the global health 'scriptural economies' that build indicators as both the description of reality and the definition of needs, which are mobilised in the end to justify interventions and create value.

Finally, successes in global health are defined with respect to specific understandings and designs, as shown by Birn (2009). What she defined as the 'stage of evidence,' powered by 'writing and calculative practices', still surprisingly defines unilaterally what is a failure after the financial crisis in 2008. This paper stresses the need to build alternative ways to represent success or failure, to practice knowledge (Feierman,

Kleinman, Stewart, Farmer, & Das, 2010), and to write about and account for reality from a broader social and political improvement perspective. This may help to avoid reinforcing global health structural inequalities that are sometimes reproduced through interventions themselves.

Acknowledgements

I am very thankful to the people in Bangui who allowed me to participate in and enter their everyday lives. I am grateful to Johanne Collin, Laurence Monnais-Rousselot and Vinh-Kim Nguyen for their comments on this part of my research. I thank the anonymous reviewers for their time, careful reading, and constructive suggestions. Any mistakes or lapses of judgement remain my sole responsibility. I am also very grateful to Session Mwamufiya for his astute comments and English revisions.

Funding

This research has been supported by a PhD fellowship from the Méos, a research group on medication as social object at the University of Montreal and a Young Researcher Fellowship from Sidaction, Paris, France.

Notes

1. The facts and biographies described in this article are the product of fieldwork (David, 2013) conducted while I was a doctoral candidate at the University of Montreal and the University of Lyon in CAR from 2005 to 2008 for my dissertation and the collection of ethnographic data on two returns in 2010 and 2011 for 2 and 3 months, respectively. Names and details have been changed to conceal the identity of the persons concerned. The project was approved by the Ethics Committee of Health Research at the University of Montreal and by the Scientific Committee of the Faculty of Health Sciences, University of Bangui.
2. This free access was implemented after international recognition that the price of antiretrovirals was a major obstacle to treatment access and treatment adherence. This is a major exception in global health international policies since the Bamako Initiative in 1987 set up the recovery of medical costs through user fees and drugs payment.
3. The material dependence of Bangui on its province is very important. For example, food dependency is evident in the popular neighbourhood, *Kodro*, a forgotten space, as described by Adrien-Rongier in 1981. ARVs would reveal new material dependencies blurring the frontier between town and country and question rural Africa as materially dependent and culturally delayed.
4. Resistance tests were rarely performed and tests for viral load were also quite rare, although enshrined in the guidelines of the Ministry of Health.
5. Indeed, these 'structured treatment interruptions' ultimately proved less effective in the long term with respect to mortality and morbidity associated with HIV (Lawrence et al., 2003). However, the toxicity of ARVs and immunological and virological parameters were not statistically different for some authors (Dybul et al., 2003). In our case, the main stress on the patient represented by an 'unstructured' treatment interruption is probably not without effect on the fate of the virus. Fortunately, this interruption is not unstructured ethically and scientifically measurable, even if it is encountered in practice. A qualitative methodology is then crucial to account for these situations.
6. One of these indicators was the rate of infected pregnant women on ARV therapy. The rate was lower than expected, but as I have described in the first part of this paper, the number of pregnant women who received a test was much higher than expected and could have resulted in more difficulties keeping the rate of pregnant women on ART, as noted in the grant.
7. Michel de Certeau defines the scriptural economy as the moment when 'writing acquires an interest in history, in order to recover, watch or educate…[it transforms] nature by registering. It is violence, cutting and slashing the irrationality of superstitious people or enchanted regions' (de Certeau, 1980/1990, p. 212).

References

Adams, V. (2013). Evidence-based global public health: Subjects, profits, erasures. In J. Biehl & A. Petryna (Eds.), *When people come first: Critical studies in global health* (pp. 54–90). Princeton, NJ: Princeton University Press.

Adams, V., Novotny, T. E., & Leslie, H. (2008). Global health diplomacy. *Medical Anthropology, 27*, 315–323. doi:10.1080/01459740802427067

Adrien-Rongier, M.-F. (1981). Les kodro de Bangui: Un espace urbain oublié [Bangui's kodro: A forgotten urban space]. *Cahiers D'études Africaines, 21*, 93–110.

Atlani-Duault, L., & Vidal, L. (2013). La santé globale, nouveau laboratoire de l'aide internationale? [Global health: A new laboratory for international aid?] *Revue Tiers Monde*, 215.

Bayart, J.-F., Mbembe, A., Toulabor, C. (2008). *Le politique par le bas en Afrique noire* [Politics from below in blak Africa]. Paris: Karthala Editions.

Biehl, J. G. (2007). Pharmaceuticalization: AIDS treatment and global health politics. *Anthropological Quarterly, 80*, 1083–1126. doi:10.1353/anq.2007.0056

Bierschenk, T., & de Sardan, J.-P. O. (1997). Local powers and a distant state in rural Central African Republic. *The Journal of Modern African Studies, 35*, 441–468. doi:10.1017/S0022278X97002504

Birn, A.-E. (2005). Gates's grandest challenge: Transcending technology as public health ideology. *Lancet, 366*, 514–519. doi:10.1016/S0140-6736(05)66479-3

Birn, A.-E. (2009). The stages of international (global) health: Histories of success or successes of history? *Global Public Health, 4*(1), 50–68. doi:10.1080/17441690802017797

Boidin, B. (2007). Aide au développement et santé comme droit humain [International aid and health as a human right]. *Éthique et économique/Ethics and Economics, 5*(1), 1–21.

Brown, T. M., Cueto, M., & Fee, E. (2006). The World Health Organization and the transition from 'international' to 'global' public health. *American Journal of Public Health, 96*(1), 62–72. doi:10.2105/AJPH.2004.050831

David, P.-M. (2011a). Asymptomatic cholesterol, 'wonderdrugs' and western forms of pharmaceutical inclusion. In S. Fainzang & C. Haxaire (Eds.), *Of bodies and symptoms* (pp. 205–222). Tarragona: Publications de la Universitat Rovira i Virgili.

David, P.-M. (2011b). La santé: un enjeu de plus en plus central dans les politiques publiques de développement international? Socio-logos [The place of health in international public policies]. *Revue de l'association française de sociologie, 6*. Retrieved from http://socio-logos.revues.org/2550

David, P.-M. (2013). *Le traitement de l'oubli. Epreuve de l'incorporation des antirétroviraux et temporalités des traitements du sida en Centrafrique* [The oblivion treatment. The ordeal of antiretroviral drugs embodiment and aids treatments temporalities in the Central African Republic] (Unpublished doctoral dissertation). Université de Montréal, Université de Lyon, France.

de Certeau, M. (1980/1990). *L'invention du quotidien: Arts de faire* [The practice of everyday life]. Paris: Éditions Gallimard.

Dybul, M., Nies-Kraske, E., Daucher, M., Hertogs, K., Hallahan, C. W., Csako, G., & Fauci, A. S. (2003). Long-cycle structured intermittent versus continuous highly active antiretroviral therapy for the treatment of chronic infection with human immunodeficiency virus: Effects on drug toxicity and on immunologic and virologic parameters. *Journal of Infectious Diseases, 188*, 388–396. doi:10.1086/376535

Eboko, F. (2013). Déterminants socio-politiques de l'accès aux antirétroviraux en Afrique: Une approche comparée de l'action publique contre le SIDA [Social determinants of antiretroviral drugs access in Africa: A comparative study of public policy against AIDS]. In C. Possas & B. Larouze (Eds.), *Propriété intellectuelle et politiques publiques pour l'accès aux antirétroviraux dans les pays du Sud* [Intellectual property rights and ARV access public policies in developing countries] (pp. 207–224). Paris: Éditions EDK.

Ecks, S. (2005). Pharmaceutical citizenship: Antidepressant marketing and the promise of demarginalization in India. *Anthropology & Medicine, 12*, 239–254. doi:10.1080/13648470500291360

Fanon, F. (2011). *Œuvres* [Works]. Paris: La Découverte.

Fassin, D. (1996). *L'espace politique de la santé: Essai de généalogie* [The political space of health]. Paris: Presses Universitaires de France.

Favret-Saada, J. (1990). Être affecté [Being affected]. *Gradhiva, 8*(8), 3–9.

Feierman, S., Kleinman, A., Stewart, K., Farmer, P., & Das, V. (2010). Anthropology, knowledge-flows and global health. *Global Public Health*, *5*(2), 122–128. doi:10.1080/17441690903401338

Ferguson, J. (2011). Toward a left art of government: from 'Foucauldian critique' to Foucauldian politics. *History of the Human Sciences*, *24*(4), 61–68. doi:10.1177/0952695111413849

Geissler, P. W., Rottenburg, R., & Zenker, J. (2012). *Rethinking biomedicine and governance in Africa: Contributions from anthropology*. Bielefeld: Transcript Verlag.

Global Fund to Fight AIDS, Tuberculosis and Malaria. (2008). *Request from the Central African Republic for the HIV/AIDS component*. Retrieved from https://www.google.com/url?q=http://www.theglobalfund.org/grantDocuments/CAF-R07-HA_Proposal_0_en/&sa=U&ei=36W3UcekG8abrAHZx4CYAg&ved=0CAcQFjAA&client=internal-uds-cse&usg=AFQjCNGBB5RlkNRiD_SNVMaDc0JsDGwr4w

Hardon, A., & Dilger, H. (2011). Global AIDS medicines in East Africa health institutions. *Medical Anthropology*, *30*, 136–157. doi:10.1080/01459740.2011.552458

Hirsch, J. S., Parker, R. G., & Aggleton, P. (2007). Social aspects of antiretroviral therapy scale-up: introduction and overview. *AIDS*, *21*(Suppl 5), S1–S4. doi:10.1097/01.aids.0000298096.51728.7d

Lawrence, J., Mayers, D. L., Hullsiek, K. H., Collins, G., Abrams, D. I., Reisler, R. B., ... Baxter, J. D. (2003). Structured treatment interruption in patients with multidrug-resistant human immunodeficiency virus. *New England Journal of Medicine*, *349*, 837–846. doi:10.1056/NEJMoa035103

Lee, K., Buse, K., & Fustukian, S. (2002). *Health policy in a globalising world*. Cambridge: Cambridge University Press.

Le Marcis, F., & Ebrahim-Vally, R. (2005). People living with HIV and AIDS in everyday conditions of township life in South Africa: Between structural constraint and individual tactics. *SAHARA-J: Journal of Social Aspects of HIV/AIDS*, *2*, 217–235. doi:10.1080/17290376.2005.9724844

Lock, M., & Nguyen, V.-K. (2010). *An anthropology of biomedicine*. Chichester: Wiley-Blackwell.

Lombard, L. N. (2012). *Raiding sovereignty in Central African borderlands* (Unpublished doctoral dissertation thesis). Duke University, Durham. Retrieved from http://dukespace.lib.duke.edu/dspace/handle/10161/5861

Marechal, V., Jauvin, V., Selekon, B., Leal, J., Pelembi, P., Fikouma, V., ... Serdouma, E. (2006). Increasing HIV type 1 polymorphic diversity but no resistance to antiretroviral drugs in untreated patients from Central African Republic: A 2005 study. *AIDS Research & Human Retroviruses*, *22*, 1036–1044. doi:10.1089/aid.2006.22.1036

Mattes, D. (2012). 'I am also a human being!' Antiretroviral treatment in local moral worlds. *Anthropology & Medicine*, *19*(1), 75–84. doi:10.1080/13648470.2012.660463

Nguyen, V.-K. (2005). Antiretroviral globalism, biopolitics, and therapeutic citizenship. In A. Ong & J. Collier (Eds.), *Global assemblages: Technology, politics, and ethics as anthropological problems* (pp. 124–144). Oxford: Blackwell Publishing.

Nguyen, V.-K. (2009). Government-by-exception: Enrolment and experimentality in mass HIV treatment programmes in Africa. *Social Theory and Health*, *7*, 196–217. doi:10.1057/sth.2009.12

Nguyen, V.-K. (2010). *The republic of therapy: Triage and sovereignty in West Africa's time of AIDS*. Durham, NC: Duke University Press.

Pandolfi, M. (2000). Une souveraineté mouvante et supracoloniale [A mobile and supracolonial sovereignty]. *Multitudes*, *3*(3), 97–105. doi:10.3917/mult.003.0097

Pandolfi, M. (2002). 'Moral entrepreneurs', souverainetés mouvantes et barbelés: Le bio-politique dans les Balkans postcommunistes [Moral entrepreneurs, migrant sovereignties and barbed wire. The biopolitics in the poscommunist Balkans]. *Anthropologie et sociétés*, *26*(1), 29–51.

Park, S. J. (2012). Stock-outs in global health: Pharmaceutical governance and uncertainties in the global supply of ARVs in Uganda. In P.W. Geissler, R. Rottenburg, & J. Zenker (Eds.), *Rethinking biomedicine and governance in Africa: Contributions from anthropology* (pp. 177–194). Bielefeld: Transcript Verlag.

Péré, H., Charpentier, C., Mbelesso, P., Dandy, M., Matta, M., Moussa, S., ... Bélec, L. (2012). Virological response and resistance profiles after 24 months of first-line antiretroviral treatment in adults living in Bangui, Central African Republic. *AIDS Research and Human Retroviruses*, *28*, 315–323. doi:10.1089/aid.2011.0127

Petryna, A. (2011). Pharmaceuticals and the right to health: Reclaiming patients and the evidence base of new drugs. *Anthropological Quarterly*, *84*, 305–329. doi:10.1353/anq.2011.0024

Povinelli, E. A. (2011). *Economies of abandonment: Social belonging and endurance in late liberalism*. Durham, NC: Duke University Press.

Rottenburg, R. (2009). Social and public experiments and new figurations of science and politics in postcolonial Africa. *Postcolonial Studies, 12*, 423–440. doi:10.1080/13688790903350666

Sanabria, E. (2010). From sub-to super-citizenship: Sex hormones and the body politic in Brazil. *Ethnos, 75*, 377–401. doi:10.1080/00141844.2010.544393

Sidibé, M., Tanaka, S., & Buse, K. (2010). People, passion and politics: Looking back and moving forward in the governance of the AIDS response. *Global Health Governance, 4*(1), 1–17.

Soulé, B. (2007). Observation participante ou participation observante? Usages et justifications de la notion de participation observante en sciences sociales [Participative observation or observant participation?]. *Recherches Qualitatives, 27*(1), 127–140.

UNAIDS. (2010). *Country report*. Retrieved from http://www.unaids.org/en/regionscountries/countries/centralafricanrepublic/

UNAIDS. (2012). *World AIDS day report*. Retrieved from http://www.unaids.org/en/resources/publications/2012/name,76120,en.asp

WHO. (2013). *National health accounts*. Retrieved from http://www.who.int/nha/country/caf/en/

Whyte, S., Whyte, M., Meinert, L., & Twebaze, J. (2013). Therapeutic clientship: Belonging in Uganda's projectified landscape of AIDS care. In J. Biehl & A. Petryna (Eds.), *When people come first: Critical studies in global health* (pp. 140–161). Princeton, NJ: Princeton University Press.

Meaningful change or more of the same? The Global Fund's new funding model and the politics of HIV scale-up

Anuj Kapilashrami[a] and Johanna Hanefeld[b]

[a]Institute for International Health and Development, Queen Margaret University, Edinburgh, UK; [b]Department of Global Health and Development, London School of Hygiene and Tropical Medicine, London, UK

As we enter the fourth decade of HIV and AIDS, sustainability of treatment and prevention programmes is a growing concern in an environment of shrinking resources. The Global Fund to Fight AIDS, Tuberculosis and Malaria (GFATM) will be critical to maintaining current trajectories of scale-up and ultimately, ensuring access to HIV treatment and prevention for people in low/middle-income countries. The authors' prior research in India, Zambia and South Africa contributed evidence on the politics and impact of new institutional and funding arrangements, revealing a 'rhetoric-reality gap' in their impact on health systems, civil society participation, and achievement of population health. With its new funding strategy and disbursement model, the Fund proposes dramatic changes to its approach, emphasising value for money, greater fund predictability and flexibility and more proactive engagement in recipient countries, while foregrounding a human rights approach. This paper reviews the Fund's new strategy and examines its potential to respond to key criticisms concerning health systems impact, particularly the elite nature of this funding mechanism that generates competition between public and private sectors and marginalises local voices. The authors analyse strategy documents against their own research and published literature and reflect on whether the changes are likely to address challenges faced in bringing HIV programmes to scale and their likely effect on AIDS politics.

Introduction: the context of scale-up

Thirty years after the first reported case of HIV, the landscape of HIV has changed in multiple ways, with a consistent slowing in the growth trajectories of the pandemic globally[1] (Kanki & Grimes, 2013). Much of the reduction in rates of new infections and associated mortality is attributed to the roll-out of large-scale treatment programmes, especially rapid scale-up of antiretroviral (ARV) coverage, reportedly reaching almost half of the population in need of such life-saving therapies in low- and middle-income countries by 2010 (WHO, UNAIDS and UNICEF, 2011). Global health initiatives, namely the Global Fund to Fight AIDS, Tuberculosis and Malaria (GFATM) and Global Alliance for Vaccines and Immunizations (GAVI), together with other multilateral, bilateral (such as the US President's Emergency Plan for AIDS Relief, PEPFAR) and philanthropic foundations (such as the Bill and Melinda Gates Foundation) are regarded as the backbone of this global response (El-Sadr et al., 2012), contributing unprecedented amounts of financial resources for scaling-up access to prevention and treatment services. The Global Fund alone is reported as placing 4.2 million people on ARV globally and disbursing approximately US$20 billion to date for its three focal diseases (Global Fund website).

The response to the pandemic has enabled a transformation of the landscape of global health financing and programming. In the last decade, available global funding for the pandemic has risen from an estimated US$2.1 billion in 2001 to US$8.7 billion in 2009 (WHO, UNAIDS and UNICEF, 2011). Increased funding for global health was accompanied by growth in new institutional actors and mechanisms, and shifts in discursive ideas surrounding effectiveness of aid and programmes supported through traditional and contemporary aid channels. In the last decade there has been a gradual move away from AIDS *exceptionalism* to integrated approaches while the long-standing debate on horizontal vs. vertical approaches has been responded to by the emerging focus on diagonal[2] approaches.

Global health initiatives have responded to criticism of their health systems impact by incorporating greater focus on health systems strengthening (HSS), and more recently, underscoring human rights across their strategic frameworks (Atun & Bataringaya, 2011). This shift is driven by a growing recognition of the complexity of contemporary global health challenges – resurgent infectious diseases alongside an emergent crisis of non-communicable diseases – exacerbated by the dramatic shift in the global economic environment in recent years.

In any environment, aid is known to be unpredictable with destabilising effects on health systems, particularly in countries with a high dependency on aid and the burden of externally funded vertical programmes (Hamann & Bulir, 2001). For example, over one-third of annual health spending among African nations may come from donor aid (Stuckler, Basu, Wang, & McKee, 2011). Some examples of volatility evident in the context of the Global Fund include: disbursement delays such as those reported in Tanzania, South Africa and India; problems with managing funding cycles that are not aligned with national planning cycles; uncertainty in the status of future grants; and suspension and withdrawal of grant rounds (Garmaise, 2012; Hamann & Bulir, 2001).

Need for and emphasis on 'scale-up' of programmes have also highlighted challenges to scaling-up including recurrent costs of medicines and human resources, which necessitate long-term and predictable financing (Samb et al., 2009), systems strengthening and macro-economic impact, including absorptive capacity and aid volatility (Mangham & Hanson, 2010). Thus, greater predictability, certainty and sustainability of finances over the long-term, goals endorsed at the third high-level forum on aid effectiveness in Accra in 2008, are key to scaling-up (Dodd & Lane, 2010; Lane & Glassman, 2007).

At the same time, the economic crisis has meant fears around shrinking resources and making access to long-term predictable channels of funding even more imminent (Dodd & Lane, 2010). While some analyses conclude that development assistance in health remains unaffected and that donor governments have maintained their commitments, more recent reports suggest that donor contributions to the largest funding mechanisms (GAVI, the Global Fund and UNAIDS) have dropped by 6% since the onset of the economic crisis in 2008 (Grépin & Sridhar, 2012).

Yet, the ethical and public health imperative of scaling-up treatment and prevention is ever more compelling. Technological advancement and increased affordability and availability of medication make achievement of such scaling-up (to populations and geographical regions) feasible.

The Global Fund, along with other financing channels, is seen as critical to maintaining current trajectories of scale-up and ultimately ensuring universal access to HIV treatment and prevention for people in low- and middle-income countries. Amidst international debates on the trade-offs between vertical programmes and integrated health care, short-term health goals and provision of life-saving therapy versus building sustainable health systems, the Global Fund is constantly evolving. In this process, it draws extensively on the growing policy consensus on aid effectiveness and HSS, while retaining a focus on rapid expansion of its programmes. Faced with triple crises – fiduciary, financial and leadership – the Global Fund launched its new funding strategy in 2012 with the aim of 'investing strategically'. It emphasises greater predictability and flexibility of funding and more proactive engagement with grant implementation in recipient countries. It proposes dramatic changes to its funding mechanism – the way countries apply for funding, obtain approval of their proposals and manage their grants. More importantly, the Fund binds itself to scale-up its commitment to a human rights approach to financing and implementation of grants. These changes crystallise in a new funding model that was adopted at the start of 2013.

This funding model is the locus of our analysis. In this paper, we examine the extent to which the new strategy offers real change in light of the wider evidence on the Fund's impact on health systems including human resources and governance, civil society participation and population health outcomes. We draw comparisons between our intensive research experiences of conducting national and sub-national qualitative research on the Global Fund and other HIV funding mechanisms in India, Zambia and South Africa in 2007 and 2010. The country contexts are not comparable – different HIV epidemics, funding levels and dependency on external aid, and different historical–political contexts. Yet, the shared study focus – on governance and institutional structures and implications for health systems and outcomes – presents a unique opportunity to reflect on the research findings as we discuss the new strategy for its potential implications for scale-up in these countries.

Methodology

We analysed and reflected on the revised Global Fund Strategy on the basis of evidence emerging from previous national-level research examining the impact of Global Fund programming at the country and community levels. Both authors independently reviewed the strategy and funding model based on common areas of impact of Global Fund funding identified through earlier country-level research. Analysis and discussion were then jointly developed through an iterative process of drafting and redrafting.

Country-level findings in Zambia and South Africa were collected as part of a wider doctoral research project that examined policy processes relating to the implementation of ART roll-out in Zambia and South Africa between 2007 and 2009. The research conducted was a qualitative policy analysis and involved over 150 in-depth interviews with policy-makers at national, provincial and district levels in the two focus countries. Actors interviewed included senior Ministry of Health officials, clinicians and health workers at all levels engaged in ART roll-out, programme managers and implementers from non-governmental organisations (NGOs), civil society representatives, representatives from global health initiatives (GHIs) and their implementing organisations at national and sub-national levels, and academics in both countries. Actors were selected using a snowballing technique following an initial set of criteria defined by an in-country advisory panel. In each country, sub-national research focused on one province and two districts (in Zambia) or sub-districts (in South Africa). In addition to interviews, a review of grey literature, newspaper reports and policy documents was conducted. Findings also draw on observations of the policy process during the data collection.

The qualitative enquiry in India was undertaken between 2007 and 2010 in five states – four southern high prevalence states (two to three districts in each) and Delhi, the epicentre of ministries, donors and Fund governance. An examination of the Global Fund governance, its underlying discourse and practice, and implications for HIV management was carried out through observation of project meetings and implementation sites; a short-term consultancy with a grant recipient; documentary analysis of coordination meetings, published and unpublished performance reports; and 70 in-depth interviews carried out with 94 respondents (as some interviews involved two or more respondents) at various levels of Fund governance – 28 decision-makers and officials at national and sub-national agencies, 41 project managers and administrators and 25 implementers across governmental and non-governmental organisations (including corporate sector). Ethics approval for both research projects was granted by respective institutional ethics committees of Queen Margaret University and the London School of Hygiene and Tropical Medicine in the UK and by ethics committees in Zambia and South Africa.

In this paper, we draw on the challenges observed in the implementation of Global Fund funding, and published by the authors, to understand the extent to which these will likely be addressed by the changes announced. We review the strategy and examine the implications of the new model under the following key areas: (1) health systems – human resources and governance, (2) civil society participation and (3) human rights and equity of health outcomes. We conclude with a discussion on potential challenges for scale-up.

Description of GFATM

The Global Fund was created in 2002 following a UN General Assembly Special Session on HIV/AIDS (UNGASS) to mobilise and provide new large-scale resources to countries facing the challenges of these three diseases seen as integral to achieving the Millennium Development Goals (Brugha & Walt, 2001).

The Global Fund was seen as part of a new breed of actors in global health, GHIs. GHIs often focus on a disease such as tuberculosis (TB) or malaria, or a specific intervention, such as childhood vaccinations, and implement a common strategy across countries. Combining more 'traditional' development actors such as multilateral and bilateral organisations with private-sector actors, foundations and civil society, GHIs were seen as bringing together a broad set of skills, providing a new approach to addressing pressing health issues, as well as mobilising new funding (Brugha, 2008).

The Global Fund is seen as core to the new world of institutionalised innovations in global health. Set up primarily as a mechanism for new funding in health rather than an implementing agency, it awards funding on the basis of country proposals submitted to the Secretariat in Geneva and reviewed by a technical review panel of experts who in turn make recommendations to the Board. The Board itself has representation of donor governments, private sector, foundations and civil society.

Over the years, the Global Fund has gained legitimacy and expanded in scope beyond that of a financing mechanism. More critical evidence has questioned the extent to which the Global Fund, through its structures, mechanisms and values, steers the process of decision-making and implementation at the country level (Kapilashrami & McPake,

2012). In the process of expansion, the Global Fund risks distorting the lines of authority and is 'likely to blur the distinction between public legitimacy and private power' (Slaughter, 2004, p. 169), raising particular concerns related to accountability.

Funding is provided to one or more 'principal recipients' within countries. Notably, recipients can include civil society organisations and are not restricted to government agencies or Ministries. Country proposals used to be developed in response to calls issued periodically by the Global Fund, so-called 'Rounds' of funding. To ensure country ownership, the Global Fund stipulates that proposals have to be developed through a Country Coordinating Mechanism (CCM), with membership of different sections of society.

Innovative aspects – in particular at the time of inception – included what was referred to as the Global Fund's demand-led nature, i.e. countries determining priorities for funding, and funding being awarded purely on technical merit of the proposal and extended on the basis of rigorous performance evaluation of recipient countries. In addition, emphasis on participation of civil society and affected communities (mainly people living with HIV and AIDS, PWHAs) is a central feature of the Global Fund model, in not only its 'design' but also its development (Kapilashrami & O'Brien, 2012), through the participation of NGOs in CCMs and voting rights on the board for community representatives (Brugha et al., 2004).

Challenges…

From the outset, the Global Fund has attracted significant attention of researchers trying to understand its role as a funding mechanism in health and the impact of its programmes. The Global Fund considers itself a 'learning organisation' and has undergone several independent evaluations to monitor its performance (Brugha et al., 2004).

As the Global Fund and other GHIs focused on disease-specific interventions began to disburse funding, it became apparent that weak health systems in recipient countries posed obstacles to achieving organisational goals, such as scaling-up treatment for HIV and AIDS and TB, or childhood vaccination (Samb et al., 2009). At the same time, evidence highlighted the role of GHIs in further weakening national and sub-national health systems (Biesma et al., 2009; Hanefeld, 2010). Challenges emerged relating to the modus operandi of the Global Fund and other GHIs. This included evidence that public sector health workers were drawn to HIV programmes, potentially averting attention away from other conditions and services. In some instances, NGOs funded by the Global Fund were attracting health workers from within the public sector through allowances and higher salaries (Hanefeld & Musheke, 2009) and a more rewarding working environment for relatively less workload (Kapilashrami & McPake, 2012). In addition, as systems and programmes became increasingly dependent on external funding, sustainability became a growing concern for planners. Policy-makers and implementers reported the time spent on coordination of different implementers and funders, including the Global Fund, as a real burden in their day-to-day work (Hanefeld, 2010). Prompted by these criticisms and responses from the field, the Global Fund began to explicitly fund HSS activities in 2006 and, in 2009 together with GAVI, the World Bank and WHO, launched the Joint Platform for Health Systems' Strengthening to ensure greater alignment of programmes (England, 2009).

The Global Fund's role in regard to fostering participation of civil society has also been complex and diverse. On one hand, through its structures, such as the CCMs, the Global Fund did create space for participation for some sections of communities that had previously been at the margins of the political process, such as men who have sex with men (MSM) in China, or people who use drugs (Brugha et al., 2004; Hanefeld, 2008). On the other hand, detailed analysis indicates that, in many countries, the quest for participation failed to take account of and reinforced more complex power structures amongst civil society, marking a shift from more critical and political to technical and managerial discourses (Caceres et al., 2010; Kapilashrami & O'Brien, 2012).

Yet these challenges did not provide the impetus for the revision of the Global Fund's strategy and funding model. Instead, this was precipitated by declining donor-funding pledges as a result of the global economic recession as well as allegations of misuse of funds by recipients. While the eventual investigation revealed that this misuse of funds was limited to a small number of countries, several donor governments suspended funding in 2011, following a story reporting on this misuse of funding by the Associated Press news service (Brown & Griekspoor, 2013).

...and changes at the Global Fund

The suspension of funding led to a series of structural and staff changes at the Global Fund, including the departure of its then Executive Director, Michel Kazatchkine, and the revision of its strategy. Following this period of change, set-off by questions around its fiduciary, financial and managerial capacity, the Global Fund emerged reconstituted in 2012 with a new Executive Director, a new strategy and an announcement of its new funding model.

The new strategy, entitled *Investing for Impact – the Global Fund Strategy 2012–2016*, calls for a more strategic, focused and sustainable impact, as well as greater efficiency alongside an explicit focus on human rights. Where previously funding was awarded to countries solely on the basis of country-led proposals submitted to the Global Fund for technical review, the strategy clearly introduces the 'potential for impact' as guiding criteria for funding, targeting resources on countries, interventions and populations where highest impact can be achieved. It sets targets for a number of people needing to be reached through its funding. It also sets out the need to fund on the basis of quality national strategies and health plans to avoid duplication and ensure alignment with national planning and partners' interventions. For greater sustainability, the Global Fund seeks to further its base of donors and to work with countries towards increasing cost-sharing. There is a clear emphasis on funding highest impact interventions and accelerating their scale-up through operational research.

Unsurprisingly, the strategy places greater emphasis on more proactive grant management from the outset, including a focus on greater quality control and better management of risk within grants. It also recognises the promotion and protection of human rights as one of its five key objectives. On paper, the strategy explicitly highlights the need to invest in strengthening human rights, to systematically include most-at-risk populations, and integrate rights principles and gender analysis throughout the grant cycle, starting from the proposal development stage, to ensure that Global Fund programmes do not negatively affect human rights. Despite this focus, it does not explicitly include equitable outcomes, for example, across the targets set for patients reached through its funding. The new funding model, announced in early 2013 to be piloted for a year, remains silent on this explicit commitment to human rights. The new model will see only a limited number of countries eligible for funding on the basis of disease profile and income status.

The previous system of 'rounds' of funding is abolished and countries are able to apply to the Global Fund on an ongoing basis. A key emphasis is placed on the iterative process of proposal development between Fund Secretariat and countries, envisaged through a 'dialogue process' with countries to avoid situations where proposals are rejected outright. Working with countries towards greater co-financing and transitioning to country funding in the future is intended to ensure greater predictability of funding, in terms of when to apply and for how much, thereby allowing countries to plan better. In this context, countries have to provide a national health plan to receive funding. Given the lack of detail on the dialogue process, it is unclear what implications this would have for Global Fund country-level operations and practice.

A new narrative and implications for scale-up

A review of the new strategy indicates an emergent narrative, which has implications for scale-up of HIV interventions. The title of the strategy paper 'investing for impact' is clearly emphasised throughout the document, extending from a focus on key countries to key populations and key interventions, in what is called 'a more focused approach'. Resonating the discursive shifts in international donor aid, the Global Fund aims to become 'a more effective and efficient funder', more 'attractive to donors'. This narrative is constructed around the following key themes:

- More rigorous performance-based funding through greater investment in data modelling, baseline and progress surveys and extensive operational research to ensure rapid scale-up of highest impact interventions.
- Fiduciary risk management, characterised by a risk-differentiated approach to manage grants, appears central to the Global Fund's efforts to improve donor confidence. This appears to be in direct response to the Fund's association with financial mismanagement and corruption in its country-level programmes. The Global Fund follows earlier footsteps of the World Bank in allocating aid on the basis of recipient rankings on international benchmarks of good governance, justified by the widely held assumption that good institutional and policy environments determine aid effectiveness (Burnside & Dollar, 2000). Though contested (Hansen & Tarp, 2000; Rajan & Subramanian, 2008), such prescriptions of selectively allocating aid according to the strength of national systems have made their way into the dominant approaches to aid reform. Strategic targeting of Global Fund investments is accompanied by recurrent calls for sustainability of the HSS programmes and services delivered through these. Using such ranking as a basis for investment between countries sets up an inherent tension to the human rights principles, including equity, to which the Global Fund commits itself.
- Financial austerity emerges as an overriding theme, with emphasis laid on 'value for money' and the need 'to do more with less'. The objective of increasing procurement and operational efficiency is dominant. Unsurprisingly, fostering and expanding private-sector collaboration is viewed as pivotal to achieving efficiency objectives, as it will allow tapping into their 'world class expertise in business processes to maximise implementation efficiency, value for money and impact' (The Global Fund, 2011, p. 17).
- More 'proactive engagement' at the country level, which implies a shift away from its earlier distinctive emphasis on 'country-led' proposals and operations as a 'finance mechanism'. The latter were the basis on which the Global Fund gained

credibility and legitimacy as an institutional innovation in its first 10 years. Consequently, the earlier emphasis on 'country ownership' appears diluted, solely addressed through greater alignment with national strategies. The Strategy document cites the high-level panel in recommending that the Global Fund 'must be more assertive about where and how money is deployed' (The Global Fund, 2011, p. 8). Greater involvement at the country level is proposed to ensure 'maximum impact and value for money while identifying and mitigating risk'. This shift is concerning for the ways in which existing governance structures will be modified and its potential impact on country-level policy processes. Again, the language employed highlights an inherent tension between human rights principles of participation at the country level and the need to guide funding and interventions towards highest impact.

Against this backdrop of a changing narrative, we examine the implications of the strategy for three key themes: health systems, civil society participation and equity of health outcomes.

Health systems

Overall health systems impact was not uniform in countries studied, but common themes did emerge. Overstretched health systems coupled with limited human resource capacities for fund absorption and grant management arguably led to some of the earlier reported failures in meeting programmatic targets and health outcomes (Samb et al., 2009). The Global Fund responded and recognised the need to strengthen health systems. However, this happened reactively and within the remit of disease-specific programmes, which had already been set up with specific aims and specific funding and reporting channels. As a result, aspects of health systems began to be funded incrementally through specific interventions, for example, by hiring a data input manager to update patient records rather than addressing systemic issues of overall shortages and vacancies in health facilities. A further feature of this funding was that it was often not channelled through government systems but rather a myriad of NGOs, thus not providing additional staff capacity in ministries of health but adding coordination burden. In India, ART was delivered primarily by and within the public health facility. However, in an endeavour to bring treatment roll-out to scale and 'innovate' public–private delivery mechanisms, a civil society consortium was established to roll-out ART through corporate-led centres. Kapilashrami and McPake (2012) discuss how the resulting competition between public and private providers fragmented service delivery, and added coordination burden at the national level.

While the strategy commits itself to HSS, the focus is largely under the remit of 'invest(ing) more strategically' (Strategic objective 1) (The Global Fund, 2011). Consequently, actions are restricted to targeting of HSS investments to most-in-need countries and high-impact interventions, and better alignment of HSS investments with national systems. There is no mention of how the donor-side coordination and alignment will occur. In the three countries studied, it was this lack of harmonisation between donor grants and multiple donor-specific targets and performance reports that posed the greatest burden on human resources and resulted in challenges at the service delivery level.

Both the strategy document and the funding model are also silent on aspects relating to human resources. The impact of Global Fund funding on human resources in health is widely documented, including in the three countries studied. Particular effects that emerged in our field research include:

- Recruitment of public sector workers, including health workers. In Zambia and South Africa especially, NGOs supporting treatment roll-out were often able to recruit health workers through higher salaries. This was not limited to the Global Fund but also particularly evident from PEPFAR funding (Hanefeld & Musheke, 2009):

What is happening is that I am training people, the way we are developing [Name of a Staff member in MoH], the next you hear he has been taken by another implementer, next you will hear that in government you have no capacity. (MoH Zambia)

- Additionally, limited funding for human resources for health was reported in all three countries. In India, this emerged strongly among sub-recipients who reported poor salary scales for laboratory and technical staff and resulting problems with recruitment and retention. Further, hospital management and health workers highlighted that no funding was made available for auxiliary staff (including janitors and cleaners) for Global Fund programmes. Given the stand-alone and vertical nature of HIV interventions (ART clinics and counselling centres) and prevalent stigma, this presented itself as a challenge since the facility was unwilling to share these resources.
- Monitoring and evaluation procedures and increased workload. The need to prove impact by GHIs, including the Global Fund, meant an increasing focus on counting the number of patients reached. While intended to enhance accountability, different monitoring and evaluation systems by different funders posed an additional burden to public sector staff, which had not been budgeted for in the support provided to countries. The annual funding cycles of the Global Fund compounded these challenges:

With those [GHIs], at times they create a problem more than helping. It becomes a challenge coordinating them. You don't know at times what they are doing. They are close to 236 partners in Lusaka just in HIV. Now to track what each one is doing is a major challenge. (National Manager in Zambia)

The more general emphasis on HSS in the strategy document leaves hope that the human resource issues, especially financing and retention, will be accounted for by better alignment with national health plans and a comparative assessment of salary scales. However, the increased emphasis on 'maximising impact' and demonstrating 'value for money' suggests greater reporting and monitoring burden on human resources which need to be considered and supported. In the absence of any additional staff, such emphasis may deepen the negative health system effects of the Global Fund. The emphasis on 'value for money' and an implicit and inevitable rise in performance measurement and management systems (and M&E officers and protocols) are likely to compound problems of transaction costs and opportunistic behaviours linked to aid mechanisms of the Global Fund. In India, at the facility level, instances were reported whereby staff manipulated figures on adherence and re-registered patients under false names to show increased utilisation of beds and care facilities. Such systems tend to result in distortions and are argued as shifting incentives and overriding process- and quality-related concerns (Gulrajani, 2011). This further highlights the tensions set up between a system incentivising ambitious targets in terms of patients reached, while also including human rights principles, such as equality and participation.

Governance

The reality of countries having to manage funding cycles and requirements of different donor agencies and strategies is now specifically addressed with the focus on funding through national health strategies and joint funding platform and assessments. The strategy framework (actions 1.2 and 1.3) as well as the funding model places great emphasis on these aspects, suggesting learning has taken place. Where no such national health plan or strategy of sufficient quality exists, countries are expected to develop a plan as part of this process. Research examining the World Bank's Multi-Country HIV and AIDS Programme found that funding requirements which led to the creation of National AIDS Councils as well as NGOs meant these were in many cases unsustainable structures (Harman, 2010). Therefore, there is a potential risk that such pre-conditions may lead countries to, instead of genuinely engaging in and trying to develop an integrated system, simply develop ambitious plans and strategies to meet a new requirement of the Global Fund. The extent to which other donor agencies, including bilateral initiatives agencies, will support the same country-level process may also largely determine whether these serve their intended purpose of more overall harmonised and aligned funding. In these contexts, the extent to which these plans will be developed through existing mechanisms, such as the CCM, are also unclear. In many countries, CCMs are independent multi-stakeholder partnerships with disproportionate representation from the three focal diseases rather than the wider health sector. In the context of India, the extent to which the Planning Commission, the High Level Expert Group on Universal Health Coverage and similar committees will play a role in this process remains to be seen.

Another criticism of the Global Fund was that its annual call for grant proposals (a rounds-based system) led countries to apply in response to funding calls rather than in-depth needs and priorities-based assessments undertaken at the country level (Kapilashrami & McPake, 2012). Under this approach, the proposals were reviewed and approved for funding based on technical merit and not necessarily their ability to attain health impact. This system disadvantaged countries (and recipient organisations) with weaker capacities for writing proposals and monitoring grants, albeit with equally compelling needs. Research in India revealed that international agencies and large national or state-funded NGOs, with better access to social, economic and political capital, were far better positioned to serve as principal and sub-recipients or participate meaningfully in the Global Fund's governance structures such as the CCM. In contrast, local community-based organisations and women's networks of PWHAs remained at the periphery of fund flows. Kapilashrami and McPake (2012) further argue that exhaustive grant application and monitoring procedures denied any opportunities for an organic and consultative decision-making process, revealing a tokenistic purpose of these mechanisms. A case in point was the sporadic CCM meetings where members met only when a new round was opened or an existing round was being evaluated.

Further, the rounds-based funding call laid particular emphasis on innovation in programmes proposed and partnerships forged. As a result, programme components proposed in one round stood isolated from previous rounds. However, considerable overlap could be observed between activities of different partners and institutions created. Either new concepts of care and support were introduced or previously established concepts were modified to demonstrate 'innovation'. Reflecting on the impact of having multiple interventions and providers within a national programme, a senior bureaucrat in the state division of an Indian AIDS agency expressed, *all these separate rounds and overlaps between them lead to confusion and chaos at the implementation level.*

These concerns are partially addressed with the abandonment of the old rounds-based model. Under the new model, the Global Fund will indicate the total amount of money they can expect at the outset of the proposal process, with an opportunity to get further funds through an additional 'incentive' funding pool. Countries may apply for funding at any time. This will potentially increase predictability of funds and allow more time for engagement with stakeholders and adequate preparation among country recipients. However, scepticism is warranted over the extent to which this would directly lead to sustained dialogue and participation of hitherto marginalised voices given the greater role to be played by the Global Fund. This theme is further explored in the next section.

Civil society participation

The new model demands broader participation by stakeholders, including government agencies, donors, civil society and affected communities. Towards this end, the Global Fund proposes a 'country dialogue' through which stakeholders draft a summary of their proposed work plan, allowing the Global Fund to work more closely with countries to develop their detailed proposals much earlier in the process. Provided such dialogue is held at both national and sub-national levels through an open process, not restricted to pre-existing Global Fund networks of civil society, there is an opportunity for the civil society to clarify and engage with the processes of application and better prepare for challenges in grant management. New budget requirements ask countries to explicitly state, at the outset, how they will spend grants, and which programmes and interventions will be prioritised. This transparency offers civil society critical information with which to hold the Global Fund and its recipients to account.

It remains to be seen how the model impacts community-level engagement in decision-making, particularly vulnerable populations and groups who have hitherto remained invisible or further marginalised in the current decision-making and grant application processes. For example, evidence from India revealed how funding mechanisms (and electronic procedures of enabling civil society participation) excluded certain community-based organisations and networks of women living with HIV. Those who did participate in such mechanisms and procedures reported lack of transparency, asymmetries in information flows and an overall disempowering experience (Kapilashrami & O'Brien, 2012). The quotes below indicate the level of awareness and processes of democratic decision-making evident in the mechanisms established for seeking participation of civil society/NGO members:

> Eight NGOs were identified and 122 were to elect them…[through an online voting system] I think the 122 are not members, nor are they on the board. You apply for membership. Once you are approved, then your name will be put up for selection, I don't know by who or how. (CCM NGO member)

> I think it [online voting] was a very democratic process although it was a little surprising that somebody had already cast a vote on our behalf. My vote was already there, even before I logged in. (CCM NGO member)

Kapilashrami and O'Brien (2012) also argue that the processes of civil society engagement often undermine power hierarchies and differences between international and local, for-profit/corporate and not-for-profit organisations:

> If you take the two principles, one vote per entity and conflict of interest into account, decision making is clearly lopsided. Government occupies 18 of 34 seats through its various entities...[including] academia. So, people who are voting and leading discussions are the government...NGOs have strings attached as majority receive funds from the government. The externals like UN agencies, WHO, and bilateral could balance but among them there is clear dissonance between what is said at the headquarter level and actions by their counterparts at the country level. (Senior Fund bureaucrat)

> we had to start CCC [care centre]. They want it 10 bedded, they tell us the place where to have it, they pass a rent of 4000/- when in reality it is 30000/- pm. They call all the 'experts' together, sit in air conditioned rooms, earn in dollars and draft something which makes no sense. What makes them think people will work for this? There is no such thing as equal partners. In any partnership, not just with government, even with others, we are always made to feel as the 'dalit' [the untouchable]. (NGO sub-recipient)

While these quotes highlight specific challenges relating to CCM processes in India, they underline the challenges inherent in facilitating genuine participation of those facing greatest marginalisation at the country level. Given the absence of detail on the country dialogue process in the funding model and strategy, it seems unclear at best and unlikely at worst that the Global Fund will succeed in facilitating wider participation, including in the even more ambitious development of national health plans.

The new strategy lays particular emphasis on taking advantage of business sector expertise to maximise implementation efficiency in areas including supply–chain management. Prior country-level experience must be carefully assessed for the role of the business sector in such partnerships and the competition and inefficiencies resulting from creating parallel delivery systems (Kapilashrami & McPake, 2012):

> While it was earlier agreed that antiretroviral will be procured by the companies, they [the corporate partners] have now expressed their reluctance in doing so. They are negotiating with NACO to provide antiretroviral for the general population while they cater only to their workforce. Therefore the corporate component has been much delayed. And since it is a component of our programme, the non-performance is reflecting on the entire program. (Senior officer, civil society consortium)

Human rights and equity in health outcomes

In terms of health outcomes, the findings from Zambia and South Africa show the role of Global Fund funding, in advance of other funders in Zambia and working with specific provinces to enable funding, despite national government opposition in South Africa. Likewise, in India the arrival of the Global Fund coincided with the roll-out of ARV provision, and the subsequent up-scaling of treatment (from high-prevalence states to high-prevalence districts in mid- and low-prevalence states; from first-line to second-line drugs) is credited to the Global Fund financing.

The urgency of providing treatment to as many people as possible has meant a focus on population-dense areas at national and sub-national levels. At the time of data collection, in Zambia some facility-level implementers were reflecting on this as an ethical dilemma:

There is treatment here now, but you wonder 100miles away ... they do not have these drugs and how do they feel when they hear their cousins have access. (Programme Manager of Global Fund project at provincial level in Zambia)

Significant investments have also meant an overemphasis on demonstrating impact to justify bringing programmes to scale, and in the process, undermining sustainability concerns and systemic issues. Research conducted in India also revealed that although a high number of people were put on ARV, poor coordination of different services and agencies providing these resulted in sub-standard care received by PWHAs. This was exacerbated by the extensive documentation mandated by the Global Fund, and the inability of facility-level implementers to manage the resulting workload together with their primary responsibility of providing care. Services that suffered were adherence counselling, treatment for opportunistic infections and community care.

Globally, the Fund is credited with providing visibility to marginalised populations in countries where the HIV burden is limited, such as MSM and people who use drugs in eastern and central Europe (Sarang, Rhodes, & Sheon, 2012). One of the five strategic objectives outlined in the strategy paper is to protect and promote human rights, attainable through withdrawing support to programmes violating human rights, encouraging investments that address rights-related barriers to access and integrating a rights perspective across all aspects of the Global Fund's work.

The strategy document is carefully balanced with reference to ensuring that populations specifically affected are not left behind. The new strategy, however, is focused on maximising impact in countries where the greatest gains can be made. Likewise, the funding model targets a small number of countries on the basis of epidemiological and governance criteria. This approach runs counter to human rights endorsement by the Global Fund, as the poorest and most stigmatised populations in countries with weak governance or lower prevalence of HIV are set to lose out on funding, and consequently, access to life-saving therapeutic drugs and preventive interventions. Where this is not an explicit priority and where funds are limited, it is often the most vulnerable who lose out. Moreover, addressing the long-term determinants of vulnerabilities or the 'upstream factors' demand a combination of approaches seeking to change individual behaviours as well as modifying the community structures, norms and structural issues that underpin these vulnerabilities. To enable long-term sustained changes, it is therefore imperative that the upstream factors be addressed through the programmes supported by the Global Fund. However, the danger is that awareness of the funding amount (through the Global Fund's indicative funding proposal) and the drive to demonstrate maximum impact may push organisations to offer less ambitious (low-risk) interventions or prioritise less stigmatised communities.

The human rights approach evident in this strategy runs somewhat counter to more comprehensive statements and human rights initiatives in relation to HIV, such as the International Guidelines on HIV and Human Rights published by UNAIDS, which highlights empowerment of groups facing marginalisation and abuses of rights as essential. The strategy's limited phrasing of human rights in terms of barriers to access and HIV-related rights abuses seems to be a more narrow focus than the recommended comprehensive approach addressing underlying economic, social and cultural rights.

In addition, the strategy and funding model are silent on wider systemic issues such as the role of religion or societal norms which have been identified as key human rights to address in the context of HIV. These include, for instance, traditional gender roles that disadvantage women putting them at greater risk of HIV infection, discrimination and stigma of sexual minorities or traditional cultural practices.

This silence extends to where trade agreements may limit access to medicines. The role of international legislation in relation to access to treatment was identified as a key human rights issue by the recent Commission on HIV and the Law. Addressing issues relating to intellectual property could be an opportunity for the Global Fund to address the dual concerns of reducing cost and addressing human rights.

Conclusion: the new model, a meaningful change or more of the same rhetoric?

There has been a clear, albeit uneven, shift within the Global Fund in the direction towards aid effectiveness and HSS. In its first 10 years, it has constantly evolved and repositioned itself in relation to mounting criticism. The new financing strategy is a case in point as it comes at a time when the Global Fund is battling to regain its credibility among funders and secure sustainability for its programmes amidst a triple crisis – financial, fiduciary and leadership (McCoy, Bruen, Hill, & Kerouedan, 2012).

While there is an explicit focus on making the funding model more flexible with commitment to the principles of aid effectiveness and HSS, the emerging narrative risks amplifying some of the earlier negative effects of the Global Fund on country-level systems and health outcomes. Specifically, proposals to strategically invest and reinvest in high-impact interventions and increase 'the authority of those that manage grants' risk making the Global Fund a more vertical and donor-centric mechanism concerned with bringing selective interventions with attributable outputs to scale, rather than those operating in more difficult but nevertheless important environments.

Amidst the debates on scaling-up prevention and treatment interventions to reach wider geographical regions and populations, focus on 'select regions' for 'greatest impact' runs counter to the proposed focus on human rights and a central aspect of Global Fund support: accessibility of such funding by marginalised populations everywhere. While basing funding decisions on governance, epidemiology or disease profile is understandable, the governance provisions are worrisome. The increased focus on maximising impact and numerical targets sets up tension with the human rights commitment, which remains unresolved in the current strategy. New provisions may also increase transactional costs and put pressure on recipient organisations to adjust reporting figures.

Moreover, there is an inherent contradiction and internal dissonance in the Global Fund's operating model that raises questions around the overall intent and credibility of its latest strategy: (1) attaining health system goals by targeting the three diseases and (2) according priority to short-term health goals, presented as indicators for selected services – such as retaining people on treatment, vaccinating children, scaling-up enrolment of PWHAs in networks, residual spraying of houses (for malaria) – rather than long-term goals and process-related markers of the interventions. The demand for efficiency enhancements, and the drive for managerial logics and technocratic solutions that underpin these, has gained new force in the new strategy. This significantly departs from the human rights focus that the strategy commits to.

Even though the new strategy attempts to marry the principles of aid effectiveness and HSS with the need for scale-up, the overwhelming focus on increasing efficiency and impact merit a better understanding and scrutiny of how far the revised strategy seeks redemption or offers systemic solutions to allow for effective scale-up. Aid effectiveness is as much about the conditions of aid and political dynamics and power relations that impinge on aid, as it is about better management. Given limited acknowledgement of these conditionalities and dynamics, the optimism inherent in the Global Fund strategy document and that shared by its commentators and advocates seeking aid-management reform appears short-lived.

Notes

1. This trend in the decline of rate of new infections has been rather consistent across Asia and Africa except Uganda, where the rate has been stable between 5% and 6%, as per the joint report by WHO, UNAIDS and UNICEF (2011) on the progress with HIV/AIDS response.
2. The term 'diagonal' is described by Julio Frenk (2006) as a strategy that utilises explicit intervention priorities to drive the required improvements into the health system across all its functions including human resource development, financing, facility planning, drug supply, rational prescription and quality assurance.

References

Atun, R., & Bataringaya, J. (2011). Building a durable response to HIV/AIDS: Implications for health systems. *Journal of Acquired Immune Deficiency Syndrome*, *57*(S2), 91–95. doi:10.1097/QAI.0b013e3182218441

Biesma, R. G., Brugha, R., Harmer, A., Walsh, A., Spicer, N., & Walt, G. (2009). The effects of global health initiatives on country health systems: A review of the evidence from HIV/AIDS control. *Health Policy Planning*, *24*, 239–252. doi:10.1093/heapol/czp025

Brown, J. C., & Griekspoor, W. (2013). Fraud at the Global Fund? A viewpoint. *International Journal of Health Planning and Management*, *28*(1), 138–143. doi:10.1002/hpm.2152

Brugha, R. (2008). Global health initiatives and public health policy. In K. Heggenhougen & S. Quah (Eds.), *International encyclopedia of public health* (pp. 72–81). San Diego, CA: Academic Press.

Brugha, R., Donoghue, M., Starling, M., Ndubani, P., Ssengooba, F., Fernandes, B., & Walt, G. (2004). The Global Fund: Managing great expectations. *Lancet*, *364*, 95–100. doi:10.1016/S0140-6736(04)16595-1

Brugha, R., & Walt, G. (2001). A global health fund: A leap of faith? *British Medical Journal*, *323*, 152–154. doi:10.1136/bmj.323.7305.152

Burnside, C., & Dollar. D. (2000). Aid, policies, and growth. *American Economic Review*, *90*, 847–868. doi:10.1257/aer.90.4.847

Caceres, C. F., Giron, J. M., Sandoval, C., Lopez, R., Valverde, R., Pajuelo, J., … Silva-Santisteban, A. (2010). Implementation effects of GFATM-supported HIV/AIDS projects on the health sector, civil society and affected communities in Peru 2004–2007. *Global Public Health*, *5*(3), 1–19. doi:10.1080/17441691003674154

Dodd, R., & Lane, C. (2010). Improving the long-term sustainability of health aid: Are global health partnerships leading the way? *Health Policy and Planning*, *25*, 363–371. doi:10.1093/heapol/czq014

El-Sadr, W. M., Holmes, C. B., Mugyenyi, P., Thirumurthy, H., Ellerbrock, T., Ferris, R., … Whiteside, A. (2012). Scale-up of HIV treatment through PEPFAR: A historic public health achievement. *Journal of Acquired Immune Deficiency Syndrome*, *60*(S3), S96–104. doi:10.1097/QAI.0b013e31825eb27b

England, R. (2009). The GAVI. Global Fund, and World Bank joint funding platform. *Lancet*, *374*, 1595–1596. doi:10.1016/S0140-6736(09)61951-6

Frenk, J. (2006). Bridging the divide: Global lessons from evidence-based health policy in Mexico. *Lancet*, *368*, 954–961. doi:10.1016/S0140-6736(06)69376-8

Garmaise, D. (2012). *Delayed disbursements related to Global Fund grant threaten future of South Africa's treatment action campaign*. AIDSPAN. Retreived from: http://www.aidspan.org/gfo_article/delayed-disbursements-related-global-fund-grant-threaten-future-south-africas-treatment-

Grépin, K. A., & Sridhar, D. (2012) Multi-bi aid and effects of the 2008–10 economic crisis on voluntary development assistance for health contributions: A time series analysis. *Lancet*, *380* (S3), 3. doi:10.1016/S0140-6736(13)60289-5

Gulrajani, N. (2011) Transcending the great foreign aid debate: Managerialism, radicalism and the search for aid effectiveness. *Third World Quarterly*, *32*, 199–216. doi:10.1080/01436597.2011. 560465

Hamann, J., & Bulir, A. (2001). *How volatile and unpredictable are aid flows, and what are the policy implications?* IMF Working Paper No. 01/167. Retreived from: http://www.imf.org/external/pubs/cat/longres.cfm?sk=15387.0

Hanefeld, J. (2008). How have global health initiatives impacted on health equity? *Promotion and Education*, *15*(1), 19–23. doi:10.1177/1025382307088094

Hanefeld, J. (2010). The impact of global health initiatives at national and sub-national level – A policy analysis of their role in implementation processes of antiretroviral treatment (ART) roll-out in Zambia and South Africa. *AIDS Care*, *22S*(1), 93–102. doi:10.1080/09540121003759919

Hanefeld, J., & Musheke, M. (2009). What impact do global health initiatives have on human resources for antiretroviral treatment roll-out? A qualitative policy analysis of implementation processes in Zambia. *Human Resources for Health*, *7*(8), 1–9. doi:10.1186/1478-4491-7-8

Hansen, H., & Tarp, F. (2000). Aid effectiveness disputed. *Journal of International Development*, *12*, 375–398. doi:10.1002/(SICI)1099-1328(200004)12:3<375::AID-JID657>3.0.CO;2-M

Harman, S. (2010). *The World Bank and HIV/AIDS: Setting a global agenda*. Abingdon: Routledge.

Kanki, P., & Grimes, D. J. (Eds.). (2013). *Infectious diseases: Selected entries from the encyclopedia of sustainability science and technology*. New York: Springer.

Kapilashrami, A., & McPake, B. (2012). Transforming governance or reinforcing hierarchies and competition: Examining the public and hidden transcripts of the Global Fund and HIV in India. *Health Policy and Planning*, *28*, 626–635. doi:10.1093/heapol/czs102

Kapilashrami, A., & O'Brien, O. (2012). The Global Fund and the re-configuration and re-emergence of 'civil society': Widening or closing the democratic deficit? *Global Public Health*, *7*, 437–451. doi:10.1080/17441692.2011.649043

Lane, C., & Glassman, A. (2007). Bigger and better? Scaling up and innovation in health aid. *Health Affairs*, *26*, 935–948. doi:10.1377/hlthaff.26.4.935

Mangham, L. J., & Hanson, K. (2010). Scaling up in international health: What are the key issues? *Health Policy and Planning*, *25*(2), 85–96. doi:10.1093/heapol/czp066

McCoy, D., Bruen, C., Hill, P., & Kerouedan, D. (2012). *The Global Fund: What next for aid effectiveness and health systems strengthening*. Nairobi: Aidspan publisher of the Global Fund Observer.

Rajan, R. G., & Subramanian, A. (2008). Aid and growth: What does the cross-country evidence really show? *Review of Economics and Statistics*, *90*, 643–665. doi:10.1162/rest.90.4.643

Samb, B., Evans, T., Dybul, M., Atun, R., Moatti, J. P., Nishtar, S., … Etienne C. (2009). An assessment of interactions between global health initiatives and country health systems. *Lancet*, *373*, 2137–2169. doi:10.1016/S0140-6736(09)60919-3

Sarang, A., Rhodes, T., & Sheon, N. (2012). Systemic barriers accessing HIV treatment among people who inject drugs in Russia: A qualitative study. *Health Policy and Planning*, *28*, 681–691. doi:10.1093/heapol/czs107

Slaughter, A-M. (2004). Disaggregated sovereignty: Towards the public accountability of global government networks. *Government and Opposition*, *39*, 159–190

Stuckler, D., Basu, S., Wang, S. W., & McKee, M. (2011). Does recession reduce global health aid? Evidence from 15 high-income countries, 1975–2007. *Bulletin of the World Health Organization*, *89*, 252–257. doi:10.2471/BLT.10.080663

The Global Fund to Fight AIDS, Tuberculosis and Malaria (2011). *The Global Fund strategy 2012–2016: Investing for impact*. Geneva, Switzerland: Author.

WHO, UNAIDS and UNICEF (2011). *Global HIV/AIDS response: Epidemic update and health sector progress towards universal access*. Progress Report 2011. Geneva: WHO Press.

After the Global Fund: Who can sustain the HIV/AIDS response in Peru and how?

Ana B. Amaya[a,b], Carlos F. Caceres[b], Neil Spicer[a] and Dina Balabanova[a]

[a]Department of Global Health and Development, London School of Hygiene and Tropical Medicine, London, UK; [b]Institute for Health, Sexuality, and Human Development, Universidad Peruana Cavetano Heredia, Lima, Peru

Peru has received around $70 million from Global Fund to fight AIDS, Tuberculosis and Malaria (Global Fund). Recent economic growth resulted in grant ineligibility, enabling greater government funding, yet doubts remain concerning programme continuity. This study examines the transition from Global Fund support to increasing national HIV/AIDS funding in Peru (2004–2012) by analysing actor roles, motivations and effects on policies, identifying recommendations to inform decision-makers on priority areas. A conceptual framework, which informed data collection, was developed. Thirty-five in-depth interviews were conducted from October to December 2011 in Lima, Peru, among key stakeholders involved in HIV/AIDS work. Findings show that Global Fund involvement led to important breakthroughs in the HIV/AIDS response, primarily concerning treatment access, focus on vulnerable populations and development of a coordination body. Nevertheless, reliance on Global Fund financing for prevention activities via non-governmental organisations, compounded by lack of government direction and weak regional governance, diluted power and caused role uncertainty. Strengthening government and regional capacity and fostering accountability mechanisms will facilitate an effective transition to government-led financing. Only then can achievements gained from the Global Fund presence be maintained, providing lessons for countries seeking to sustain programmes following donor exit.

Introduction

A large number of low- and middle-income countries currently receive considerable amounts of aid to support their HIV/AIDS programmes, thus making the question of how to sustain these programmes central to the international development agenda (Joint United Nations Programme on HIV/AIDS (UNAIDS), 2013). There are many definitions for sustainability, usually associated with words such as 'continuity' (Scheirer, 2005; United Nations Children's Fund (UNICEF), 1992), 'maintenance' (Gruen et al., 2008; LaPelle, Zapka, & Ockene, 2006; Shediac-Rizkallah & Bone, 1998) or 'incorporation/implementation' (Bracht et al., 1994; Pluye, Potvin, & Denis, 2004; Stefanini & Ruck, 1992). In this paper, sustainability is defined as the capability of a government to manage health programmes long term without depending on the intervention of external bodies for technical or financial support within a given social, political and economic environment.

Until 2010, Peru financed a large portion of HIV/AIDS programmes through external assistance. From 2005 to 2010, 48.6% of the funding for HIV/AIDS was provided by international organisations, 36.5% was financed by the government and 14.9% was financed by the private sector (Navarro de Acosta, 2011). Bilateral donors such as US Agency for International Development (USAID), Department for International Development (DFID), German Society for International Development (GiZ) and international organisations such as Doctors without Borders and UNAIDS played a key role in providing aid in the past (Ministerio de Salud del Peru, 2006). However, since its entry in 2004, the Global Fund to fight AIDS, Tuberculosis and Malaria (Global Fund) has been the most important financial donor for HIV/AIDS (Cabrera, 2010), providing over US$70 million in the 2004–2012 period via four approved rounds (Table 1) for the implementation of HIV/AIDS projects, primarily supporting prevention activities (Global Fund to Fight AIDS, Tuberculosis and Malaria, 2012). The percentage of Global Fund funding as a share of total HIV/AIDS expenditure fluctuated in the 2005–2010 period, the lowest point reached in 2005 with an 11% contribution and the highest in 2008 with 28% of total HIV funding (Ministerio de Salud del Peru, 2012).

Country recipients of Global Fund assistance are expected to create national structures called Country Coordination Mechanisms (CCMs) to identify priorities, develop and submit proposals according to the specific priorities and harmonise disease-specific programmes with national policies and programmes. They also act as overseers of grant implementation and liaise on emerging issues with the Global Fund (Global Fund to Fight AIDS, Tuberculosis and Malaria, 2011b). Peru established such a body of country actors in 2004, namely, the National Multisectoral Coordinating Centre in Health (CONAMUSA: Coordinadora Nacional Multisectorial de Salud), with representation of different government sectors, civil society and international stakeholders. The committee has sought to decentralise some of its functions in line with the country administrative decentralisation process and created Regional Multisectoral Coordinating Agencies for Health (CORE-MUSAs) (Buffardi, Cabello & Garcia, 2011). However, these regional coordination centres have yet to be formally registered and lack access to resources (Caceres et al., 2009).

The context of external assistance in Peru has changed. In 2011, the HIV/AIDS programmes were included into a national results-based budget, a strategy that seeks to focus government resources on key populations and achieve impact (Cabrera, 2010). Indeed, between 2011 and 2012, government investment in HIV/AIDS and tuberculosis activities grew from 0.2% of the total budget to almost 0.4% (Ministerio de Economia y Finanzas del Peru, 2012). Furthermore, Peru became an upper middle-income country due to strong economic growth in the past years (World Bank, 2013a). However, inequality levels remain high, with the World Bank (2013b) reporting a Gini coefficient index in 2010 of 48.1. Additionally, due to this upper middle-income status, Peru can now only apply for smaller Global Fund grants focused on key affected populations, as is the case for round 10 (Global Fund to Fight AIDS, Tuberculosis and Malaria, 2012). This is due to a Global Fund eligibility criterion that rates countries according to their disease burden, political commitment, effectiveness of their CCM and the poverty situation in the country (Global Fund to Fight AIDS, Tuberculosis and Malaria, 2011a).

However, there is a lack of clarity about the continuity of specific dimensions of the national HIV/AIDS response (particularly if they have been successful and are still deemed necessary) and the roles and responsibilities of different country actors. There have been justifiable concerns about the sustainability of HIV/AIDS programmes and achievements, as well as other health programmes that were created to address genuine need. In some cases, donor interest may be prematurely discontinued (Gruen et al., 2008).

Table 1. HIV/AIDS Global Fund-approved grants.

Round	Grant title	Total approved	Principal recipient	Main activities
2	'Strengthening prevention and control of AIDS in Peru'. (2004–2008)	$21,347,134	CARE Peru	• Increasing access to diagnosis, treatment and prevention of vertical transmission • Prevention actions such as prevention of mother-to-child transmission (PMTCT), sex workers and men who have sex with men (MSM) • Care among people living with HIV/AIDS (PLHA) • Prevention activities such as behavioural interventions and condom distribution programmes • Strengthening civil society and reducing stigma
5	'Closing gaps to achieve Millennium Development Goals for HIV/AIDS in Peru'. (2006–2010)	$11,702,911	CARE Peru	• Strengthen objectives set in round two with exception of antiretroviral therapy (ART) treatment which by 2007 was funded by the government
6	'National Multi-sectoral plans: Integrating resources for the Fight against HIV/AIDS in Peru'. (2007–2011).	$31,827,512	CARE Peru	• Strengthen objectives set in round five • Proposal was centred around developing decentralised activities at the national level, identifying three macro-regions: North, South-Central and Eastern
10	'Building social capital to prevent HIV and improve access to comprehensive health care without transphobia or homophobia for the transsexual, gay/MSM population in Peru'. (2012–2013).	$4,344,113 (Phase I) Phase II to be submitted in August 2013	Instituto Peruano de Paternidad Responsable (note that Phase II will be administered by PARSALUD as PR)	• Strengthening capacity among key populations of MSM and transgendered • Training community agents for prevention and care • Sensitising law enforcement officials
Total		$69,221,670		

Source: Global Fund to Fight AIDS, Tuberculosis and Malaria (2012). Peru Portfolio.

Discontinuation of programmes not only leaves unmet needs, but it can also be wasteful of human, monetary and technical investments and can decrease community trust and support for future programmes (Shediac-Tizkallah & Bone, 1998). Moreover, actor incentives and asymmetries in access to knowledge about the context in which projects are being implemented have been found to hinder sustainable development outcomes, following development assistance (Ostrom, Gibson, Shivakumar, & Andersson, 2001).

While the end goal of sustainability is relevant to many countries, the economic development of a particular country frequently determines its ability to continue to fund activities once a donor leaves (Lu, Michaud, Khan, & Murray, 2006; Ooms, 2006). Moreover, sustainability also requires the political commitment to continue to prioritise these programmes (Atun, McKee, Drobniewski, & Coker, 2005; Schell et al., 2013). A clear example is Russia, now an upper middle-income country (World Bank, 2013a), and no longer eligible for Global Fund grants, where after the end of Global Fund grants, the government reneged its commitment to continue funding for HIV prevention activities among drug users due to pressure from the church and political lobbing (Twigg, 2007). Due to this, the Global Fund convened a meeting to discuss the case and decided to provide funding for a further two years (Global Fund to Fight AIDS, Tuberculosis and Malaria, 2009; International AIDS Society, 2009). In this case, disruption is not due to scarce resources but resistance to internationally accepted best practices and state policies excluding groups that are not seen as socially deserving.

Existing evidence shows that programmes that are primarily donor-driven jeopardise the sustainability of country health programmes since they often ignore the original priorities of a country and disrupt investment in training health workers to continue the projects (Dickinson, 2008; Lele, Sarna, Govindaraj, & Konstantopoulos, 2004), creating aid dependence in the long term.

This paper seeks to enrich current knowledge on these important issues by means of a historical case study designed to capture the transition from Global Fund entry in 2004 through increased financing of HIV/AIDS programmes by the government, until 2012. This type of study is particularly relevant in the current context of fiscal constraints, where donors are targeting funding to countries that need it the most, as well as the increasing number of countries graduating from aid as their income increases (Glassman, Duran, & Sumner, 2012). Thus, the 2012–2016 Global Fund funding model focuses on investing in areas with high potential for impact and increasing the sustainability of funded programmes (Global Fund to Fight AIDS, Tuberculosis and Malaria, 2011c). The paper examines the enabling and limiting factors during this process, with a focus on actor motivation and influence on programme implementation. Furthermore, this study is based on the proposition that the Global Fund investment in the HIV response in Peru has developed the necessary structures and processes for a coordinated and sustained response from all actors towards the continuity of successful policies and interventions led by the government. The recommendations derived from this study seek to inform countries becoming less dependent on external assistance but facing similar constraints, and to contribute to the global policy debate on the effects of donor assistance on national health policies.

Framework

This study employed a historical case study approach – it involved policy analysis and was guided by a conceptual framework. A number of frameworks have sought to conceptualise sustainability of policy and programmes in the health sector (Gruen et al., 2008; LaPelle et al., 2006; Olsen, 1998; Torpey, Mwenda, Thompson, Wamuwi, & van

Damme, 2010). These vary in terms of the aspects of sustainability they refer to and the explanatory factors considered regarding how countries cope after funding ends. LaPelle et al. (2006) provide a framework based on two strategies that are based on redefining the scope of services and creatively using limited resources, yet their focus on finding funding and creating demand for services is already defined in our case. Torpey et al.'s (2010) framework is useful in differentiating between technical, programmatic, social and financial sustainability, though they concentrate on service delivery, rather than explaining the policies that made the outcome possible, which is the objective of the present study. Gruen et al.'s (2008) framework represents health programme functions as a complex system that depends on the interactions between health concerns, programme components and the programme drivers, within a specific sociocultural, political and geographical context, which are also shaped by health system characteristics and available resources. Still, this framework does not capture comparisons over time periods or inputs that make the relationships happen. Olsen's (1998) framework focuses on health services in low-income countries, based on contextual factors, activity profile and organisational capacity. Again, the model does not support the study of complex processes and the interactions between different components.

For this study, a hybrid model (Figure 1) was developed drawing on the strengths of Olsen's (1998) and Gruen et al.'s framework (2008).

This framework represents an open system (a system that functions by constantly interacting with its surroundings) where organisations are exposed to the social, political and economic context in the country and must adapt to it in order to function ('external environment'). This external environment is composed by those factors that affect health but are not part of the health system, including government policies, social indicators such as inequality and employment levels, as well as the economic context that in the case of Peru is a favourable economic environment. Moreover, this framework looks at

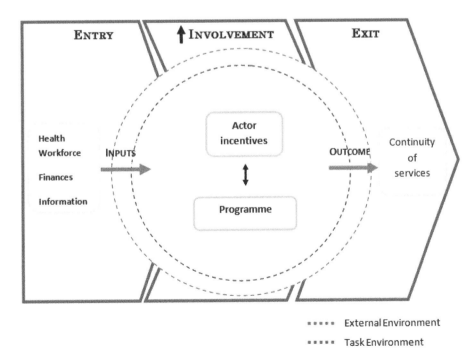

Figure 1.   Framework based on Gruen et al. (2008) and Olsen's (1998) sustainability frameworks.

inputs (resources invested in programmes), actor incentives, programme response and the outcome, which is a continuity of activities. The inputs such as the country capacity, finances and data available on the disease burden are essential for an appropriate response. These resources shape how programmes will be implemented and which actors will plan and implement these programmes. The actors and the programme are both found within the 'task environment', which are those factors related to health and HIV/AIDS that have an effect on how actors behave in the programme.

The programme component includes the HIV/AIDS policies (including financing arrangements) and activities in place, and the perceived effectiveness of the response. If actions are to take place and be sustained, it is critical to consider the incentives and the roles of the key actors including their leadership, mutual relationships and coordination of tasks, which have a direct impact on the programme. As the figure demonstrates, this relationship is bidirectional, given that actors develop programmes according to the inputs and their own priorities of what is needed, but at the same time, the programme also has an effect on actor incentives, according to the weaknesses and strengths identified when implementing the programme.

All of this has an effect on the outcome of interest, which is the continuity of activities. The framework allows these elements to be captured over time, with key phases being: (1) Global Fund entry in Peru in 2004, (2) full-blown involvement and (3) preparation for exit in 2012. Interpreting the outcomes, programmes and actor roles as they are now requires an understanding of the history of current policies and relationships.

This framework was used to identify themes and relationships emerging from the data. Given the central role of actors in the implementation of the programme, this paper specifically focused on the actor incentives and programme response components as key explanatory factors for ensuring policy and programme sustainability.

Methods

A historical case study approach was adopted for analysing the period of 2004–2012, focusing on how the behaviour of different actors enabled or hampered the move towards sustainability of national financing for HIV/AIDS programmes. The case study involved conducting 35 in-depth interviews in Lima, Peru (October–December 2011), guided by the framework, among four types of national and international stakeholders currently or formerly responsible for HIV work (Table 2). The in-depth interviews allowed us to explore predefined themes while giving the respondent freedom to bring in new perspectives and to make linkages between events and outcomes (Yin, 2003). Moreover, interview questions were adapted, if necessary, according to the respondent's expertise and decision-level in order to obtain responses that were compared to other similar respondents. Respondents were selected on the basis of their involvement in HIV work or expertise during the period of study, as well as direct or indirect participation in Global Fund projects. 'Chain sampling', a method that involved asking stakeholders to nominate other potential respondents (Mays & Pope, 2000), was also used to ensure diverse representation of relevant actors within the study.

This was complemented by a documentary review, which entailed a review of grey literature, policy documents, peer-reviewed articles and national laws and local news articles in Spanish and English on issues surrounding the HIV/AIDS programme in the country, the results-based budgeting strategy and the Global Fund proposals, published in the 2000–2012 period. Key terms included 'HIV', 'AIDS', 'financing', 'sustainability',

Table 2.   Respondent characteristics.

Sector	Number of interviews	Institutions	Positions
Government	10	Ministries of health; education; women and social development; finance and economics; foreign affairs; justice. CONAMUSA and COREMUSA leaders. Regional health leaders.	• High-level and middle-level management at the central level • Regional and local-level leaders • Coordinating mechanism leaders
International organisations	7	Bilateral (3) Multilateral (4)	• High-level and middle-level management • Programme officers
NGOs and CSOs	14	National-level NGOs and CSOs (9) Regional-level NGOs and CSOs (5)	• CSO and NGO leaders • Project implementers • Coordinating mechanism members
Academia	4	Three universities	• Heads of research units • University professors
Total	35		

'coordination', 'aid', 'decentralisation', 'Global Fund' and 'Peru'. Databases searched included MEDLINE/Pubmed, LILACS, Web of Science, Global Health, EMBASE and Google Scholar. This data provided the contextual basis for the study and informed the interpretation of main emerging themes, enabling triangulation.

Ethical approval was obtained from the Universidad Peruana Cayetano Heredia (approved 11 October 2011, Reference Number 058954) and the London School of Hygiene and Tropical Medicine (approved 7 September 2011, Reference Number 6022). Participants were provided with information, guaranteed confidentiality and asked to sign a consent form.

Following data collection, the documentary data and the interviews were analysed using the original framework mentioned in the previous section. Thematic analysis (Green & Thorogood, 2004) was used to examine the interviews and the qualitative software NVivo (version 10), provided a space to organise and code emerging themes. Specific attention was paid to interpreting the actors' roles, the meaning of the relationships and their impact on programmes and their sustainability. These interpretations were triangulated with the documentary review and analytical field notes, to arrive at policy recommendations.

Findings

A number of themes emerged from the interviews as central to explaining the process of an expanded role of national actors and moving towards sustainable HIV response. These relate first, to actor incentives (mechanisms for joint work and the power and position of civil society); second, to the nature of programme implementation (government prioritisation of the HIV response, the effect of Global Fund on policy and practice and the impact of country decentralisation as a key contextual factor affecting sustainability); and finally, the perception of the future positioning of these actors in programmes sustained at the national level. Table 3 provides an overview of the main actor roles.

Actor incentives

The Non-Governmental Organisation (NGO) dilemma

NGOs emerged as important actors due to their strong CONAMUSA representation and important role as programme implementers, especially in HIV prevention. The Global Fund funding led to the emergence and participation of many new NGOs together with older ones, which was seen (both by donor and NGOs representatives) as a positive development since it might contribute, in theory, to a more effective way of reaching vulnerable groups, strengthened the political position of these groups and increased their training and overall capacity. However, respondents from other sectors argued that the role of NGOs primarily as project executers hindered the NGOs' ability to advocate for their constituents and make the government accountable to agreements made due to NGOs' commitment to producing results. NGOs' ability to assure government accountability was identified as a key element to guarantee that successful Global Fund-funded activities would be continued:

> People Living with HIV/AIDS' organisations should return to what they should have never left, their role of social oversight … from the moment they became involved as project executers, I think they lost this role. [Academia respondent]

Moreover, the pattern of direct funding of NGOs as sub-recipients has affected the steering role of the Ministry of Health, with a government official stating that Global Fund NGO subrecipients frequently made unilateral decisions without consulting government bodies.

On the one hand, NGO leaders reported that they are organised into networks to coordinate their work towards common goals, such as demanding greater access to medications. However, on the other hand, a concern voiced by members of academia was that NGO involvement in these networks is on an adjunct basis, meaning they are not held accountable. A more important side effect has been that isolated and uncoordinated programmes led by NGOs resulted in insufficient political activism to ensure access to HIV services for all. This lack of coordination with the HIV strategy office was seen as a hindrance to a coherent response to HIV/AIDS, as well as a detriment to the constituencies these NGOs represent.

Effective coordination yet dwindling commitments

Central to the continuity of activities is the ability and commitment of the different actors to work together in a coordinated and coherent manner towards common goals. It is a widely supported view that the CONAMUSA since its constitution in 2004 has been instrumental in bringing together the main actors working with HIV and developing proposals:

> When people meet each other and develop trust, they work better together; I think this is what the Global Fund has been able to do. [NGO respondent]

However, a frequent criticism both from national and regional actors is that decision-making has been concentrated at the national level, with little input from regional leaders, as well as the lack of active involvement of other ministries besides the Ministry of

Table 3. Main actor roles.

	Main responsibilities in HIV/AIDS policies and programmes	Involvement with other actors	Level of participation in CONAMUSA	Received money from the Global Fund	Role change after Global Fund entry	Relationship with Global Fund
Government						
STI and HIV strategy office	• Leading and coordinating the HIV/AIDS response • Development of policies and plans	All sectors	High	Yes (indirectly)	None	Country counterparts; Implement certain activities
Other Ministry of Health offices (such as National Institute of Health; General Epidemiology Bureau and the National Health Insurance)	• Diagnosis • Surveillance of the epidemic • Monitoring and evaluation of activities (in part) • Funding of treatment and care (National Health Ins.)	Primarily STI & HIV strategy	Mainly delegated to the HIV strategy though the Minister of Health alternates as the head of CONAMUSA.	No (except in special cases, e.g. studies)	None	Country counterparts
Other ministries (such as the Ministries of Education; Foreign Affairs; Labour; Tourism, Women; and Social Affairs and Justice)	• The ministry of education: participates in activities related to the promotion of healthy lifestyles in adolescents and young people • The armed and police forces: contribute to the prevention and control of HIV/AIDS among their populations.	Primarily the government, NGOs and CSOs, as well as some UN agencies.	Low/medium	Yes (indirectly, primarily: education and justice)	Increased involvement in HIV activities	Country counterparts; Implement certain activities

Table 3 (*Continued*)

	Main responsibilities in HIV/AIDS policies and programmes	Involvement with other actors	Level of participation in CONAMUSA	Received money from the Global Fund	Role change after Global Fund entry	Relationship with Global Fund
•	• Others have very limited participation					
Non-Governmental Organisations (NGOs)						
HIV/AIDS service organisations	• Social advocacy to increase prevention and access to treatment and care • Main implementers for Global Fund projects	All sectors	High	Yes	Switched their role from advocacy to project implementation	Principal and sub-recipients of projects (some)
PLHA Organisations	• Support and training of their constituents • Advocate for access to treatment and improvement in care • Implementation of activities	All sectors	High	Yes	Switched their role from advocacy to project implementation	Subrecipients of projects (some)
Lesbian, gay, bisexual, and transgender (LGBT), MSM, TS and sex worker organisations	• Social advocacy • Representing their peers at the policy-level • Educating their peers • Implementation of activities	All sectors	High	Yes	Switched their role from advocacy to project implementation	Subrecipients of projects (some)

Table 3 (*Continued*)

	Main responsibilities in HIV/AIDS policies and programmes	Involvement with other actors	Level of participation in CONAMUSA	Received money from the Global Fund	Role change after Global Fund entry	Relationship with Global Fund
Faith-based organisations	• Primarily involved in the care of children and women living with HIV/AIDS	State, other NGOs and PLHA	Low	Indirectly	Increased involvement in HIV activities	None
International NGOs (e.g. CARE, Pathfinder, local International Planned Parenthood Federation [IPPF] Affiliate)	• Managing Global Fund projects • Involved in implementation of activities	All sectors	Low	Yes	Increased involvement in HIV activities	Principal and sub-recipients of projects
International Organisations						
UN agencies	• Providing technical assistance • Funding training and projects	All sectors	Low	No	Decreased funding	Supports Global Fund projects
Other bilateral organisations	• Technical assistance • Provision of funding to support government projects and research	State, NGOs and CSOs.	Low	No	Decreased funding	Supports Global Fund projects
Academia	• Conducting research • Capacity building • Contributing to the development of policy • Serving as external reviewers for Global Fund projects	All other sectors directly or indirectly.	Low	Occasionally (activity-based)	None	External reviewer of projects; occasionally as consultants

Health. Thus, many respondents from the NGO sector stated that there is no real 'multisectoral' response. This multisectoral response was an important factor for all of the actors, since it meant HIV/AIDS would be seen as a national policy priority and not only one for the health sector. This would, in their view, ensure that the HIV/AIDS response would continue to receive funding in the long term. Moreover, some respondents with health systems expertise viewed the preparation of proposals to the Global Fund as insufficiently reflective of population need but corresponding to the interests of the principal recipient or the organisations that participated in the CONAMUSA assembly.

As stated by the majority of the respondents, the work of the COREMUSAs (regional coordinating bodies) has varied in terms of performance mostly due to overburdened staff and lack of resources. However, Callao, one of the regions most strongly affected by HIV, was frequently noted by subnational respondents as an example of success mainly due to their multisectoral efforts convened through their regional committee. This was explained as resulting from committed individuals who met regularly and understood the needs in the region. In addition, round six of the Global Fund was seen among NGO leaders as having established a different way of working, from implementing projects in the regions directed from the central-level, to developing macro-region (groupings of regions)-led projects so local capacities could be strengthened; this was seen as a positive legacy of inter-regional work.

In comparison, a common perception of respondents about the relationship between the stakeholders in the long term was that a lack of commitment for collaborative work:

> There is a divorce between the State and the organisations to intervene. When it does happen it is because the funders force them to or it is part of the requirements for funding but it is not because the State wants to work closely with NGOs. [NGO respondent]

Indeed, respondents at all levels saw the rules for receiving a Global Fund grant as fostering better accountability and collaborative work across sectors and requiring political will at the government level by promoting HIV as a priority. In this sense, NGO respondents saw the Global Fund proposal process as laying the ground for stronger political commitment. This point of view was shared by several government respondents, which reported that their actions are driven not only by the need to continue the response to HIV but also to take a formal responsibility to sustain the commitments expressed in their grant proposals.

Programme implementation

The changes in actor incentives and behaviour have had a direct impact on programme implementation, both in terms of strategies and policies for HIV/AIDS and the effects of the sociopolitical decentralisation. This has been a gradual process, with complete transfer of health functions to the regions concluding in 2008.

HIV/AIDS: a national priority but with a weak strategy

Themes around planning and strategy emerged as key in the analysis of the potential for sustainability. Central to effective programming is the ability to develop and enact a strategy reflecting national priorities including the priority of HIV/AIDS in the country. All respondents agreed that a single national HIV strategy is the best approach to integrate the health, education, development and law enforcement sectors working in this area, thereby building the foundations for lasting and effective actions:

> The Multisectoral Strategic Plan has undoubtedly been an important tool for planning, but in this new government we need to build on this knowledge and motivation of the government to develop a new multisectoral plan. [NGO respondent]

However, the development of this strategy has not been easy. Respondents recalled that following a first frustrated attempt for the 2001–2003 period, the 2007–2011 Multisectoral Strategic Plan for the Prevention and Control of STIs and HIV/AIDS was approved. This strategic plan signalled that a concerted effort from different sectors would be needed to increase HIV/AIDS treatment and prevention under the leadership of the Ministry of Health (Ministerio de Salud del Peru, 2006). The shared opinion with regards to this plan was that the participation of the various actors in its development meant they were invested in working within this framework. Yet a view from the NGO sector was that the plan objectives were too ambitious both in terms of results and funding required within this time period, as well as having weak prevention strategies, especially among the most vulnerable populations, including MSM and transgender women.

Though at the time of the interviews in 2011, the appointment of the president was fairly recent, the predominant view among the respondents as compared to prior, more conservative administrations, was that HIV was a higher priority for the central government than before and was expected to continue as such. This was supported with the fact that the government included HIV/AIDS, together with TB, as a national health strategic line of the results-based budgetary strategy in 2011. This meant that HIV/AIDS programmes were given a separate budget instead of being aggregated within the general health budget, as was previously the case.

As stated by NGO leaders, although a limited number of regions have developed Regional Multisectoral Strategic Plans for HIV/AIDS, where they do exist, they are seen as more successful than the National Multisectoral Strategic Plan for STI and HIV/AIDS due to the smaller number of actors involved.

An issue negatively affecting the sustainability of actions and progress in the response was the lack of a national strategic plan for 2012–2016, which is yet to be approved. This was frequently seen as a major concern since it essentially implied that the different sectors involved continue to work under guidelines and indicators set over six years ago.

Global Fund as a facilitator for new models of working

The process of applying for and implementing Global Fund grants emerged as important preparation for setting long-term sustainable policies. The Global Fund proposals both affected and were affected by national planning processes. The development of the round six Global Fund grant in line with the objectives of the multisectoral plan was considered as key by the majority of the respondents, and this was seen as a measure of significant progress in aligning donor activities with national policy. Furthermore, although one of the objectives within the plan was to strengthen the monitoring and evaluation mechanisms to follow up on the results of the plan itself, the lack of updated and quality data remains a major concern among all of the sectors interviewed, especially within academia.

Additionally, two of the most common views among respondents of the influence of the Global Fund in long-term planning are: (1) in requiring the creation of the CONAMUSA, which has become the main multisectoral policy space to discuss HIV issues; and (2) in serving as a catalyst to implement new strategies. In this sense, it was seen as a useful mechanism to begin to pilot or expand strategies proposed by the

Ministry of Health and also an opportunity to study the cost-effectiveness of certain activities, with one respondent stating that international cooperation has the tools to operationalise plans faster and in a more effective manner than the government itself:

> There are things that operationally the international cooperation can do faster, in a more effective and efficient manner than the State itself. [NGO respondent]

The most commonly cited example by respondents of the piloting of strategies was the first phase of the Global Fund's round two grant in 2004 which was identified at that moment as an important driver for implementing health promotion activities and most importantly, increasing access to ART. By 2006, the provision of free ART was fully funded by the government, which had a positive effect on coverage and was seen to mark a first step towards sustaining the results of the Global Fund programmes. Yet this is somewhat contested by respondents from NGOs who expressed concerns that the distribution of ART often does not reach the most vulnerable populations, and the issues are compounded by the lengthy tender of the medications frequently resulting in disrupted supply.

Round 10 (approved in 2011) was seen as an important success for the NGOs since it was specifically formulated to increase access to services and decrease stigma and discrimination among MSM and transwomen, again placing greater attention on addressing this issue at the national level.

Rapid decentralisation hampering leadership and governance

The governance capacity in Peru is an essential component of ensuring continuity of successful HIV programmes. The process of decentralisation emerged as having a large effect on the central-level leadership in HIV. It was a predominant view that decentralisation took place rapidly, with insufficient preparation and without verifying capacities of different actors to act, given the transfer of responsibilities from central to regional level:

> There are still difficulties in the management capacity, which means that even though the resources are available, they may not all be planned for or implemented at the regional level. [Academia respondent]

Meanwhile, at the central level, the STI and HIV programme in the Ministry of Health was transformed in 2004 into an STI and HIV strategy office. According to government officials, this resulted in a major change in responsibilities. The head of the HIV programme who was previously director of the programme became a facilitator of HIV activities within what is now deemed a 'strategy' department.

According to some respondents, this strategy office should coordinate the work around HIV in the country. In practice, its position has at times been limited. A key source of this, identified in interviews with those working outside the government, was the technical capacity of the strategy team, which was seen as smaller compared to the one found in other larger organisations. According to academia and NGO actors, this weakness has been compounded by the significant number of personnel within the strategy team hired with Global Fund money. This was confirmed by several government officials who reported that in 2005 there were officially 3 people hired by the Ministry of Health and 10 more people hired with Global Fund support. Up until the moment the interviews were being conducted, several of those 10 people were still being funded by the Global Fund, though they were seeking to be incorporated into the regular Ministry of Health budget. Nonetheless, while certain procedures such as the purchase of ART still take place at the central level, within the present context of decentralisation, it is the regions that develop the plans and the budgets.

The prior experience with the Global Fund, which is also based on indicators and results, was expressed by members of the CONAMUSA as an important strength in transitioning to results-based budget. However, the tension between planning and managing and how the funding was implemented in the regions were evident from the beginning. It was suggested that this was primarily in terms of poorly developed plans given the budgets available, not allocating all of the funding available or deviating funds for other purposes and also what some deemed 'cultural and political' motivations.

> We have had to travel to the regions to explain that the results-based budget is to reach targets; that they can diversify a little, taking advantage of this push to fix other things that aren't working, but first they have to reach the goals...this has been an important challenge, explaining to these people who are used to the immediate political moment, the world of political campaigning, who [think that] if everything is ok right now, tomorrow is not as important. [Government respondent]

Four areas emerged among the respondents in government, academia and NGOs as the most important causes for this poor execution of budget plans for HIV activities; the plan was prematurely rolled out without proper planning, monitoring mechanisms and lack of training, which led to inappropriate identification of needs and funding requirements with short timelines. In one instance, a region had to develop the budget in four days, with very little dialogue between the central, regional and local levels and with no access to up-to-date data on health indicators and human resources distribution to inform planning. This lack of quality data also had an important effect on accountability, with respondents from academia and NGOs noting that this hampers tracking and corroborating results.

Looking towards the future: perceived contribution to sustainable programming

The perception of the actors on what sustainability entailed and their contribution to it demonstrates both their vision for the future and what they consider priority areas that need to be addressed for a sustained HIV response. It is a widely shared view that although the basic prevention activities and universal treatment would continue, there is also a need to maintain other successful prevention activities such as NGO-managed peer-promoters for health promotion and micro-finance projects – an activity the other sectors disagreed with, seeing it as a failed project – as well as ensuring the political will to continue to see HIV/AIDS as a priority issue in the long term, also linked to the financial resources from the government. The need to enhance country governance and capacity was also a concern among respondents in various sectors, given the issues in the initial years of the results-based budget. Furthermore, a common thread throughout all the interviews was that for sustainable planning, there was a need for greater advocacy and accountability of government activities on behalf of NGOs, a role that until that moment was perceived as weakened. One respondent went as far as suggesting that NGOs had to transition from a focus on their constituents to support a shared goal of increasing access to the population in general.

Yet when asked about their future roles in the post-Global Fund environment, most stakeholders believed their roles would not change. The NGO respondents were divided in their opinion, with some stating they would continue their advocacy work, albeit with less resources, while the majority were concerned about the uncertainty of how to continue their activities and supporting the need for a continued research and peer-promoter projects among their constituents. At that time they had not been approached by the Ministry of Health in participating in the results-based budget, though they expressed an interest in continuing their roles as project implementers.

The role of CONAMUSA as a space to convene different actors would end with the exit of the Global Fund, according to actors belonging to sectors outside of the government, unless efforts are made to reconfigure its mandate or a separate mechanism is created. Although some government respondents saw the CONAMUSA as a valuable mechanism, they suggested that in the long term it would no longer be necessary, given that the regions would take over the majority of planning and NGOs would cease implementing projects. Even so, many others believed the COREMUSAs, which in some regions have gained political support and have a more operational role, would likely continue to exist.

Discussion

This paper sought to examine the process of promoting sustainability of HIV programmes following the exit of a major donor, the Global Fund. This issue has received surprisingly little attention in the literature despite its relevance to multiple settings. The roles and behaviours of the main country stakeholders were analysed during the transition of Global Fund entry in 2004, with subsequent implementation of four grants, and then the increased role of national institutions in 2012, associated with the scaling down of the Global Fund involvement and how they impact and promote the sustainability of the HIV response.

Certain limitations have to be acknowledged. Some recall bias of the respondents may have occurred, given that they were asked about the history of current initiatives and policies. However, there was an effort to signpost and remind the respondents about the basic timeline of events. Inevitably, the personal interests and position of the respondents may have influenced their responses, however, this was offset by interviewing a wide-range of respondents and using triangulation to cross-examine findings. The study employed a case study methodology tailored to the unique characteristics of the country; nonetheless, there is a level of conceptual generalisability and identifying lessons that are relevant to other countries in terms of useful structures and mechanisms for sustainability.

According to the definition for sustainability employed in this study, namely, the ability of the government to manage health programmes long term without depending on the intervention of external bodies for technical or financial support, our findings demonstrate that Peru has made significant steps towards sustainability of the HIV/AIDS response. The creation of partnerships and early alignment of Global Fund activities with national policies were found to be enabling factors for sustainability. Moreover, the use of the CONAMUSA and the decentralised COREMUSAs as spaces for intersectoral discussion suggests that these working relationships can carry on in the long term. Furthermore, the inclusion of HIV/AIDS in the results-based budget and the transfer of the responsibilities to the regions demonstrate that the country is focused on improving the performance of their HIV programme and increasing access to care by maintaining some of the previous activities. A sustainable HIV/AIDS response in Peru is highly dependent on policies ensuring the continuity of successful activities. The literature shows that aligning donor activities with government policies promotes a sustainable and coherent national response (Bossert, 1990; Hay & Williams, 2005; Johnson, Hays,

Center, & Daley, 2004; Organisation for Economic Cooperation and Development (OECD), 2008, 2011; Scheirer, 2005; Tibbits, Bumbarger, Kyler, & Perkins, 2010). Furthermore, the existence of an alignment plan among different actors demonstrates that there is a demand for these activities and facilitates the institution building and strategies required by phasing-out of funding (Slob & Jerve, 2008). Peru started the process of aligning Global Fund activities with local priorities early on. This ensured that activities were integrated within the national response. However, our findings also show that prevention activities implemented by NGOs were still being prioritised.

On the other hand, the literature also shows that effective partnerships among country stakeholders is an important element of a coherent strategy and coordinated response (Johnson et al., 2004; Scheirer, 2005), as well as their ability to hold members accountable (Walsh, Mulambia, Brugha, & Hanefeld, 2012). Peru has made important progress in this area. The wide representation of actors in the CONAMUSA and their use as the main policy spaces for intersectoral dialogue on HIV issues are an important legacy of the Global Fund in the country. Despite relatively weak coordination by the HIV strategy office, these partnerships have flourished due to positive personal working relationships between actors. The use of the CONAMUSA to discuss the 2007–2011 Multisectoral Strategic Plan for the Prevention and Control of STIs and HIV/AIDS demonstrates that the CONAMUSA's contribution to policy goes beyond developing proposals for the Global Fund.

However, if these gains are to be sustained, the coordinating mechanisms will have to be promoted and strengthened and an increased focus on improving the capacities at the Ministry of Health and regional level is essential. Other major limiting factors to this sustainability are posed by the predominant role of NGOs in implementing prevention activities, at times threatening a coherent response and the still weak accountability role of NGOs as overseer of government commitments.

Consequently, in 2004–2012, the nature of the Global Fund funding in Peru has changed dramatically, with increasing participation of the government in financing the HIV programme (Ministerio de Salud del Peru, 2012). This has occurred amidst a decentralisation process and a problematic process of planning and implementing the results-based budget in the regions, pointing to the need to train the health professionals in the regions on these changes. This need for strengthening local health capacity following decentralisation is not unique to Peru. Brazil and Russia, large federal states, have faced similar challenges during their process of decentralisation primarily in ensuring role clarity (Collins, Araujo, & Barbosa, 2000) and effective decision-making (Danishevski, Balabanova, McKee, & Atkinson, 2006), though in the Russian case decision-making power is associated with historical political ties and a complex hierarchical system.

Unlike other countries, such as Ghana (Atun & Kwansah, 2011) and Mozambique (Ooms, Van Damme, & Tammermann, 2007), Peru does not require Global Fund financing to expand their ART programme, given that the government has fully financed ART provision since 2006. However, in Peru, the Global Fund has financed most HIV prevention efforts, similar to Kazakhstan (UNAIDS, 2013) and Kenya, where the majority of health promotion activities are donor funded and implemented by NGOs (Wamani, 2004). Moreover, though the basic prevention activities are included in the results-based budgets, there is still uncertainty about the targeted prevention work focused on vulnerable populations, particularly since there is no national precedent of contracting NGOs to deliver services paid by public budgets. Some of the problems that emerge have parallels in India, experiencing rapid economical growth and involving NGOs in project implementation (Chakma, 2013) but facing challenges in ensuring efficient monitoring mechanisms and accountability structures to ensure that public grants are reaching the most vulnerable populations.

Indeed, Peru is unique in many ways due to the ongoing process of decentralisation and increased economic growth, yet there are a number of patterns that emerge and can inform other settings. The difficulty in reaching vulnerable populations is relevant for other countries, particularly those that are also experiencing economic growth, given that this growth has frequently been associated with increased social and economic inequality (Kuznets, 1955; Morrison, 2000). This is concerning for stakeholders working in the HIV/AIDS field, given the rise in prevalence in many countries among traditionally socially excluded groups, making it crucial to consider the effects of both economic and social inequality on the HIV/AIDS response and generate strategies to address these effects.

Additionally, the predominant role of NGOs in Peru in prevention programmes at times making unilateral decisions threatened a coherent programme response and undermined the coordinating role of the Ministry of Health-based HIV strategy office. Similar governance issues as a result of new partnership models have been found in multiple settings (Caines et al., 2004; Kapilashrami & McPake, 2013; Oomman, Bernstein, & Rosenzweig, 2008; Spicer et al., 2010; World Health Organization Maximizing Positive Synergies Collaborative Group (WHOMPS), 2009). An example of this is found in Zambia where US President's Emergency Plan for AIDS Relief (PEPFAR) support of civil society was observed to be at the cost of building government capacity (Oomman et al., 2008). Moreover, the literature shows that this focus of NGOs on project implementation may have negative effects on the vulnerable populations these organisations are meant to serve, which, in their work with international bodies, refocus their agendas on short-term interventions (Kapilashrami & O'Brien, 2012; Seckinelgin, 2005), also resulting in a loss of legitimacy of their original role (Doyle & Patel, 2008; Kapilashrami & O'Brien, 2012; Spicer et al., 2011).

However, the transitional period where Global Fund support was phased out also presents an opportunity for NGOs to retake this social accountability role. Similar to the agreements signed at CONAMUSA to remain independent of decision-making when applying for funding (Ministerio de Salud del Peru, 2006), NGOs should also commit to being accountable themselves in the long-term, via self-regulation with a supporting enforcement structure either at the sectoral or national level, or through independent assessments (Lloyd, 2005). However, this study clearly demonstrates that the role of the HIV/AIDS strategy office – through its central coordinating, oversight and advisory role in relation to the regions – is key in ensuring sustainable HIV policy and programmes.

Conclusion

The study findings demonstrate some of the enabling and limiting factors for sustainability of the HIV/AIDS response in Peru. Important enabling factors identified for sustainability of the HIV/AIDS programme in the country have been the creation of spaces for intersectoral work, early alignment of grant activities with local policies, focus on most-at-risk populations and (in theory) universal access to treatment. The inclusion of HIV/AIDS activities into the new budgetary strategy based on results also points to increased political willingness to allocate an appropriate budget to address the HIV/AIDS epidemic according to need. However, factors limiting the sustainability of the response were found to be associated with poor technical capacity at the central and regional level, the weakened social advocacy and accountability role of all actors and the threat posed by a predominant role of NGOs in prevention activities to a coherent HIV/AIDS response.

Addressing the weaknesses in the HIV strategy office will not only support the overall response to HIV/AIDS by improving the coordination of activities and the provision of guidance for the regions but will also result in generating more productive and effective partnerships. This requires both investing in training policy-makers on managerial and technical skills, as well as increasing their budget, so they have the resources necessary to respond to the demanding task of liaising with 25 regions. Increasing the advocacy and social accountability role of the NGOs and CSOs is critical to ensure that government commitments are maintained and that HIV/AIDS continues to be a political priority, according to needs.

Moreover, as our findings demonstrate, sustainability is not only about continuing prior activities but also evolving strategies which respond to new evidence, resources and need. The changes brought about by economic growth and increased social inequality, which can result in greater difficulty reaching most-at-risk populations, are examples of possible future challenges that the government will need to tackle. However, this will only be successful if the foundations for sustainability are in place; the nine-year presence of the Global Fund has catalysed some of these processes, but it is now the responsibility of the country actors to sustain and build on these gains.

References

Atun, R., & Kwansah, J. (2011). Critical interactions between the global fund-supported HIV programs and the health system in Ghana. *Journal of Acquired Immune Deficiency Syndrome, 57*, S72–S76. doi:10.1097/QAI.0b013e318221842a

Atun, R., McKee, M., Drobniewski, F., & Coker, R. (2005). Analysis of how the health systems context shapes responses to the control of human immunodeficiency virus: Case studies from the Russian Federation. *Bulletin of the World Health Organization, 83*, 730–738.

Bossert, T. J. (1990). Can they get along without us? Sustainability of donor-supported health projects in Central America and Africa. *Social Sciences of Medicine, 30*, 1015–1023. doi:10.1016/0277-9536(90)90148-L

Bracht, N., Finnegan, J. R., Rissel, C., Weisbrod, R., Gleason, J., Corbett, J., & Veblen-Mortenson, S. (1994). Community ownership and program continuation following a health demonstration project. *Health Education Research, 9*, 243–255. doi:10.1093/her/9.2.243

Buffardi, A., Cabello, R., & Garcia, P. (2011, March). *The chronicles of CONAMUSA: Institutional strategies to overcome shared governance challenges*. Paper presented at the Annual Convention of the International Studies Association, Montreal.

Cabrera, A. (2010). *Propuesta de alineamiento de los planes de sostenbilidad y transferencia de los objetivos del programa de la ronda 6 con el presupuesto por resultados del programa estrategico de prevencion y control del VIH y SIDA y otros instrumentos del marco rector nacional* [Proposal for the alignment of the sustainability and transfer plans of the round 6 objectives with the results-based budget of the strategic programme for the prevention and control of HIV/AIDS and other national policies]. Lima: ONUSIDA.

Caceres, C., Giron, M., Sandoval, C., Lopez, R., Pajuelo, J., Valverde, R., ... Rosasco, A.M. (2009). Effects of the implementation of global fund-supported HIV/AIDS projects on health systems, civil society and affected communities, 2004–2007. In The Maximizing Positive Synergies Academic Consortium (Ed.), *Interactions between global health initiatives and health systems: Evidence from countries* (pp. 134–143). Geneva: World Health Organization.

Caines, K., Buse, K., Carlson, C., de-Loor, R., Druce, N., Grace, C., ... Sadanandan, R. (2004). *Assessing the impact of global health partnerships*. London: DFID Health Resource Centre.

Chakma, S. (2013). *India's funds to NGOs squandered*. New Delhi: Asian Centre for Human Rights.

Collins, C., Araujo, J., & Barbosa, J. (2000). Decentralising the health sector: Issues in Brazil. *Health Policy, 52*, 113–127. doi:10.1016/S0168-8510(00)00069-5

Danishevski, K., Balabanova, D., McKee, M., & Atkinson, S. (2006). The fragmentary federation: Experiences with the decentralized health system in Russia. *Health Policy and Planning, 21*, 183–194. doi:10.1093/heapol/czl002

Dickinson, C. (2008). *Global health initiatives and health system strengthening: The challenges of providing technical support.* London: HLSP Institute.

Doyle, C., & Patel, P. (2008). Civil society organizations and global health initiatives: Problems of legitimacy. *Social Science and Medicine, 66*, 1928–1938. doi:10.1016/j.socscimed.2007.12.029

Glassman, A., Duran, D., & Sumner, A. (2012). Global health and the new bottom billion: What do shifts in global poverty and disease burden mean for donor agencies? *Global Policy, 4*, 1–14. doi:10.1111/j.1758-5899.2012.00176.x

Global Fund to Fight AIDS, Tuberculosis and Malaria. (2009). *Global Fund to provide $24 million of new funding to fight HIV/AIDS in Russia [Press release].* Retrieved from http://www.theglobalfund.org/en/mediacenter/newsreleases/2009-11-13_Global_Fund_to_provide_USD_24_million_of_new_funding_to_fight_HIV_AIDS_in_Russia/

Global Fund to Fight AIDS, Tuberculosis and Malaria. (2011a). *Policy on eligibility criteria, counterpart financing requirements, and prioritization of proposals for funding from the global fund.* Geneva: Author.

Global Fund to Fight AIDS, Tuberculosis and Malaria. (2011b). *Guidelines and requirements for country coordinating mechanisms.* Retrieved from http://www.theglobalfund.org/en/ccm/guidelines/

Global Fund to Fight AIDS, Tuberculosis and Malaria. (2011c). *The global fund strategy 2012–2016: Investing for Impact.* Geneva: Author.

Global Fund to Fight AIDS, Tuberculosis and Malaria. (2012). *Peru – Grant portfolio.* Retrieved from http://portfolio.theglobalfund.org/en/Grant/List/PER

Green, J., & Thorogood, N. (2004). *Qualitative methods for health research.* London: Sage.

Gruen, R., Elliot, J., Nolan, M., Lawton, P., Parkhill, A., McLaren, C., & Lavis, J. (2008). Sustainability science: An integrated approach for health-programme planning. *The Lancet, 372*, 1579–1589. doi:10.1016/S0140-6736(08)61659-1

Hay, R., & Williams, G. (2005). *Fiscal space and sustainability from the perspective of the health sector.* In High Level Forum on the Health Millennium Development Goals, K. Cahill, World Health Organization, World Bank (Eds.), *High-level forum on the health millennium development goals: Selected papers 2003–2005* (pp. 44–66). Geneva: World Health Organization.

International AIDS Society. (2009). *Global Fund extension of HIV prevention programmes for people at high risk for HIV in Russia will save thousands of young lives* [Press release]. Retrieved from http://www.iasociety.org/Default.aspx?pageId=383

Johnson, K., Hays, C., Center, H., & Daley, C. (2004). Building capacity and sustainable prevention innovations: A sustainability planning model. *Evaluation and Program Planning, 27*, 135–149. doi:10.1016/j.evalprogplan.2004.01.002

Joint United Nations Programme on HIV/AIDS (UNAIDS). (2013). *Efficient and sustainable HIV responses: Case studies on country progress.* Geneva: Author.

Kapilashrami, A., & McPake, B. (2013). Transforming governance or reinforcing hierarchies and competition: Examining the public and hidden transcripts of the global fund and HIV in India. *Health Policy and Planning, 28*, 626–635. doi:10.1093/heapol/czs102

Kapilashrami, A., & O'Brien, O. (2012). The global fund and the re-configuration and re-emergence of 'civil society': Widening or closing the democratic deficit? *Global Public Health, 7*, 437–451. doi:10.1080/17441692.2011.649043

Kuznets, S. (1955). Economic growth and income inequality. *American Economic Review, 65*, 1–28.

LaPelle, N., Zapka, J., & Ockene, J. (2006). Sustainability of public health programs: The example of tobacco treatment services in Massachusetts. *American Journal of Public Health, 96*, 1363–1369. doi:10.2105/AJPH.2005.067124

Lele, U., Sarna, N., Govindaraj, R., & Konstantopoulos, Y. (2004). *Global health programs, millennium development goals and the World Bank's role.* Addressing challenges of globalization: An independent evaluation of the World Bank's approach to global programs. Washington, DC: World Bank.

Lloyd, R. (2005). *The role of NGO self-regulation in increasing stakeholder accountability.* London: One World Trust.

Lu, C., Michaud, C., Khan, K., & Murray, C. (2006). Absorptive capacity and disbursements by the Global Fund to fight AIDS, Tuberculosis and Malaria: Analysis of grant implementation. *The Lancet, 368*, 483–488. doi:10.1016/S0140-6736(06)69156-3

Mays, N., & Pope, C. (2000). Qualitative research in health care: Assessing quality in qualitative research. *British Medical Journal, 320*, 50–52. doi:10.1136/bmj.320.7226.50

Ministerio de Economia y Finanzas del Peru. (2012). *Consulta amigable: Consulta de ejecucion del gasto* [Friendly query: Data on spending] [Data set]. Retrieved from http://ofi.mef.gob.pe/transparencia/Navegador/default.aspx?*y*=2011&ap=ActProy

Ministerio de Salud del Peru. (2006). *Plan estrategico multisectorial para la prevencion y control de las ITS y el VIH/SIDA en el Peru (2007–2011)* [Strategic multisectoral plan for the prevention and control of STIs and HIV/AIDS in Peru (2007–2011)]. Lima: Author.

Ministerio de Salud del Peru. (2012). *Informe nacional sobre los progresos realizados en el país* [National report on country progress]. Lima: Author.

Morrison, C. (2000). Historical perspectives on income distribution: The case of Europe. In A. B. Atkinson & F. Bourguignon (Eds.), *Handbook of income distribution* (pp. 220–259). Amsterdam: North-Holland.

Navarro de Acosta, M. (2011). *Medicion del gasto en SIDA – MEGAS* [Measuring spending in AIDS]. Lima: Ministerio de Salud.

Olsen, I. (1998). Sustainability of health care: A framework for analysis. *Health Policy and Planning, 13*, 287–295. doi:10.1093/heapol/13.3.287

Oomman, N., Bernstein, M., & Rosenzweig, S. (2008). *The numbers behind the stories*. Washington, DC: Center for Global Development.

Ooms, G. (2006). Health development versus medical relief: The illusion versus the irrelevance of sustainability. *PloS Medicine, 3*, e345. doi:10.1371/journal.pmed.0030345

Ooms, G., Van Damme, W., & Temmermann, M. (2007). Medicines without doctors: Why the Global Fund must fund salaries of health workers to expand AIDS treatment. *PloS Medicine, 4*, e128. doi:10.1371/journal.pmed.0040128

Organisation for Economic Cooperation and Development (OECD). (2008). *Paris declaration and Accra Plan of action*. Paris: Author.

Organisation for Economic Cooperation and Development (OECD). (2011). *Busan partnership for effective development co-operation*. Retrieved from http://www.oecd.org/dac/effectiveness/49650173.pdf

Ostrom, E., Gibson, C., Shivakumar, S., & Andersson, K. (2001). *Aid, incentives and sustainability: An institutional analysis of development cooperation*. Stockholm: SIDA.

Pluye, P., Potvin, L., & Denis, J. L. (2004). Making public health programs last: Conceptualizing sustainability. *Evaluation and Program Planning, 27*, 121–133. doi:10.1016/j.evalprogplan.2004.01.001

Scheirer, M. A. (2005). Is sustainability possible? A review and commentary on empirical studies of program sustainability. *American Journal of Evaluation, 26*, 320–347. doi:10.1177/1098214005278752

Schell, S., Luke, D., Schooley, M., Elliot, M., Herbers, S., Mueller, N., & Bunger, A. (2013). Public health program capacity for sustainability: A new framework. *Implementation Science, 8*, 15. doi:10.1186/1748-5908-8-15

Seckinelgin, H. (2005). Time to stop and think: HIV/AIDS, global civil society, and people's politics. In H. Anheir, M. Glasius, & M. Calder (Eds.), *Global civil society* (pp. 109–136). Oxford: Oxford University Press.

Shediac-Rizkallah, M., & Bone, L. (1998). Planning for sustainability of community-based health programs: Conceptual frameworks and future directions for research, practice and policy. *Health Education Research, 13*, 87–108. doi:10.1093/her/13.1.87

Slob, A., & Jerve, A. M. (2008). *Managing aid exit and transformation: Lessons from Botswana, Eritrea, India, Malawi and South Africa: Synthesis report*. Joint donor evaluation. Stockholm: Sida.

Spicer, N., Aleshkina, J., Biesma, R., Brugha, R., Caceres, C., Chilundo, B., … Zhang, X. (2010). National and subnational HIV/AIDS coordination: Are global health initiatives closing the gap between intent and practice? *Globalization and Health, 6*(1), 3. doi:10.1186/1744-8603-6-3

Spicer, N., Harmer, A., Aleshkina, J., Bogdan, D., Chkhatarashvili, K., Murzalieva, G., … Walt, G. (2011). Circus monkeys or change agents? Civil society advocacy for HIV/AIDS in adverse policy environments. *Social Science and Medicine*, *73*, 1748–1755. doi:10.1016/j.socscimed. 2011.08.024

Stefanini, A., & Ruck, N. (1992). *Managing externally assisted health projects for sustainability – A framework for assessment*. Leeds: University of Leeds.

Tibbits, M. K., Bumbarger, B. K., Kyler, S. J., & Perkins, D. F. (2010). Sustaining evidence-based interventions under real-world conditions: Results from a large-scale diffusion project. *Prevention Science*, *11*, 252–262. doi:10.1007/s11121-010-0170-9

Torpey, K., Mwenda L., Thompson, C., Wamuwi, E., & van Damme, W. (2010). From project aid to sustainable HIV services: A case study from Zambia. *Journal of the International AIDS Society*, *13*, 19. doi:10.1186/1758-2652-13-19

Twigg, J. (2007). *HIV/AIDS in Russia: Commitment, resources, momentum, challenges*. Washington, DC: Centre for Strategic and International Studies.

United Nations Children's Fund (UNICEF). (1992). *Health policies and strategies, sustainability, integration and national capacity-building*. New York, NY: Author.

Walsh, A., Mulambia, C., Brugha, R., & Hanefeld, J. (2012). "The problem is ours, it is not CRAIDS". Evaluating sustainability of community based organisations for HIV/AIDS in a rural district in Zambia. *Globalization and Health*, *8*, 40. doi:10.1186/1744-8603-8-40

Wamani, R. (2004). *NGO and public health systems: Comparative trends in transforming health systems in Kenya and Finland*. Paper presented at the International Society for third sector research, Toronto, July 2004.

World Bank. (2013a). *Country and lending groups*. Retrieved from http://data.worldbank.org/about/ country-classifications/country-and-lending-groups#Upper_middle_income

World Bank. (2013b). *Data: GINI index*. Retrieved from http://data.worldbank.org/indicator/SI. POV.GINI

World Health Organization Maximizing Positive Synergies Collaborative Group (WHOMPS). (2009). An assessment of interactions between global health initiatives and country health systems. *The Lancet*, *373*, 2137–69. doi:10.1016/S0140-6736(09)60919-3

Yin, R. (2003). *Case study research: Design and methods*. Thousand Oaks, CA: Sage.

Confronting 'scale-down': Assessing Namibia's human resource strategies in the context of decreased HIV/AIDS funding

Liita-Iyaloo Cairney[a] and Anuj Kapilashrami[b]

[a]Global Public Health Unit, Social Policy, School of Social & Political Sciences, University of Edinburgh, Edinburgh, UK; [b]Institute for International Health & Development, Queen Margaret University, Edinburgh, UK

In Namibia, support through the Global Fund and President's Emergency Plan for AIDS Relief has facilitated an increase in access to HIV and AIDS services over the past 10 years. In collaboration with the Namibian government, these institutions have enabled the rapid scale-up of prevention, treatment and care services. Inadequate human resources capacity in the public sector was cited as a key challenge to initial scale-up; and a substantial portion of donor funding has gone towards the recruitment of new health workers. However, a recent scale-down of donor funding to the Namibian health sector has taken place, despite the country's high HIV and AIDS burden. With a specific focus on human resources, this paper examines the extent to which management processes that were adopted at scale-up have proven sustainable in the context of scale-down. Drawing on data from 43 semi-structured interviews, we argue that human resources planning and management decisions made at the onset of the country's relationship with the two institutions appear to be primarily driven by the demands of rapid scale-up and counter-productive to the sustainability of interventions.

Introduction

The Global Fund to Fight AIDS, Tuberculosis and Malaria (Global Fund) and the President's Emergency Plan for AIDS Relief (PEPFAR) emerged in the wake of the Millennium Development Goals (MDGs). Both initially had the objective to facilitate the rapid scale-up of HIV and AIDS interventions in countries that had not proven to be able to do so by themselves (The Global Fund, 2013b; United States AIDS, Leadership Against HIV/AIDS, Tuberculosis, and Malaria Act of Tuberculosis, and Malaria Act, 2003). Commonly referred to as Global Health Initiatives (GHIs), the Global Fund and PEPFAR have been the international actors most credited for the significant increase in access to HIV and AIDS prevention, treatment and care services that has occurred in sub-Saharan Africa within the past 10 years (Banati, 2008; Biesma et al., 2009; Caines et al., 2004; Dodd & Lane, 2010; Hanefeld & Musheke, 2009; Ravishankar et al., 2009; World Health Organization (WHO) Maximizing Positive Synergies Collaborative Group, 2009).

As has been the case in other African countries, human resources capacity was found to be a limiting factor to the initial Global Fund and PEPFAR supported scale-up of AIDS interventions in Namibia (Banteyerga, Brugha & Stillman, 2006; Biesma et al., 2009; Drager, Gedik, & Dal Poz, 2006; Gaye & Nelson, 2009; Hanefeld & Musheke, 2009; Mtonya, Mwapasa, & Kadzandira, 2005; Oomman, Bernstein, Center for Global Development, & HIV/AIDS Monitor, 2008). At the onset of the Namibian government's relationship with the GHIs, the country's public health sector was found to lack the adequate number of health workers who were also sufficiently skilled to handle a quick rise in HIV and AIDS services. To address these deficits, a large portion of Global Fund and PEPFAR funding to the government went towards recruiting new health workers.

In 2011, the World Bank (2013) increased Namibia's economic ranking from middle-income to upper middle-income status. Concurrently, both the Global Fund and PEPFAR have also experienced shifts in their global funding priorities. Countries such as Namibia, which are viewed as having the ability pay for their own HIV and AIDS interventions, are now expected to take on a greater share of the financial burden that had been previously borne by GHIs. As a result of these funding shifts, the Namibian health system has experienced a reduction in Global Fund and PEPFAR funding to human resources in the past two years.

GHIs and human resources in the literature

Although funding from the Global Fund and PEPFAR has been credited for expanding human resources capacity in recipient countries, both GHIs have also been criticised for not doing so in a sustainable manner. Research has shown that their gains are often achieved through grant management and service provision processes parallel to those that already exist in the countries that they fund. As a result, GHI funding for HIV and AIDS has been found to undermine the health systems of recipient countries, some of which were already weak to begin with (Atun, de Jongh, Secci, Kelechi, & Adeyi, 2009; Banati, 2008; Banteyerga et al., 2006; Biesma et al., 2009; Brugha et al., 2005; Dodd & Lane, 2010; Hanefeld, 2010; Le Loup, Fleury, Camargo, & Larouzé, 2009; WHO Maximizing Positive Synergies Collaborative Group, 2009).

With regard to human resources, the literature on the health system impacts of GHIs has predominantly focused on the tensions that parallel structures create at the service delivery level. In countries such as Ethiopia, Benin, Mozambique, Zambia and Uganda, funding from both the Global Fund and PEPFAR initiatives has been used to exclusively train and pay health workers to provide HIV and AIDS interventions in parallel to those that already exist. GHI-funded staff often earn more attractive employment benefits, including higher salaries, than their public sector counterparts. Thus Global Fund and PEPFAR increases in human resources capacity have been found to occur at the expense of wider health system strengthening of recipient countries, by siphoning away workers from often under-staffed government-supported interventions (Banteyerga et al., 2006; Brugha, Simbaya, Walsh, Dicker, & Ndubani, 2010; Caines et al., 2004; Carlson, Druce, Sadanandan, Sancho, & De Loor, 2004; Dickinson, Attawell, & Druce, 2009; Drager et al., 2006; Hanefeld & Musheke, 2009; Mtonya et al., 2005; Oomman et al., 2008; WHO Maximizing Positive Synergies Collaborative Group, 2009).

This paper focuses on the grant management level of GHI operations with regard to human resources. Using Namibia as a case study, it presents a historical and longitudinal analysis of how funding through the Global Fund and PEPFAR initiatives has influenced health worker capacity in the country. We draw on data from 43 semi-structured interviews carried out between 2012 and 2013 with respondents associated with the AIDS programme in Namibia. Through case study data on salary-level changes in response to the Global Fund and PEPFAR's influence on recruitment practices, we evaluate the extent to which the human resources tensions evident in the time of financial scale-down are a reflection of management and planning decisions made at scale-up by the GHIs and the Namibian government.

Policy context and HIV/AIDS in Namibia

Since the country's independence in 1990, the Namibian government, through the Ministry of Health and Social Services (MoHSS), has been the primary provider of health services. The country has one of the highest total government health expenditures per capita and the lowest out-of-pocket payments for patients in Africa (Leive & Xu, 2008; MoHSS, 2005). On average, Namibians pay less than 10% of overall health visit costs in out-of-pocket payments, as opposed to 40% in many other African countries, and over 60% in the Ivory Coast and Chad (Leive & Xu, 2008). Namibia, however, has high inequalities in income, which means that government initiatives aimed at extending universal and affordable access to health care are diluted by the poverty in which many people live (Iipinge, Hofnie, van der Westhuizen, & Pendukeni, 2006; MoHSS, 2010; Zere et al., 2006).

Health system expenditures in Namibia have also been impacted by the rise of the HIV and AIDS epidemic. The country currently has a generalised, mature HIV and AIDS epidemic, which is primarily marked by heterosexual transmission of the HIV virus (MoHSS & ICF Macro, 2010; MoHSS, 2008, 2009). The first reported incident of HIV/AIDS in Namibia was in 1986. Between 1992 and 2000, overall rates of HIV infection in the country rose from 4% to 22.3% (MoHSS, 2010; MoHSS: Directorate of Special Programs, 2008).

Through its own contributions and support from the Global Fund and PEPFAR, the Namibian government undertook a rapid scale-up of HIV treatment. In 2002–2003, it piloted free prevention of mother-to-child transmission (PMTCT) and free antiretroviral therapy (ART). By 2010, it had scaled up to all 34 district hospitals and 250 health facilities and clinics (MoHSS 2010). As a result, the ART coverage rate in Namibia rose from 3% in 2003 to 90% by 2010 (MoHSS 2010; PEPFAR Namibia 2012). Due to a wide range of HIV/AIDS services, including behavioural interventions, the general HIV prevalence rate in Namibia also decreased to 13.3% by 2010, and has since plateaued (MoHSS, 2010; PEPFAR Namibia, 2012).

Global Fund and PEPFAR contributions to HIV/AIDS in Namibia

To date, Namibia has been a recipient of grants in five different rounds of Global Fund funding, two of which have been for HIV and AIDS. The country first received funding for HIV and AIDS in January 2004 under Round 2 (Kaiser Family Foundation, 2012; The Global Fund, 2004). The country was then invited to apply for a continuation of its Round 2 HIV and AIDS grant under the Rolling Continuation Channel (RCC); for which it began to receive funding in June 2010. At the time of this research, in early 2012, the RCC grant was in its second year of a six-year grant agreement. In total, the Global Fund has approved US$323,696,364 for HIV and AIDS interventions in Namibia (Kaiser Family Foundation, 2012).

For PEPFAR, Namibia has been a recipient of both Phase 1 and Phase 2 funding, which was authorised by the United States Congress in 2003 and 2008, respectively (PEPFAR Namibia, 2012). Due to its high HIV and AIDS burden at the time, Namibia was chosen as 1 of the 15 'focus countries' that received a bulk of the funding under Phase 1. In Phase 2, the 'focus country' category was removed, but Namibia has remained in the top 10 highest recipients of PEPFAR funding. Between 2004 and 2011, the country received a total of approximately US$102,600,000 PEPFAR funds for HIV and AIDS interventions (Kaiser Family Foundation, 2011; PEPFAR, 2011; PEPFAR Namibia, 2012).

The Ministry of Health has been the single largest recipient of PEPFAR and Global Fund revenues in Namibia. It was the sole principle recipient (PR) and a sub-recipient for Global Fund Round 2; and one of two PRs and a sub-recipient for RCC. As a result, it has served as both a principal funding agent and service provider for Global Fund resources in the country. The Ministry has received PEPFAR funds through its partnership with the US Centres for Disease Control and Prevention (CDC) in Namibia, which has mainly gone towards the provision of clinical HIV and AIDS services at government-run facilities (MoHSS and CDC, 2010; PEPFAR Namibia, 2012).

Overview of GHI impacts on the Namibian health and funding shifts

In the budget year 2001/2002, 2 years prior to the arrival of GHI funding, the Namibian government accounted for 63.3% of funding to the Namibian health sector, while donors only contributed 3.8% (MoHSS, 2008). When the Global Fund and PEPFAR arrived in Namibia, the country had witnessed a change in its economic ranking from low-income to middle-income status (MoHSS, 2005, 2008). Notwithstanding this transition, within 2 years of their arrival, in 2006/2007, the proportion of government funding to the health sector had declined to 44%, while donor contributions had increased to 22.4%. The Ministry of Health's share of donor funding, in turn, also increased from 5% in 2001/ 2002 to 14% in 2006/2007 (MoHSS, 2008).

The proportional changes in total donor funding to the health sector imply reduced financial commitments by the Namibian government. Global Fund and PEPFAR funding to the country have in fact been 'in addition' to increased investments by the government. In 2000/2001, the Namibian government contributed US$165 million out of the total US $261 million total funding to the health sector for that year. By 2006/2007 the government's contributions had increased by approximately 30% to US$241 million. Due to GHI contributions total health sector spending for 2006/2007 had also increased to US$549 million (MoHSS, 2008). Increased government investments in the Namibian health system appeared proportionately lower due to the higher allocations from the Global Fund and PEPFAR.

In 2011, the World Bank (2013) further increased Namibia's economic ranking from middle-income to upper middle-income status. Concurrently, the 2008 global financial crisis combined with resource constraints within the GHIs, especially Global Fund, led to a decline in funding availability and shift in donor priorities. As a result, after approving grants for Round 8, the Global Fund (2011) called for a 10% reduction in all approved budgets. In 2011, at the onset of Round 11, the Global Fund again cancelled funding for all countries (Health Gap, 2011). In 2013, the Global Fund released its new funding model, which aims to gives priority to low-income countries with high burden of HIV. Although Namibia has one of the highest burdens of HIV and AIDS globally, the Global Fund considers it as having a high ability to pay for its own interventions due to its economic ranking (The Global Fund, 2013a). Under the new funding model, the Global Fund will allocate resources to countries such as Namibia based on their willingness to pay for their own interventions rather than their demonstrated burden of disease, as had previously been the case.

PEPFAR's global transformation was reflected in the difference between the objectives of the 2003 and 2008 funding authorisations. The legislation for the second phase of funding emphasised a focus on 'sustainability', when compared to Phase 1. The Phase 1 PEPFAR legislation and strategy documents emphasised the emergency nature of the AIDS epidemic at the time and sought to fund the rapid scale-up of existing interventions. The goals of phase 2, on the other hand, were defined as seeking to 'maintain, sustain and expand' upon the successes from phase 1 (Tom Lantos and Henry J. Hyde United States Global Leadership Against HIV/ AIDS, Tuberculosis, and Malaria Reauthorization Act, 2008; United States AIDS, Leadership Against HIV/AIDS, Tuberculosis, and Malaria Act of Tuberculosis, and Malaria Act, 2003).

According to PEPFAR officials in Namibia, the country was considered a rapid scale-up success, particularly in relation to the GHI's partnership with the Ministry of Health. In 2011, the US Government made the decision to phase out PEPFAR funding from the country by 2015. Thus although both Global Fund and PEPFAR resources have enabled the expansion of HIV interventions in Namibia, there is growing impetus from both GHIs for Namibia to take on a greater portion of the financing of the interventions.

GHI influences on human resources scale-up in the Ministry of Health

When the Ministry of Health began its relationship with the Global Fund and PEPFAR, the Ministry of Health was perceived to lack the necessary human resources capacity to absorb the level of funding provided by the GHIs. In the year 2000, for Namibia as a whole, there were about 7500 people per public service doctor, and about 950 people per registered nurse for the total population of 2 million (El Obeid, 2001). Of the medical officers who were available to the public sector, more than 55% of doctors in Namibia were expatriates (El Obeid, 2001). Namibia did not have a medical school until 2010, and the indigenous doctors were all trained abroad. As a result, GHI resources arrived in a context where there was a general shortage of skilled personnel in the public health system in terms of doctors, senior managers and other specialists.

According to a CDC technical adviser associated with the PEPFAR programme in Namibia, 'there were too many vacancies in the field and the government was simply unable to recruit and hire people fast enough to allow for the rapid scale-up of the ART services'. Building health worker capacity, both in terms of increasing the number of workers available and improving the skill set of existing staff, was treated as a critical component of PEPFAR and Global Fund interventions in Namibia. For all the Ministry of Health's grants from Global Fund and PEPFAR, human resources has been the highest cost category (K. Kahuure, personal communication, December 11, 2011; MoHSS, 2009; MoHSS and CDC, 2010; Office of the Inspector General: USAID, 2011).

In terms of human resources, GHI funding has mainly gone towards the recruitment of additional staff to support the public sector's roll-out of the ART and PMTCT services (Global Fund OIG, 2012). The Ministry of Health has also used GHI funds to implement a task-shifting model for service delivery. This approach progressively equips nurses to initiate ART at health care sites with clinical support supervision from medical officers (Global Fund OIG, 2012). Global Fund and PEPFAR resources were, however, used to establish human resources management structures, alongside those that already existed for the Ministry of Health.

Salary levels at Global Fund scale-up and their impacts at scale-down

When the Ministry of Health first became a PR to Global Fund resources under Round 2, it was required to establish a Programme Management Unit (PMU) to oversee the programme. The creation of the PMU was justified on the basis that the Ministry did not have the appropriate health expertise to oversee the Global Fund programme by itself. Since it came into operation in 2004, senior positions within the PMU have mainly been staffed with non-Namibian expatriates. The PMU has been responsible for managing a wide range of national functions of the Global Fund grant, including hiring and managing all intervention staff. It has carried out its human resources functions independently of and in addition to all other Ministry of Health human resources functions, which are usually managed through the Directorate of Policy, Planning and Human Resources Development (PPHRD).

From the onset of the Round 2 grant, individuals paid by the Global Fund in Namibia earned more than their Ministry of Health counterparts who had similar jobs. In November 2011, following an in-country salary survey earlier in the same year, the Global Fund mandated across-the-board salary cuts for all the health workers that it funded in Namibia. After more than six years of providing funding to the country, the Geneva Secretariat concluded that the salaries that it supported were too high when compared to those earned by other health workers in the Namibian health sector. It therefore mandated salary cuts for more than 1000 expatriate and indigenous health workers who were based within government health facilities, some of whom had their salaries decreased by more than 50% of their pre-survey earnings (V. Bampoe, personal communication, November 16, 2011).

In learning of the salary cuts, the national media mainly focused on how they impacted PMU staff. As reported at the time of data collection, the Ministry of Health had replied to the salary directive by requesting that the Global Fund allow it to retain PMU staff at their pre-survey salary levels. The Minister of Health at the time argued that this would be the best way to avoid disruption to the government's HIV and AIDS programmes. According to the media, the minister apparently then received a phone call from the Geneva Secretariat informing the minister that it 'would not release funds to Namibia if the Ministry did not correct the situation' with regard to high PMU salaries (Jaramito, 2012; Nghidengwa, 2012).

At the start of February 2012, senior PMU employees received notices that their contracts would be terminated by the end of March 2012. Due to these salary tensions, the top five PMU positions were barely functioning for the month of March. As soon as they received their notices, the Finance and Monitoring and Evaluation (M&E) managers chose to leave their posts. They avoided working to the end of their contracts by applying their remaining annual leave to the rest of March. The Operations Manager had chosen to ignore the termination letter and had declared through the media that she would take the Ministry of Health to the Namibian Labour Court for breaching their contract with her (Poolman, 2012). At the service-delivery level, there was also anecdotal evidence that the salary decreases had resulted in a disruption of services as employees funded by the Global Fund neglected their responsibilities to seek more secure employment.

PEPFAR-funded recruitment at scale-up and impacts at scale-down

Similar to the Global Fund, PEPFAR funding has been used to address human resources weaknesses in the Namibian public sector independent of existing Ministry of Health processes. At the start of its partnership with the Ministry of Health, CDC Namibia contracted a third-party human resources Consultancy company called Potentia to 'provide management and recruitment services' (Department of Health and Human Services, Office of the Inspector General, 2013). Since 2006, Potentia has been responsible for recruiting all health workers employed to work on PEPFAR-funded interventions in government-run facilities.

Whereas the PMU is closely associated with the Ministry of Health, Potentia's contractual relationship has been exclusively with CDC. Thus through its contract with CDC, Potentia has been a substantial direct recipient of PEPFAR funding in Namibia. An US government audit of CDC's relationship with the consultancy for the budget period 1 April 2009 through 31 March 2010, found that out of a total $39.5 million that CDC awarded to 4 PEPFAR recipients in Namibia that year, a total of $14,486,635 went to Potentia: approximately 38% of total funding (Department of Health and Human Services, 2013). The US government views Potentia as having been a successful strategy for addressing human resources deficits in Namibia, and has sought to encourage its PEPFAR operations in other countries to adopt a similar model (PEPFAR, 2006).

In 2011, following the decision to phase out PEPFAR funding from the country, PEPFAR administrators informed the Ministry of Health that it would immediately start experiencing annual 10% cuts in its previously approved budget for human resources. Ministry of Health officials found the decision to reduce the budget problematic for a number of reasons. In particular, senior Ministry of Health officials associated with the PEPFAR programme informed us that the decision was made without the input of the Namibian government. They argued that the Ministry was not given enough time to develop a strategy for absorbing all the health workers that had been recruited through Potentia.

The Ministry of Health had an opportunity to reflect on Potentia's implications for sustainability when the Ministry of Labour introduced a new Legislation in 2007, which prohibited the use of third-party contracting companies in Namibia (Jauch, 2008; Maletsky, 2009; Sasman, 2009). However, as reported within the local papers, the acting Permanent Secretary of the Ministry of Health at the time, was quoted as saying that Potentia was a 'technicality' that needed to be sorted out between the ministries because of the health sector's reliance on the specialists hired with PEPFAR funding (Sasman, 2009). The Ministry of Health did not seek to transition Potentia staff away from GHI funding until it been informed of the reduction in PEPFAR funding to human resources.

Impact of GHI scale-up funding on Ministry of Health human resources operations

Typically, the Ministry of Health recruits on the basis of a public servants list or 'Staff Establishment', approved by the Namibian government's Public Services Commission (PSC). This defines the categories and number of health workers deemed necessary for the Ministry's operations. The Ministry then receives its annual budget for human resources based on the established positions. Health workers can only be part of the Ministry's payroll following an approval from the Namibian Parliament. According to a respondent from the Ministry of Health, getting Cabinet approval for staff positions 'is a lengthy process, which takes between two to five years'.

Many of the positions funded by Global Fund and PEPFAR were not on the Staff Establishment, either in terms of specific specialisations or in terms of the number of pre-approved positions. They belonged to a special category, called 'in addition to Staff Establishment'. This category was developed especially to accommodate the various positions funded by the Global Fund and PEPFAR. Until the Ministry of Health established a Human Resources for Health (HRH) taskforce in 2011 there was no long-term strategy for

Global Fund and PEPFAR-funded health workers in Namibia. This only happened in the wake of indications from the two GHIs that they would be scaling down funding to the country.

The HRH taskforce was given the responsibility to oversee the transition of human resources from being GHI-funded to becoming government-funded by fiscal year 2014/2015. By March 2012, the taskforce had only transitioned 41 medical doctors that had been previously funded by either Global Fund or PEPFAR. According to respondents, the medical doctors were the only ones transitioned because they were already on the staff establishment. The ministry has declared intentions to eventually transition all critical positions. However, a monitoring and evaluation official from the Ministry of Health, who viewed the division as having been critical to the success of GHI-supported interventions, pointed out that it was not clear when this might happen given the need for Cabinet approval of Ministry of Health positions.

Reflections on the impact of Global Fund and PEPFAR scale-down on human resources

In Namibia, Global Fund and PEPFAR funding was used to increase the human resources capacity in government-run facilities. This increase has, however, occurred on an ad hoc basis, which bypassed existing institutions and procedures. The structures of Global Fund and PEPFAR have been justified due to the 'emergency' nature of HIV/AIDS, coupled with the perceived weaknesses and inefficiencies in the health systems of many African countries (Biesma et al., 2009; Hanefeld & Musheke, 2009; Ooms, Van Damme, Baker, Zeitz, & Schrecker, 2008; WHO Maximizing Positive Synergies Collaborative Group, 2009). While parallel GHI structures may allow for the immediate translation of donor resources into easily measurable results, they often have negative implications for overall health system strengthening and sustainability of HIV and AIDS interventions (Dodd & Lane, 2010; Dräger, Gedik, & Dal Poz, 2006; Drager et al., 2006; Hanefeld & Musheke, 2009; Kapilashrami & O'Brien, 2012). Sustained impacts of interventions require strengthened human resource capacities and coherent long-term strategies into which the GHIs can feed (Banteyerga et al. 2006; Drager et al., 2006).

In findings reflective of both Global Fund and PEPFAR operations in Namibia, a 2011 US government audit of PEPFAR funds in Namibia found two critical elements missing in relation to human resources (Office of the Inspector General, USAID, 2011). The first was a lack of transition plan for shifting the cost of workers' salaries to Namibian entities. The second was the lack of baseline data, indicators and targets for HRH activities. These weaknesses were defined as limiting Namibia's ability to sustain its HIV efforts and gains in the event of total withdrawal of PEPFAR funding. The report was produced before PEPFAR administrators informed the Ministry of Health that it would be reducing human resources by 10% on an annual basis. It concluded that without a transition plan, the US government 'will continue paying health worker costs indefinitely, which is unsustainable' (Office of the Inspector General, USAID, 2011).

When asked to reflect on the salary crisis in relation to the Global Fund, a former senior PMU official argued that tensions associated with scale-down were not necessarily unexpected. She characterised the Global Fund as having 'broad guidelines' that allow recipient countries to define their human resource needs as they saw fit. Had the Global Fund been more specific about how Namibia should have increased its health worker capacity at scale-up, it would not have needed to require the country to reduce the salary of staff in the middle of grant implementation.

As an initial boost to human resources, the Potentia decision made sense given the perceived weak national human resources infrastructure, as well as the known weaknesses of the Ministry of Health in terms of recruitment. However, for the purposes of sustainability, strengthening systems and human resource capacities, Potentia should have only been a temporary measure. Yet, it was not treated as such. Changes in the labour law were a missed opportunity for the Ministry of Health and a potential check for the two GHIs. Rather than waiting until PEPFAR had communicated the decrease in funding, the labour law should have been the first sign of potential challenges in sustaining GHI-funded human resources capacity in Namibia.

In many countries, interventions and corresponding health worker positions did not predate the entry of GHIs. Global Fund and PEPFAR resources enabled the introduction of interventions such as ART roll out, community care and other 'innovative' models. These were largely achieved through third-party contracts and performance monitoring of grant recipients. There was an urgency with which these programmes were established, which was used to justify their delivery through an independent cadre of human resources. The pace, scale and processes through which this was undertaken in Namibia did not allow space for dialogue and planning with the Namibian government, until funding became scarce.

Marchal, Cavalli, and Kegels (2009) suggest that initiatives such as the Global Fund and PEPFAR could best address human resources challenges in recipient countries by developing and adhering to a 'code of recruitment'. This argument, however, places the onus on the donors to decide what would be an appropriate approach to human resources capacity building. The answer does not alone lie in creating more uniform approaches to disbursing aid. The emphasis should be on ensuring that donor aid is based on cautious assessments by recipient governments of country-level human resources environments and systems in which donor aid can be integrated.

Once services were up and running, and over the 10 years of GHI operations in Namibia, there were opportunities for serious reflection on the parts of GHIs and the Namibian Government to work towards effective management and greater sustainability of HIV interventions. The Global Fund and PEPFAR cannot be held to account for limitations in the human resources capacities in Namibia that predate their entry. However, the case studies illustrate that the mechanisms and processes instituted by the GHIs in the process of scaling-up their interventions did not explicitly incorporate sustainability considerations. Were sustainability taken more seriously, the efforts to transition human resources ownership to the Namibian Government might have occurred earlier and in a more strategic manner. As it is, preparations for the decrease in funding appear to be occurring in a state of panic.

Conclusion

Both Global Fund and PEPFAR were established with the intent to provide surplus funding to recipient countries. They started with the ultimate goal of rapidly scaling-up resources and efforts to prevent and mitigate the impact of HIV and AIDS. As the case of Namibia demonstrates, both GHIs were able to show an impact in the form of a decreased and now stabilized HIV prevalence rate, as well as wide access to prevention, treatment and care services. In the case of Namibia, the human resources case studies just presented, however, indicate that rapid scale-up has at times occurred at the expense of sustainable thinking.

When both the Global Fund and PEPFAR resources arrived in Namibia, it was widely accepted that the country did not have the human resources capacity to absorb the substantial funding that was available from the GHIs. Thus both GHIs emphasised human resources as a critical component of their budgets. In order to meet their health services objectives rapidly, intervention staff were recruited independent of Ministry of Health procedures. However, such a model was not sustainable. Following the scale-down of Global Fund and PEPFAR funding at the global and national level, the Ministry of Health was expected to prioritise sustainability as an objective (while retaining the focus on scale-up) and re-adjust its approach to human resources in relation to the two GHIs.

This paper has sought to provide a longitudinal view of how human resources management decisions made while bringing GHI interventions to scale can play out negatively when financial resources are being scaled-down. The findings show that structures that might be suitable for scale-up are not necessarily suitable for ensuring sustainability of programmes. The partnership between the two GHIs and the Ministry of Health has not operated in a manner that positioned the Namibian government to become self-sufficient in the event of total withdrawal of its highest donors from the health sector. These findings, though specific to the Namibian context, have wider implications for other middle- and low-income countries that face the risk of depleting resources from their largest donors. Notwithstanding the burden that HIV poses in its third decade, these countries may witness an exacerbated human resource crisis if their relationships with the GHIs do not adequately take issues of health system sustainability into account.

References

Atun, R., de Jongh, T., Secci, F. V., Kelechi, O., & Adeyi, O. (2009). *Clearing the global health fog: A systematic review of the evidence on integration of health systems and targeted interventions* (Report No. 166, p. 80). Washington, DC: The World Bank.

Banati, P. (2008). The positive contributions of global health initatives. *Bulletin of the World Health Organization, 86*, 820–820. doi:10.2471/BLT.07.049361

Banteyerga, H., Kidanu, A., & Stillman, K. (2006). *The systemwide effects of the Global Fund in Ethiopia: Final study report*. Bethesda, MD: Abt Associates.

Biesma, R. G., Brugha, R., Harmer, A., Walsh, A., Spicer, N., & Walt, G. (2009). The effects of global health initiatives on country health systems: A review of the evidence from HIV/AIDS control. *Health Policy and Planning, 24*, 239–252. doi:10.1093/heapol/czp025

Brugha, R., Donoghue, M., Starling, M., Walt, G., Cliff, J., Fernandes, B., ... Ndubani, P. (2005). *Global Fund tracking study: A cross-country comparative analysis*. London: London School of Hygiene and Tropical Medicine (LSHTM).

Brugha, R., Simbaya, J., Walsh, A., Dicker, P., & Ndubani, P. (2010). How HIV/AIDS scale-up has impacted on non-HIV priority services in Zambia. *BMC Public Health, 10*, 540–551. doi:10.1186/1471-2458-10-540

Caines, K., Buse, K., De Loor, R.-M., Druce, N., Grace, C., Pearson, M., ... Sadanandan, R. (2004). *Assessing the impact of global health partnerships*. London: DFID Health Resource Centre.

Carlson, C., Druce, N., Sadanandan, R., Sancho, J., & De Loor, R.-M. (2004). *Assessing the impact of global health partnerships: Country case study report (India, Sierra Leone, Uganda)* (Report No. 7). London: DFID Health Resource Centre.

Department of Health and Human Services, Office of the Inspector General. (2013). Potentia Namibia recruitment consultancy generally managed the President's emergency plan for AIDS relief funds and met program goals in accordance with award requirements (Audit Report No. A--06--11--00056, p. 19). Washington, DC: Author.

Dickinson, C., Attawell, K., & Druce, N. (2009). Progress on scaling up integrated services for sexual and reproductive health and HIV. *Bulletin of the World Health Organization, 87*, 846–851. doi:10.2471/BLT.08.059279

Dodd, R., & Lane, C. (2010). Improving the long-term sustainability of health aid: Are global health partnerships leading the way? *Health Policy and Planning*, *25*, 363–371. doi:10.1093/heapol/czq014

Drager, S., Gedik, G., & Dal Poz, M. R. (2006). Health workforce issues and the Global Fund to fight AIDS, Tuberculosis and Malaria: An analytical review. *Human Resources for Health*, *4*, 23–35. Retrieved from http://www.human-resources-health.com/content/4/1/23

El Obeid, S. (2001). *Health in Namibia: Progress and challenges*. Windhoek: Research and Information Services of Namibia.

Gaye, P. A., & Nelson, D. (2009). Effective scale-up: Avoiding the same old traps. *Human Resources for Health*, *7*(1), 2. doi:10.1186/1478-4491-7-2

Hanefeld, J. (2010). The impact of global health initiatives at national and sub-national level – A policy analysis of their role in implementation processes of antiretroviral treatment (ART) roll-out in Zambia and South Africa. *AIDS Care*, *22*, 93–102. doi:10.1080/09540121003759919

Hanefeld, J., & Musheke, M. (2009). What impact do global health initiatives have on human resources for antiretroviral treatment roll-out? A qualitative policy analysis of implementation processes in Zambia. *Human Resources for Health*, *7*(1), 8. doi:10.1186/1478-4491-7-8

Health Gap. (2011). *Global fund round 11 canceled*. Retrieved from http://www.healthgap.org/press/gfatm_round11.html

Iipinge, S. N., Hofnie, K., van der Westhuizen, L., & Pendukeni, M. (2006). *Perceptions health workers about conditions of service: A Namibian case study*. Windhoek: Regional Network for Equity in Health in Southern Africa (EQUINET).

Jaramito, G. (2012, March 10). Official jeapordise global fund money. *Windhoek Observer*, 1–2.

Jauch, H. (2008, November). *Namibia bans labour hire. Fos-socialist solidarity*. Retrieved from http://www.fos-socsol.be/tools/zuidnieuws/pdf/Namibia%20bans%20labour%20hire%20-%20by%20Herbert%20Jauch.pdf

Kaiser Family Foundation. (2011). *PEPFAR approved funding (US$)*. Retrieved from http://kff.org/global-indicator/pepfar-funding/

Kaiser Family Foundation. (2012, November). *Global fund to fight AIDS, Tuberculosis and Malaria – Cumulative disbursements for HIV/AIDS grants (US$)*. Retrieved from http://kff.org/global-indicator/global-fund-disbursements-hivaids-grants/

Kapilashrami, A., & O'Brien, O. (2012). The global fund and the re-configuration and re-emergence of 'civil society': Widening or closing the democratic deficit? *Global Public Health*, *7*, 437–451. doi:10.1080/17441692.2011.649043

Le Loup, G., Fleury, S., Camargo, K., & Larouzé, B. (2009). International institutions, Global health initiatives and the challenge of sustainability: Lessons from the Brazilian AIDS programme. *Tropical Medicine & International Health*, *15*(1), 5–10. doi:10.1111/j.1365-3156.2009.02411.x

Leive, A., & Xu, K. (2008). Coping with out-of-pocket health payments: Empirical evidence from 15 African countries. *Bulletin of the World Health Organization*, *86*, 849–856. doi:10.2471/BLT.07.049403

Maletsky, C. (2009, January 27). Labour-hire ban sparks health crisis. *The Namibian*, p. 1–2.

Marchal, B., Cavalli, A., & Kegels, G. (2009). Global health actors claim to support health system strengthening – Is this reality or rhetoric? *PLoS Medicine*, *6*, e1000059. doi:10.1371/journal.pmed.1000059

Ministry of Health and Social Services. (MoHSS). (2005). *Follow-up to the declaration of commitment on HIV/AIDS: Namibia country report* 2005. Windhoek: Ministry of Health and Social Services (MoHSS): Directorate of Special Programmes.

Ministry of Health and Social Services. (MoHSS). (2008). *Health and social services system review*. Windhoek: Author.

Ministry of Health and Social Services (MoHSS). (2009). *Strategic plan 2009–2013*. Windhoek: Author.

Ministry of Health and Social Services. (MoHSS). (2010). *2010 review of universal access progress in Namibia*. Windhoek: Author.

Ministry of Health and Social Services (MoHSS), & ICF Macro. (2010). *Namibia health facility census (HFC) 2009*. Windhoek: Author.

Ministry of Health and Social Services: Directorate of Special Programs. (2008). *Estimates and projections of the impact of HIV/AIDS in Namibia* (p. 36). Windhoek: Author.

Ministry of Health and Social Services (MoHSS) and Centers for Disease Control and Prevention (CDC). (2010). *CDC-RFA-PS10-1095 - Expanded support for healthcare systems strengthening activities within the Ministry of Health and Social Services in the Republic of Namibia under the President's Emergency Plan for AIDS Relief (PEPFAR)*. Retrieved from CDC website: http://www.cdc.gov

Mtonya, B., Mwapasa, V., & Kadzandira, J. (2005). *System-wide effects of global fund in Malawi: Baseline study report (The partners for health reformplus project)*. Bethesda, MD: Abt Associates.

Nghidengwa, M. (2012, March 8). Kamwi accused of conspiring against his own ministry. *Confidente*, p. 1–2.

Office of the Inspector General, USAID. (2011). *Audit of USAID/Namibia's HIV/AIDS efforts to build health workforce capacity* (Audi Report No. 9-000-11-001-P, p. 15). Washington, DC: Author.

Oomman, N., Bernstein, M., Center for Global Development, & HIV/AIDS Monitor. (2008). *Seizing the opportunity on AIDS and health system: A comparison of donor interactions with national health systems in Mozambique, Uganda, and Zambia, focusing on the US President's Emergency Plan for AIDS relief, the Global Fund to fight AIDS, Tuberculosis and Malaria, and the World Bank's Africa multi-country AIDS program*. Washington, DC: Author.

Ooms, G., Van Damme, W., Baker, B. K., Zeitz, P., & Schrecker, T. (2008). The 'diagonal' approach to Global Fund financing: A cure for the broader malaise of health systems? *Globalization and Health, 4*(1), 6. doi:10.1186/1744-8603-4-6

PEPFAR. (2006). *Chapter 4 – Building capacity: Partnerships for sustainability*. Retrieved from http://www.pepfar.gov/press/81202.htm

PEPFAR. (2011). *PEPFAR: Partnership to fight HIV/AIDS in Namibia*. Retrieved from http://www.pepfar.gov/documents/organization/199600.pdf

PEPFAR Namibia. (2012). *PEPFAR program Namibia*. Namibia: Author.

Poolman, J. (2012, May 15). *Kamwi dismisses Global Fund managers*. Retrieved from http://allafrica.com/stories/201205150669.html

Ravishankar, N., Gubbins, P., Cooley, R. J., Leach-Kemon, K., Michaud, C. M., Jamison, D. T., & Murray, C. J. L. (2009). Financing of global health: Tracking development assistance for health from 1990 to 2007. *The Lancet, 373*, 2113–2124. doi:10.1016/S0140-6736(09)60881-3

Sasman, C. (2009, January 27). Can prohibition on labour hire affect health sector? *New Era*. Retrieved from http://allafrica.com/stories/200901270466.html.

The Global Fund. (2004). *The program grant agreement between the Global Fund to fight AIDS, Tuberculosis and Malaria (Global Fund) and the Ministry of Health and Social Services of the Government of Namibia PR (Principal Recipient)*. Geneva, Switzerland: Author.

The Global Fund. (2011). *The Global Fund annual report 2011* (Annual report). Geneva, Switzerland: Author.

The Global Fund. (2013a). *New funding model*. Retrieved from http://www.theglobalfund.org/en/about/grantmanagement/fundingmodel/

The Global Fund. (2013b). *Who we are. The Global Fund to fight AIDS, Tuberculosis and Malaria*. Retrieved from http://www.theglobalfund.org/en/about/whoweare/

The Global Fund: The Office of the Inspector General (OIG). (2012). *Audit of Global Fund grants to the Republic of Namibia* (Report No. GF-OIG-11-006). Geneva, Switzerland: Author.

The World Bank. (2013). *Namibia at a glance*. Retrieved from http://www.worldbank.org/en/country/namibia

Tom Lantos and Henry J. Hyde United States Global Leadership Against HIV/ AIDS, Tuberculosis, and Malaria Reauthorization Act of 2008, 181 U.S.C § 22 (2008).

United States AIDS, Leadership Against HIV/AIDS, Tuberculosis, and Malaria Act of Tuberculosis, and Malaria Act of 2003, 181 U.S.C § 22 40 (2003).

World Health Organization Maximizing Positive Synergies Collaborative Group. (2009). An assessment of interactions between global health initiatives and country health systems. *The Lancet, 373*, 2137–2167. doi:10.1016/S0140-6736(09)60919-3

Zere, E., Mbeeli, T., Shangula, K., Mandlhate, C., Mutirua, K., Tjivambi, B., & Kapenambili, W. (2006). Technical efficiency of district hospitals: Evidence from Namibia using data envelopment analysis. *Cost Effectiveness and Resource Allocation, 4*, 5–14. Retrieved from http://www.resource-allocation.com/content/4/1/5

HIV scale-up in Mozambique: Exceptionalism, normalisation and global health

Erling Høg[a,b]

[a]LSE Health, London School of Economics and Political Science, London, UK; [b]Department of International Health, Immunology and Microbiology, University of Copenhagen, København K, Denmark

The large-scale introduction of HIV and AIDS services in Mozambique from 2000 onwards occurred in the context of deep political commitment to sovereign nation-building and an important transition in the nation's health system. Simultaneously, the international community encountered a willing state partner that recognised the need to take action against the HIV epidemic. This article examines two critical policy shifts: sustained international funding and public health system integration (the move from parallel to integrated HIV services). The Mozambican government struggles to support its national health system against privatisation, NGO competition and internal brain drain. This is a sovereignty issue. However, the dominant discourse on self-determination shows a contradictory twist: it is part of the political rhetoric to keep the sovereignty discourse alive, while the real challenge is coordination, not partnerships. Nevertheless, we need more anthropological studies to understand the political implications of global health funding and governance. Other studies need to examine the consequences of public health system integration for the quality of access to health care.

Introduction

Free large-scale antiretroviral (ARV) treatment through the public health system began in Mozambique in June 2004. The Mozambican government and supportive donors favoured a decentralised model in which HIV and AIDS services would be integrated into the public health system. However, services provided by NGOs began in 2001 according to the 'exceptional' HIV and AIDS model in which infrastructure, including voluntary counselling and testing centres and day hospitals, was established separately from normal health services, an effort supported by large increases in international *disease-specific* funding (Pfeiffer et al., 2010). This scenario generated the still ongoing service integration process marked by power discourses (sovereignty, ownership, national self-determination) and partnership encounters (coordination, capacity, respect and trust). Drawing on ethnographic research in Mozambique, I argue that Mozambican health care remains highly politicised with roots in post-independence priorities foremost implying sovereign self-determination. However, I will show that it is part of the political rhetoric to keep the sovereignty discourse alive and dominant, while in practical terms the real challenge is coordination, not partnerships. Yet, the move from AIDS exceptionalism towards normalised AIDS services in Mozambique's public health system strengthened by exceptional *sustained* international funding produces thought-provoking political questions for the governance of global health: will this create *global health exceptionalism*? Does this implicate *exceptional global health governance*? What are the political implications for 'local government ownership' in terms of self-determination and sovereignty, when *de facto* foreign powers decide and pay?

Notably, during the first decade of the epidemic, *HIV* exceptionalism referred to a departure from classic public health measures (compulsory testing, name reporting, compulsory treatment and quarantine) and a re-orientation towards a rights-based approach (informed and voluntary consent and testing under confidential or anonymous conditions). The shift was championed by an alliance of gay leaders, civil libertarians, physicians and public health officials (Bayer, 1991). Later, *AIDS* exceptionalism came to describe the disease-specific global response and the resources dedicated to addressing the epidemic (Smith & Whiteside, 2010).

Indeed, HIV and AIDS have received disproportionate funding relative to many other epidemics. Ironically, though, this exceptional funding of HIV and AIDS initiatives has also brought about a process of *normalisation* in many countries with regard to the provision of HIV testing (e.g. Bayer & Fairchild, 2006; De Cock, 2005) and AIDS treatment (disease integration, decentralisation) (e.g. Boyer et al., 2010; Decroo et al., 2009), in which these services have become increasingly routine and are integrated into the broader system of health-care services. While exceptionality affords sustained 'reliance on open-ended international solidarity', normalisation implies an extension of this funding relationship to the broader health system of the poorest countries of the world (Ooms et al., 2010). Normalisation also includes the integration of NGOs into the public-health sector as part of *health systems strengthening efforts*. Global health proponents, recipient governments, foreign governments, donors and other stakeholders widely recommend and support this horizontal approach. Most notably, the Global Fund, GAVI Alliance, the World Bank and the World Health Organisation have recently joined forces to create the Health Systems Funding Platform. Does this signal the end of AIDS exceptionalism, both in terms of exceptional funding and exceptional scale-up?

Importantly, the Mozambican case provides a third perspective on HIV and AIDS exceptionalism. Even while the Mozambican government strove to reduce aid dependency, HIV and AIDS funding became an exception. This *political exceptionalism* required a negotiation over the framing of the epidemic and the objectives of HIV and AIDS programming (Ooms, 2006, 2008). The Mozambican government has portrayed scale-up simultaneously as an emergency response and an opportunity to resurrect the weak public health-care system ruined during the country's recent civil war.

What are the implications of this negotiation for health governance? As anthropologist Vinh-Kim Nguyen eloquently asks, how we can understand massive interventions into the lives of populations defined by their medical conditions? Does it implicate 'global' or 'foreign' government-by-exception or government-by-rule? The significance of such interventions is economic, socio-demographic and political (Nguyen, 2009). They entail massive economic commitments into the undefined future. The end of AIDS funding exceptionalism demands economic commitment to the entire burden of disease on a global scale. The line of patients is growing rapidly in countries with meagre state budgets that cannot afford the cost of health care. Will this burden create *global health exceptionalism*? In other words, will the emergency rhetoric survive, when targeting multiple diseases? As Nguyen reflects, 'As a humanitarian emergency, AIDS now defines exception in political terms, as an issue that may in fragmented and partial ways suspend national sovereignty' (Nguyen, 2009, 201–202).

Methods

To address these questions, I draw on 15 months of multi-sited fieldwork conducted in 2005–2006 to explore the experiences, limitations and politics of ARV treatment in Mozambique (Høg, 2008a). I interviewed hospital and health-centre country coordinators (5), expatriate and Mozambican health workers in 5 NGO-driven Day Hospitals and 1 state hospital (75), patients living with HIV and AIDS (30), Ministry of Health (MoH) staff and ARV Committee members (10), and national and international NGO advocacy workers (20). I also participated in numerous meetings, seminars and conferences, involving civil society, government and international community representatives. Fieldwork involved full-time participant observation, including office space hospitably offered by two advocacy organisations. Additionally, I collected more than 1300 policy and data documents. Epidemiological and antiretroviral treatment (ART) data were obtained from the MoH until 2010. Interviews, conducted in Portuguese with Mozambicans and English with foreigners, were transcribed and analysed using the TAMS qualitative research software.

Exceptional event or structural problem

Initially, the Mozambican government had two choices for financing the response to HIV: the *health development paradigm* (*sustainability, domestic resources, self-determination* and *sovereignty*) or the *medical relief paradigm* (*dependency, foreign aid, humanitarian assistance* and *an exceptional response*) (Ooms, 2006, 2008). Should HIV be classified as a *structural, emergency* or *exceptional* problem? Should *domestic budgets* or *international funding* solve the problem? There was no third way. Only exceptional problems allow the use of the medical relief paradigm. The health development paradigm would aid the Mozambican process, but the government had limited finances for action in favour of its own agenda within its state budget. Money for antiretrovirals would take away scarce resources from other expenditures. The government was not in a position to borrow the money or to raise taxes to create financial space for AIDS medicines. Ooms shows how the third way *new health paradigm* appeared (exceptional sustained international funding for antiretrovirals). The Mozambican government pushed the 'calamity button' under the given circumstances, which is common practice in a country with recurrent natural disasters. Calamity funding relates to *exceptional* events with no limit to foreign assistance (Ooms, 2008, 93). Disaster funding means that large sums of money enter the country, but it also means more dependency on foreign aid. The calamity compromise specified that when you cannot have access to basic health care for all and access to AIDS treatment for some, paid by the state budget, then relief money is welcome, though this means more dependency (Ooms, 2008, 93, 116, 130). This may sound contradictory to the government policy attempting to reduce donor dependency. The AIDS treatment programme became a *political exception*, adding a new dimension to AIDS exceptionalism.

Tracking scale-up in Mozambique

Exceptional scale-up

The lowering of generic drug prices in 2001 changed the scene in Mozambique. The cost of ARV drugs per patient dropped from around 10,000 US dollars per year to around 350 dollars in early 2001, down to 132 dollars in July 2006 (MSF, 2006). In Mozambique, the Clinton Foundation successfully negotiated lower drug prices from generic producers, which provided the final motivation for Mozambique to introduce ART (Pfeiffer, 2013, 169) after much government reluctance in the Ministerial decree on AIDS treatment (Ministry of Health, 2001). The ART 'business plan' was developed during 2002–2003 by the MoH, supported by the Clinton Foundation, Health Alliance International (HAI) and others, with initial funding from the Global Fund (Republic of Mozambique and Clinton Foundation, 2003). This was the original ART plan for nationwide scale-up with MoH leadership. Meanwhile, Sant'Egidio and MSF Luxembourg had started small-scale parallel NGO HIV and AIDS structures in 2001, followed by MSF Switzerland, ASIDH Spain, HAI, ICAP and about 10 additional minor organisations.

Free large-scale ARV treatment through the public health system started in June 2004, initially drawing on the WHO 'public health' approach in resource-poor settings (Gilks et al., 2006), supported by the World Bank, the Clinton Foundation, PEPFAR, the Global Fund, the governments of Ireland and Canada, and more (Høg, 2008a; Pfeiffer, 2013). The 2003 'business plan' designated this public health system approach to health services delivery, but since parallel HIV and AIDS structures were already in operation, the *normalisation* process was necessary. Additionally, significant funding from PEPFAR created parallel structures that bypassed the government health system to directly fund NGO partners (Pfeiffer, 2013, 169). The priorities of the Mozambican government and the push by donors and global health stakeholders decided the relatively quick move towards integrating HIV and AIDS services into the Mozambican public health system. This move rested much on timing and circumstances. Its implementation is still in progress in the fourth HIV decade.

Normalisation

The first steps to integrate HIV and AIDS care into the public health system began in 2005. The MoH intended to harmonise all aspects of the process, but different work philosophies among the international treatment providers, different levels of technical and human resources capacities, and general work overload all complicated its achievement. In August 2006, Benedito, a member of the MoH ARV Committee, described ART provided by NGOs as a 'heavy machine' out of proportions with reality in Mozambique:

> The NGOs are working in a very heavy structure in terms of human resources. You will notice that an NGO ART unit probably has 20–30 people working there. Administrator, logistician, physician, laboratory technician, activist—a heavy machine that no African country is under the condition to replicate. If we were to utilise the same strategy like the NGOs, no African country would have the capacity to expand ART. We have to adapt to our reality, our conditions. Our position from 2005 was the following: From now on as we get involved with ART, we begin to target the whole process. We have started to create our own models. We want to resolve the emergency problem. That is, with the conditions we have in the [health] system – let's start ART.

The MoH introduced its own model: *health* counselling centres[1] and AIDS care within the public health system. This was a complicated, difficult, yet necessary challenge, considering the priorities of the Mozambican government. Benedito said:

> ART for us is a double challenge, because it is a disease that challenges the conditions that we consider specialised at the primary level, and we are not prepared. And today we are working in all of the system at the same time, trying to improve the quality of our existing system.

In May 2008, the Mozambican government decided that *all* AIDS treatment services should be integrated into the public health system. This meant closing down all parallel NGO facilities with four objectives in mind: (a) *Equity* in access of services (for all patients), (b) *Efficiency*, rationalisation and optimisation (health workers, infrastructure, etc.), (c) *Overall strengthening* of the National Health Service and (d) *Increased access* for AIDS patients (due to integration of services) (Health Partners Group, 2009).

Normalisation of HIV and AIDS services means the end of HIV exceptionalism in terms of extraordinary care compared to other patient care. It means equal attention to all diseases. Disease normalisation is part of the government's post-independence struggle to establish a National Health System – without parallel *non*-governmental structures that are not under the legislative mandate of the MoH.

Epidemiology doubtfully motivated normalisation in health. The numbers are daunting. The national 2007 adult HIV prevalence was estimated at 16%, with regional variation: South (21%), Centre (18%) and North (9%) (Ministry of Health, 2008b). While new UNAIDS assumptions have lowered prevalence rates to approximately 0.8 times the prevalence found in antenatal clinic surveillance in countries like Mozambique without population-based surveys to provide a more accurate estimate of the number of HIV infected people, the estimated figures would, nevertheless, foresee a collapse of the health system in the case of disease integration: UNAIDS suggests that 1.4 million Mozambicans (range 1.2–1.6 million) were living with HIV by the end of 2010 (UNAIDS, 2011) (Figure 1).

Likewise, the political and technical challenges of normalising AIDS treatment remain enormous. The numbers escalated rapidly during 2004–2008: testing sites (359/2006), treatment sites (213/2008), AIDS patients (128,000/2008), patients in need of AIDS treatment (370,000/2007) (Ministry of Health, 2006, 2008a; UNAIDS, 2008). But the exceptional focus on AIDS diverted scarce resources away from the primary health-care system (Pfeiffer et al., 2010). Recent data reveal that the number of AIDS patients

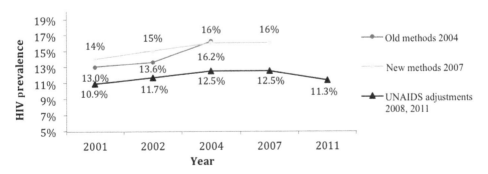

Figure 1. HIV prevalence, 2001–2011. Sources: Ministry of Health (2005c, 2008b) and UNAIDS (2008, 2011).

more than doubled from 128,000 in 2008 to 270,000 in 2012 (GFATM, 2013), while the ones in need of treatment lamentably also doubled to 600,000 (UNAIDS, 2012).

Moreover, the health system already faced a high disease burden. Malaria has been declared a national emergency. Nearly 6 million of the country's 20 million people suffered from this disease in 2005 (GFATM, 2006). Tuberculosis affects more than 30,000 people every year, which makes Mozambique one of the worst affected countries in the world (GFATM, 2007). Moreover, the burden of disease also includes diarrhoea, measles, cholera, tetanus, pneumonia, rabies, whooping cough, polio, meningitis, plague and sleeping sickness. It comes as no surprise that the *efficiency* objective overwhelms the limited carrying capacity of the health system (Decroo et al., 2009).

However, the new funding paid for drugs, and not for the recruitment and training of health workers. The human resource question posed an identical dilemma, since neither emergency nor state funding could solve it (not an exception and insufficient state budgetary room). Ooms coined this the *Medicines Without Doctors Paradox* (Ooms, 2008; Ooms, van Damme, & Temmerman, 2007). Health workers were forgotten under the principle of AIDS exceptionalism, which exclusively paid for the medicines. A recent study conducted in Central Mozambique showed how human resource shortages negatively affected the risk of patient dropout (Lambdin et al., 2011). There are not enough health workers and infrastructure to deal with the influx of new patients to the integrated services, though task shifting to non-physician providers has proven successful (Sherr et al., 2009).

Public health and the discourse of sovereignty and nationhood
Intimate and distant partners

Benedito said with sincerity: 'All these people that are coming to work for the country need to understand that they come to work within a system.' 'Common funds', 'sector wide approaches to health'[2] and central drug procurement and distribution were established as harmonisation procedures towards this end. This happens in accordance with the UN 'Three Ones' principles, defined as One National AIDS Coordinating Body, One Monitoring and Evaluation Framework and One Agreed AIDS Action Framework. Indeed, international funding and global health governance stakeholders have also pushed for national ownership – with reference to the 'Three Ones', The Paris Declaration, the Accra Agenda and decentralisation (World Bank, UNAIDS, PEPFAR, USAID and WHO). But I maintain that the Mozambican government strategically appropriates these calls into its discourse of political power. The political process is pre-eminently about respect for the Mozambican nation-building project and the longstanding goal of one unique public health system.

In general, the Mozambican government welcomes those international organisations that approve the goal of public health systems strengthening, but it embraces the ones that agree to end AIDS exceptionalism to improve overall health-care delivery. The government does not salute affirmative action for AIDS under the circumstances of high disease burden.

I distinguish between *intimate* and *distant* government partners. Intimate partners are those that agree to the national health project and have worked for many years in Mozambique as government *cooperantes*. Prime examples include HAI, MSF Luxembourg and Sant'Egidio that worked in Mozambique many years before the response to HIV. Distant partners are those that do not enjoy the trust of the government, as they construct parallel health structures. The government perceives them as unruly trouble-makers, when and if they do not abide by the rules of integration and one public health system without parallel competition. I have elsewhere introduced the introduction of

PEPFAR as an example (Høg, 2008b). The Mozambican government initially perceived the Bush administration as arrogant and neo-colonial as it ignored negotiation. However, upon insistence, they produced an agreement that honoured Mozambican priorities (Sontag, 2004). But the process turned out to be muddy during the early days of 'partnerships' and 'multi-sectoral' approaches. According to Pfeiffer, PEPFAR was the outlier among donors, avoiding 'basket funding', while insisting on NGO targets for support. Yet, PEPFAR could not completely avoid the public system, since the MoH provided most services. PEPFAR was awkwardly attached to the public health system (Pfeiffer, 2013, 169).

Health care in Mozambique: a native reserve

In other words, health care in Mozambique remains an ideological fortress. I invoke two events that took place during 2006 to develop this argument: the first national meeting on STI/HIV/AIDS and the third signing of the Kaya Kwanga Commitment between the MoH and NGOs. Health care represents the very identity and success of the reigning party. I have already said that foreign-sponsored ART challenges this ideological position: it is therefore a test of capability and autonomy in the government's relation with bilateral and multilateral donor partners. I draw four lessons from this analysis, which may seem idiosyncratic and even contradictory: (1) the problem is coordination, not partnerships, (2) the problem is diminished sovereignty, caused by partnerships, (3) the government insists on national leadership of the development process and (4) the Mozambican government will depend on foreign aid for many years, aggravated by the increasing need for sustained financial and human resources to scale up HIV, AIDS and all other health services.

The ambivalence of partnerships

The first (five-day) national meeting on STDs and HIV/AIDS was held at the MoH in March 2006. Participants included representatives from Sant'Egidio, HAI, MSF, Clinton Foundation, CDC, DFID, Columbia University, National Institute of Health, MONASO, Médicos Mundi, provincial health managers, MoH staff, the National STI/HIV/AIDS Program and the National AIDS Council.

NAP Director Alfredo Mac-Arthur opened the meeting. He addressed the issue of partnerships in a sympathetic yet vexed manner by saying 'We can't close the doors.' However, from his facial expression I wondered whether he was celebrating or lamenting this fact, as I imagined him continue: 'even if we wanted to'. After all, I had heard the politicisation of HIV by the Minister of Health, the President and the Prime Minister: they insist on national sovereignty. At least rhetorically, less in practice, as pragmatism and contradictions characterise the Mozambican government. I had also noticed the issue of foreign human resources as one of the most politically sensitive issues of the HIV epidemic. The HIV epidemic not only brought another infectious disease problem to the general population: it initiated a new unprecedented era of foreign aid dependence that the government would prefer to do without, in the continued struggle for political and economic independence.

Mac-Arthur addressed the challenges on how to progressively integrate HIV and AIDS into the National Health System by emphasising that 'The problem is not financing and it is not partnerships. The challenge is coordination'. This reminded me of an interview at UNDP, where I was told 'We see a sector wide SWAP coordination recommended, but each sector still works on its own. They are not ready for this level of coordination'. It also echoed decades-long policy debates about the large number of external agencies involved in health sectors of developing countries (Buse & Walt, 1997) and the particular issue of unwanted parallel *non*-governmental structures and vertical funding in Mozambique (Mussa, Pfeiffer, Gloyd, & Sherr, 2013; Pfeiffer, 2003, 2013; Pfeiffer et al., 2008; Sherr et al., 2013). Therefore, the major objective of the National STI/HIV/AIDS Program was to review and adjust the Mozambican response and targets in relation to accumulated experience and the reality within the country. The final meeting produced 14 decisions. Four important decisions that relate to the purpose of this article are (1) nationwide ART expansion, (2) integrate HIV/AIDS services into the public health system, (3) increase training of MoH health workers and (4) no HIV testing facility outside MoH facilities (USAID, 2006).

Mozambican leadership

The MoH leads the process to regulate its relations with its partners. This is called the Kaya Kwanga Commitment. This process began in 1999, after nearly a decade of freedom of association that produced a heavy presence of NGOs. The first code of conduct related the following: (1) commitment to the health reform process, (2) no legal implications, (3) existing bilateral and multilateral agreements remain intact and (4) development of 'a sector wide approach to health' (Ministry of Health, 2000). The second code of conduct was signed in July 2003 (Ministry of Health, 2003), and the third in August 2006 (Ministry of Health, 2005a).

The three agreements compare in terms of *purposes*, *commitments*, *principles* and *mechanisms* for the relation between the MoH and its external partners in the pursuit of Mozambican policy goals (Ministry of Health, 2000). The key objectives are *public health* (health of the population), *capacity* (sustainable health care) and *idealism* (gradual access to health care for all citizens). In other words, idealistic objectives should be taken with a grain of salt: action is essentially pragmatic. Nonetheless, the three codes of conduct strongly emphasise Mozambican leadership: *sovereignty, empowerment, trust* and *capacity*. To this end, the MoH sets the agenda for all strategies, plans and guidelines in line with the ideal type of governance defined by Foucault as an interdependent triangular modus of *sovereignty-discipline-government* (Foucault, 1979).

National self-determination

This assertion can be supported by discourse analysis of the meeting in which the 2006 Kaya Kwanga Commitment was signed. The meeting gathered about 120 participants, who represented the MoH and international and national NGOs. The Minister talked for 50 minutes about health and cooperation in Mozambique: (1) *coordination* between the MoH and NGOs, (2) *respect* for the dignity of Mozambique and Mozambicans and (3) *authorisation* to work in Mozambique.

Garrido initially emphasised: 'We need to work in an organized manner. Someone has to lead the process'. Garrido referred to the 'problem of coordination between hundreds of NGOs', their 'inefficiency' and the 'confusion' that it produced. A reoccurring problem was the 'foreign personnel that work within the National Health System without permission from the Ministry of Health'. Garrido repeated the rules of the process and emphasised that foreigners need 'government authorisation' to work in Mozambique. Garrido thundered: 'It's a matter of sovereignty. It's about respect for human beings'.

This was a loud and serious monologue. The audience listened in complete silence, somewhat perplexed.

Leadership, discipline and sovereignty

The Minister implied that foreign health workers *do not* respect the Mozambican government and Mozambicans, and that they *do not* have sufficient qualifications to work in Mozambique. Garrido followed the nationalistic supposedly uncompromising way of doing politics, which dictates retention of sovereign power to show who is in control governing the Mozambican nation. This is not far from the first president Samora Machel's way with words during the 1970s (Machel, 1985, 163).

Colonial legacies

Contemporary discourse eloquently epitomises the past, even as the government portrays the old Mozambican system as 'centralized and obsolete, which belongs to a state apparatus model conceived at a different point in history' (Ministry of Health, 2005b). In my experience, a discourse has emerged within the political and health system transition characterised by opposing signifiers, pointing to the future, looking to the past. Indeed, a culture of contradictions remains an intrinsic feature of Mozambican politics (Mackintosh & Wuyts, 1988; Saul, 1985; Sidaway, 1992), but what is power in such a situation? Today, an ideological hodgepodge surrounds the government. Think of HAI, World Bank, PEPFAR, GFATM, Sant'Egidio, ASIDH, MSF, UNAIDS, Humana People to People, DANIDA, CARE, HOPE, and many more: one government against '1001 actors' from all corners of the political spectrum. The varying roles of donors, governments and non-state providers, what Palmer calls 'an awkward threesome' (Palmer, 2006), influence the emerging mix of ART delivery models in African countries (Harries, Makombe, Schouten, Ben-Smith, & Jahn, 2008).

Though much has changed and is still changing in Mozambique, through political and health systems transition, its colonial legacy nevertheless plays an important role for its national responses to infectious disease epidemics, including HIV. Mozambique retains key elements of the Portuguese 'vertical' administration along a fusion of socialist, modernist and nationalist ideologies (Pitcher, 2002). In this sense, Mozambique remains an African ideological chameleon with historical and contemporary political ties to its colonial power, socialism and communism, neoliberalism (promotion of free markets, privatisation, small government, and economic deregulation (Pfeiffer & Chapman, 2010, 150)), welfare states and the Portuguese-speaking community.

In my experience, the double discourse prevails: the government remains against privatisation and parallel structures. However, it cannot save its health-care system without external donor support and it cannot pay its health workers salaries that compare to international standards. Health workers lose their motivation to stay within the public health system: they seek greener grass with the NGOs. According to Garrido, 'The UN and the NGOs are sucking my blood!' (Lewis, 2006).

The Minister of Health finally gave some credit to the international and national *non-governmental* organisations: 'In general we have good and professional relations with NGOs. We highly value the collaboration with NGOs. Let us continue to improve this relation, with respect for the dignity of Mozambicans in mind'.

This was to me a surprising change of tone considering the long talk about sovereignty and disrespect. It would have made more sense to begin the meeting giving praise to partnerships considering its nature. The ministry had already set the welcoming tone during the preparatory meeting in November 2005:

> We need general norms to improve the relation between NGOs and MoH. Contracting opens the possibility for MoH funding. But NGOs are not obliged to contract MoH. At the same time, contracts will not change the way each NGO works. We do not want to speak about conditionality. It is not what it is about. Complementarity is the general principle. I want to emphasise that we do not intend to create difficulties for the work of NGOs. People are dying and they need your intervention.

Anthropologist James Pfeiffer followed the early *Kaya Kwanga* process during the 1990s. I agree with Pfeiffer's uncertainty as to why the code of conduct was necessary: it could imply a certain level of *mis*conduct and it could be an empty strategic gesture considering its non-legal nature (Pfeiffer, 2004). However, it could signal an ideological compromise between the government, the donors and implementers.

Who calls the shots?

The Mozambican government continues to demand full sovereignty as set out at independence. It therefore maintains an ambivalent position towards foreign aid, ART funding and foreign health workers. Politicians call for national self-determination, in my interpretation, *with* or *without* the HIV epidemic. Such a call for sovereignty would be irrelevant in an apolitical world for the response to the HIV epidemic. Economic and human resources would ideally come from anywhere in the world. However, the real world is different: it remains questionable whether international organisations could recruit the number of health workers needed in Southern Africa. Yet, the Mozambican government experiences the impact of external threats to Mozambican sovereignty: NGO competition, privatisation and the internal brain drain. Nevertheless, I have shown the contradictory twist to this phenomenon: it is part of the political rhetoric to keep the sovereignty discourse alive and dominant, while in practical terms the real challenge is coordination, not partnerships. In other words, the government produces the sovereignty and nation-building discourses through political strategy with public health implications. These are some of the key factors that must be kept in mind, when we try to understand statements such as 'it's about sovereignty' and 'respect the dignity of Mozambicans'.

But the most striking feature of the government discourse targeted at Mozambican citizens is the *absence* of reference to global health initiatives related to health systems strengthening and decentralisation of AIDS care. Yet, the schism presented by Ooms between the health development paradigm and the medical relief paradigm shows intrinsic struggles over ownership of the development process. HIV increases aid dependency, which adds to the progressive demise of the government development agenda. However, the problem cannot be solved without external funding. This creates a 'culture of political contradictions', which helps us to understand the politics of HIV scale-up in terms of nation-building and self-determination.

The policy shifts presented in this article towards exceptional sustained international funding for HIV and the normalisation of access to health care in the public health system pose challenging questions for the politics of global health in the fourth decade. What are the political implications of global health governance considering the (diminishing) role of the nation-state? What are the implications of an alleged growing local rhetoric and insistence on local government ownership of decentralisation in health, when arguably the real decision makers belong to foreign governments and donors that at the end of the day also pay all the bills? 'Who calls the shots', as Hanlon asked more than two decades ago (Hanlon, 1991), implying that the ultimate decision-making power locates outside Mozambique. Do the new funding trends implicate 'global' or 'foreign' government-by-exception or government-by-rule, thinking with Nguyen (Nguyen, 2009)? Will it create *global health exceptionalism*? What is the fate of the exceptional funding introduced here as the third way between state budgets and donor aid? Ooms and colleagues advocate a Global *Health* Fund, but fear the lack of donor commitments (Ooms, Van Damme, Baker, Zeitz, & Schrecker, 2008). The nature, future and politics of global health funding and implementation still need to be explored, evidenced in the current literature (e.g. Ingram, 2013; Sundewall et al., 2011). As we have seen, the Mozambican government wants sovereign nation-building and less dependency on foreign donor aid, yet it pragmatically welcomes external sponsorship. Global health governance tends to be depoliticised, but in the long run nation states and the global health community *will* be faced by questions of sovereignty, power, domination and the politics of interference with the health of populations of other states.

Notes

1. I visited a pilot CTH clinic in 2006: The consultation is a normal clinic with no specific disease-related indications why the patient seeks health care (e.g. AIDS ribbon, posters). The doctor performs several health tests, including HIV, yet with patient consent. This pilot test showed a rapid increase in the number of people testing for HIV.
2. Unfortunately, I did not gain access to participate in Health SWAP meetings, due to the dynamic political situation within the MoH. The SWAP HIV Working Group did not feel it prudent to allow an outside observer to attend their meetings.

References

Bayer, R. (1991). Public-health policy and the AIDS Epidemic—An end to HIV exceptionalism? *New England Journal of Medicine*, *324*, 1500–1504. doi:10.1056/NEJM199105233242111

Bayer, R., & Fairchild, A. L. (2006). Changing the paradigm for HIV testing—The end of exceptionalism. *New England Journal of Medicine*, *355*, 647–649. doi:10.1056/NEJMp068153

Boyer, S., Eboko, F., Camara, M., Abé, C., Nguini, M. E. O., Koulla-Shiro, S., & Moatti, J.-P. (2010). Scaling up access to antiretroviral treatment for HIV infection: The impact of decentralization of healthcare delivery in Cameroon. *AIDS*, *24*, S5–S15. doi:10.1097/01. aids.0000366078.45451.46

Buse, K., & Walt, G. (1997). An unruly mélange? Coordinating external resources to the health sector: A review. *Social Science & Medicine*, *45*, 449–463. doi:10.1016/S0277-9536(96)00365-6

De Cock, K. M. (2005). HIV testing in the era of treatment scale up. *Health and Human Rights*, *8*(2), 31–35. Retrieved from http://www.hhrjournal.org/archives-pdf/4065331.pdf.bannered.pdf

Decroo, T., Panunzi, I., das Dores, C., Maldonado, F., Biot, M., Ford, N., & Chu, K. (2009). Lessons learned during down referral of antiretroviral treatment in Tete, Mozambique. *Journal of the International AIDS Society*, *12*(1), 6. doi:10.1186/1758-2652-12-6

Foucault, M. (1979). On governmentality. *Ideology & Consciousness*, *6*(Autumn), 5–21.

GFATM. (2006). *Sixth call for proposals. Component section malaria*. The Global Fund to Fight AIDS, Tuberculosis and Malaria. Retrieved January 28, 2010, from http://www.theglobalfund. org/en/

GFATM. (2007). *Seventh call for proposals. Component section tuberculosis*. The Global Fund to Fight AIDS, Tuberculosis and Malaria. Retrieved January 28, 2010, from http://www. theglobalfund.org/en/

GFATM. (2013). *Global fund portfolio Mozambique*. The Global Fund to Fight AIDS, Tuberculosis and Malaria. Retrieved June 13, 2013, from http://portfolio.theglobalfund.org/en/Country/ Index/MOZ

Gilks, C. F., Crowley, S., Ekpini, R., Gove, S., Perriens, J., Souteyrand, Y., ... De Cock, K. M. (2006). The WHO public-health approach to antiretroviral treatment against HIV in resource-limited settings. *Lancet, 368*, 505–510. doi:10.1016/S0140-6736(06)69158-7

Hanlon, J. (1991). *Mozambique: Who calls the shots?* London: James Currey.

Harries, A. D., Makombe, S. D., Schouten, E. J., Ben-Smith, A., & Jahn, A. (2008). Different delivery models for antiretroviral therapy in sub-Saharan Africa in the context of 'Universal Access'. *Transactions of the Royal Society of Tropical Medicine and Hygiene, 102*, 310–311. doi:10.1016/j.trstmh.2008.01.005

Health Partners Group. (2009). *Technical note: Decentralization of ART services.* Maputo: Health Partners Group.

Høg, E. (2008a). *The process: Experiences, limitations, and politics of ARV treatment in Mozambique* (PhD dissertation). London School of Economics and Political Science, London.

Høg, E. (2008b). *States of HIV fragility: Capacity, vulnerabilities, and epidemic evolution in Mozambique.* ASCI Research Report, AIDS, Security and Conflict Initiative, Social Science Research Council, New York & Clingendael Institute, The Hague. New York.

Ingram, A. (2013). After the exception: HIV/AIDS beyond salvation and scarcity. *Antipode, 45*, 436–454. doi:10.1111/j.1467-8330.2012.01008.x

Lambdin, B. H., Micek, M. A., Koepsell, T. D., Hughes, J. P., Sherr, K., Pfeiffer, J., ... Stergachis, A. (2011). Patient volume, human resource levels, and attrition from HIV treatment programs in central Mozambique. *Journal of Acquired Immune Deficiency Syndromes, 57*(3), e33–e39. doi:10.1097/QAI.0b013e3182167e90

Lewis, S. (2006). *Report on the mission of Stephen Lewis, UN secretary-general's special envoy on HIV/AIDS in Africa, to Mozambique, 3rd July–7th July, 2006.* Maputo: United Nations, 13.

Machel, S. (1985). We must strengthen people's power in our hospitals. In B. Munslow (Ed.), *Samora Machel: An African revolutionary: Selected speeches and writings* (pp. 156–168). London: Zed Books.

Mackintosh, M., & Wuyts, M. (1988). Accumulation, social services and socialist transition in the third world: Reflections on decentralised planning based on Mozambican experience. *Journal of Development Studies, 24*(4), 136–179. doi:10.1080/00220388808422086

Ministry of Health. (2000). *The Kaya Kwanga commitment: A code of conduct to guide the partnership for health development in Mozambique.* Maputo: Ministry of Health.

Ministry of Health. (2001). *Dignidade e satisfação do doente são o termómetro da nossa prestação* [Dignity and satisfaction are the thermometers of our performance]. Maputo: Ministry of Health.

Ministry of Health. (2003). *The Kaya Kwanga commitment: A code of conduct to guide the partnership for health development in Mozambique.* Maputo: Ministry of Health, 13.

Ministry of Health. (2005a). *Código de conduta para orientar a parceira entre o Ministério da Saúde e as organizações não governmentais* [Code of conduct to inform the partnership between the Ministry of Health and non governmental organisations]. Maputo: Ministry of Health.

Ministry of Health. (2005b). *Plano de desenvolvimento de recursos humanos período 2006–2010* [Human resource development plan 2006–2010]. Maputo: Ministry of Health.

Ministry of Health. (2005c). *Report on the update of the epidemiological surveillance data—2004 round.* Maputo: Ministry of Health.

Ministry of Health. (2006). *Relatório Anual da informação do aconselhamento e testagem em saúde* [Annual report on information about counselling and testing for health]. Maputo: Ministry of Health.

Ministry of Health. (2008a). *ARV data, 2004–2008.* Maputo: Ministry of Health.

Ministry of Health. (2008b). *Report on the revision of the data from HIV Epidemiological surveillance—round 2007.* Maputo: Ministry of Health, 46.

MSF. (2006). *Untangling the web of price reductions: A pricing guide for the purchase of ARVs in developing countries*, 9th edition. Médicins Sans Frontières. Retrieved December 16, 2013, from http://www.doctorswithoutborders.org/news/hiv-aids/untangled.pdf

Mussa, A. H., Pfeiffer, J., Gloyd, S. S., & Sherr, K. (2013). Vertical funding, non-governmental organizations, and health system strengthening: Perspectives of public sector health workers in Mozambique. *Human Resources for Health, 11*(1), 26. doi:10.1186/1478-4491-11-26

Nguyen, V.-K. (2009). Government-by-exception: Enrolment and experimentality in mass HIV treatment programmes in Africa. *Social Theory & Health, 7*, 196–217. doi:10.1057/sth.2009.12

Ooms, G. (2006). Health development versus medical relief: The illusion versus the irrelevance of sustainability. *PLoS Medicine, 3*(8), e345. doi:10.1371/journal.pmed.0030345

Ooms, G. (2008). *The right to health and the sustainability of healthcare: Why a new global health aid paradigm is needed* (PhD dissertation). Ghent University, Ghent.

Ooms, G., Hill, P. S., Hammonds, R., Leemput, L. V., Assefa, Y., Miti, K., & van Damme, W. (2010). Applying the principles of AIDS 'Exceptionality' to global health: Challenges for global health governance. *Global Health Governance, 4*(1), 1–9. Retrieved from http://ghgj.org/Ooms_final.pdf

Ooms, G., van Damme, W., Baker, B. K., Zeitz, P., & Schrecker, T. (2008). The 'diagonal' approach to Global Fund financing: A cure for the broader malaise of health systems? *Global Health, 4*, 6. doi:10.1186/1744-8603-4-6

Ooms, G., van Damme, W., & Temmerman, M. (2007). Medicines without doctors: Why the global fund must fund salaries of health workers to expand AIDS treatment. *PLoS Medicine, 4*, 605–608. doi:10.1371/journal.pmed.0040128

Palmer, N. (2006). An awkward threesome—Donors, governments and non-state providers of health in low income countries. *Public Administration and Development, 26*, 231–240. doi:10.1002/pad.421

Pfeiffer, J. (2003). International NGOs and primary health care in Mozambique: The need for a new model of collaboration. *Social Science & Medicine, 56*, 725–738. doi:10.1016/S0277-9536(02)00068-0

Pfeiffer, J. (2004). International NGOs in the Mozambique health sector: The 'The Velvet Glove' of privatization. In A. Castro & M. Singer (Eds.), *Unhealthy health policies* (pp. 43–62). Oxford: Altamira Press.

Pfeiffer, J. (2013). The struggle for a public sector. In A. Petryna & J. Biehl (Eds.), *When people come first: Critical studies in global health* (pp. 166–181). Princeton: Princeton University Press.

Pfeiffer, J., & Chapman, R. (2010). Anthropological perspectives on structural adjustment and public health. *Annual Review of Anthropology, 39*, 149–165. doi:10.1146/annurev.anthro.012809.105101

Pfeiffer, J., Johnson, W., Fort, M., Shakow, A., Hagopian, A., Gloyd, S., & Gimbel-Sherr, K. (2008). Strengthening health systems in poor countries: A code of conduct for nongovernmental organizations. *American Journal of Public Health, 98*, 2134–2140. doi:10.2105/AJPH.2007.125989

Pfeiffer, J., Montoya, P., Baptista, A., Karagianis, M., Pugas, M.d. M., Micek, M., ... Gloyd, S. (2010). Integration of HIV/AIDS services into African primary health care: Lessons learned for health system strengthening in Mozambique—A case study. *Journal of the International AIDS Society, 13*(1), 3. doi:10.1186/1758-2652-13-3

Pitcher, M. A. (2002). *Transforming Mozambique: The politics of privatization, 1975–2000.* Cambridge: Cambridge University Press. doi:10.1017/CBO9780511491085

Republic of Mozambique and Clinton Foundation. (2003). *Strategic plan for scaling-up HIV/AIDS care and treatment in Mozambique.* Business Plan 6.0. 25 May ed., Republic of Mozambique and Clinton Foundation.

Saul, J. S. (1985). *A difficult road: The transition to socialism in Mozambique.* New York: Monthly Review Press.

Sherr, K., Cuembelo, F., Michel, C., Gimbel, S., Micek, M., Kariaganis, M., ... Gloyd, S. (2013). Strengthening integrated primary health care in Sofala, Mozambique. *BMC Health Services Research, 13*(Suppl. 2), S4. doi:10.1186/1472-6963-13-S2-S4

Sherr, K., Pfeiffer, J., Mussa, A., Vio, F., Gimbel, S., Micek, M., & Gloyd, S. (2009). The role of nonphysician clinicians in the rapid expansion of HIV care in Mozambique. *Journal of Acquired Immune Deficiency Syndromes, 52* (Suppl. 1), S20–S23. doi:10.1097/QAI.0b013e3181bbc9c0

Sidaway, J. D. (1992). Mozambique: Destabilization, state, society and space. *Political Geography, 11*, 239–258. doi:10.1016/0962-6298(92)90028-R

Smith, J. H., & Whiteside, A. (2010). The history of AIDS exceptionalism. *Journal of the International AIDS Society, 13*, 47. doi:10.1186/1758-2652-13-47

Sontag, D. (2004). Early tests for U.S. in its global fight on AIDS. *New York Times*, 14 July.

Sundewall, J., Swanson, R. C., Betigeri, A., Sanders, D., Collins, T. E., Shakarishvili, G., & Brugha, R. (2011). Health-systems strengthening: Current and future activities. *Lancet, 377*, 1222–1223. doi:10.1016/S0140-6736(10)60679-4

UNAIDS. (2008). *Epidemiological fact sheet on HIV and AIDS. Core data on epidemiology and response.* Mozambique 2008 update. UNAIDS. Retrieved January 30, 2010, from http://www.unaids.org

UNAIDS. (2011). *HIV estimates with uncertainty bounds 2011*. UNAIDS. Retrieved November 5, 2013, from http://www.unaids.org

UNAIDS. (2012). *UNAIDS report on the global AIDS epidemic 2012*. UNAIDS. Retrieved December 16, 2013, from http://www.unaids.org

USAID. (2006). *Decisions taken at the national HIV/AIDS meeting as summarized by the minister 11 March 2006*. Maputo: USAID/Mozambique.

AIDS policy responsiveness in Africa: Evidence from opinion surveys

Ashley M. Fox

Department of Health Evidence and Policy, Mount Sinai School of Medicine, New York, NY, USA

As a result of massive scale-up efforts in developing countries, millions of people living with HIV are now receiving antiretroviral therapy (ART). However, countries have been uneven in their scale-up efforts with ART coverage rates exceeding expectations in some places and lagging behind expectation in others. This paper develops a model that explains ART scale-up as a function of the responsiveness of political parties to their primary constituents. Specifically, the paper argues that, faced with a perilous 'threat to the nation', countries responded in one of two ways, both of which were designed to appeal to their primary constituents – either adopting a 'Geneva Consensus' response, or depicting the epidemic as a Western disease and adopting a 'pan-African' response. The article tests this theory using Afrobarometer data for eleven countries. The paper finds that HIV/AIDS is generally a non-partisan issue in most countries. However, the analysis does uncover some differences in partisan support for HIV/AIDS responses in both countries that have adopted Geneva Consensus and pan-African responses, though not in the direction hypothesised. The lack of congruence in policy preferences between the public and their governments suggests a democratic deficit in that these governments have acted independently of the preferences of core constituents.

Introduction

Some in our common world consider the questions I and the rest of our government have raised around the HIV-AIDS issue … as akin to grave criminal and genocidal misconduct.

Former President of South Africa, Thabo Mbeki, Durban, 2000

Some 26,000 people in this country of less than 1.6 million died from AIDS-related illnesses last year alone … We are threatened with extinction … People are dying in chillingly high numbers. It is a crisis of the first magnitude.

Former President of Botswana, Festus Mogae, UN General Assembly, 2002

The HIV/AIDS pandemic that has ravaged parts of sub-Saharan Africa and is continuing to mount in other parts of the world has spurred a surprising array of responses from national governments, including universal treatment access in Brazil and 'zero grazing' in Uganda to denial and defiance in South Africa. Despite an international consensus on best practices, there has been wide variation in the policies adopted across countries and the strength of efforts to implement recommended responses. While treatment access has been made near universal in certain countries, others have lagged behind in their provision of needed treatment and services in spite of large donor infusions to facilitate treatment scale-up.

In countries with skyrocketing HIV/AIDS prevalence rates and generalised, hetero-sexual epidemics that threaten the prosperity of the country as a whole, one would expect the public to demand an aggressive response from their governments and for their governments to have a strong incentive to signal their commitment to combating the epidemic through treatment provision. Yet, in Southern and Eastern Africa, some of the countries with the greatest empirical need to respond swiftly and efficaciously to HIV/ AIDS have been perceived as policy laggards (e.g., South Africa, Zimbabwe, Swaziland) while other countries with a similar empirical need and state capacity have responded in a manner that has garnered international praise (e.g., Botswana, Uganda). What accounts for the different degrees of HIV/AIDS policy effort amongst similarly situated countries?

A theory of government policy responsiveness: when, why and how do governments respond to HIV/AIDS?

This paper argues that countries have generally responded to the epidemic in one of two ways: embracing a 'Geneva Consensus' approach,[1] accepting 'mainstream' global scientific discourse on the disease, or taking a 'pan-African' approach,[2] depicting HIV/ AIDS as a foreign disease with appeals to tradition, nation and crafting an 'African response to an African epidemic' (Cassidy & Leach, 2009). The paper hypothesises that both responses are attempts to be responsive to core constituents of voters.

Both Geneva Consensus and pan-African rhetoric about HIV/AIDS may be deployed to accomplish the same goal in that both bring about a sense of national unity – the former against a common epidemic threat to the nation – 'la patrie en danger' (Nathanson, 2007), and the latter against foreign hegemony. The strategy that the government chooses depends on which the incumbent thinks will resonate most strongly with a majority of constituents and the ideological leaning of the party in power. While researchers and advocates have depicted leaders espousing pan-African rhetoric as backwards and retrograde in their beliefs, this critical, post-colonial discourse should not necessarily be viewed as irrational. Rather, countries that adopt a pan-African response may do so because they believe this framing will resonate with the public. Previous studies have shown that HIV/AIDS does not rank highly among the priorities of Africans, even in high prevalence countries, and public support for government HIV/AIDS responses is stronger than would be expected in several countries that have received international criticism for their HIV/AIDS responses (Dionne, 2012; Youde, 2009, 2012). Together, these findings indicate that African electorates may be wary of Western constructions of HIV/AIDS and broadly supportive of pan-African solutions. Likewise, countries adopting the Geneva Consensus response may do so at their own peril if these responses do not resonate with the public.

Pan-Africanism and oppositional HIV/AIDS theories

As a result of many dominant parties in Africa coming to power via anti-colonial struggles inspired by neo-Marxist, African socialist and post-colonial thought, a central ideological platform of African governments has been at times to portray themselves as wary of Western intervention (Butler, 2005; Phillips, 2004; Schneider, 2002). While HIV/

AIDS has the potential to be framed in terms of a non-partisan threat to the nation, early associations of the virus as originating in Africa and the high rates among African populations have been portrayed through Western media outlets as another example of all things negative emanating from Africa (Washington, 2007). Many governments may have initially rejected HIV/AIDS as a Western disease and African origin theories as another example of racist biomedicine (Washington, 2007).

In the clearest case of this ideologically driven response, South Africa's muted HIV/AIDS response has been attributed to the personal idiosyncrasies of former president Mbeki, who embraced dissident HIV/AIDS theory and appointed a health minister with similar views – a clear example of the potentially deadly consequences of a failure to employ evidence-based policy – which has been discussed at length elsewhere (e.g., Butler 2005; Schneider, 2002; Youde, 2007). However, Mbeki is not alone in his quizzical views of the disease. Other leaders, such as current South African president Jacob Zuma and King Mswati III of Swaziland, have been more indirect in their opposition to HIV/AIDS orthodoxy through an open and flaunting failure to lead by example in their personal lives, controversially taking multiple wives in addition to various sexual indiscretions. Other African leaders, such as Mugabe in Zimbabwe, have embedded their responses to HIV/AIDS in larger tensions over the politics of sexual identity, labelling HIV/AIDS a 'white-man's disease' and associating HIV primarily with Western homosexuality (Phillips, 1997, 2004). Still others have embraced the disease but under the mantra of 'African solutions to African problems' – Gambia's president claims to have found a cure for HIV/AIDS based on herbal, Islamic, and traditional medicine, and is requesting all patients to replace their ARVs with this official state remedy (Cassidy & Leach, 2009). Gambia's attempt at home grown cures is reminiscent of South Africa's early virodene scandal and later attempts to promote traditional home remedies for HIV/AIDS as well as Kenya's claim to have found a cure under former president Arap Moi in the 90s (Mbali, 2013; Nattrass, 2003). Due to the recalcitrance of many African leaders to take on the issue of treatment access, much of the credit for treatment scale-up has been placed on the success of grassroots social movements, notably the Treatment Action Campaign. This movement helped spur the development of the global treatment access architecture, including the Global Fund and President's Emergency Plan for AIDS Relief (PEPFAR), which now provide affordable ARVs to millions in developing countries, who a decade earlier had little to no prospects of receiving these medicines (Mbali, 2013). Part of the success of the treatment access movement, arguably, rests on the social justice claims against these recalcitrant states, particularly South Africa.

How these oppositional HIV/AIDS messages resonate with the public is unclear. As a media attendee to the First International Conference on Virus-Related Cancers in Dakar, Senegal explains,

> to a people who, barely 20 years earlier were under the yoke of Western colonialism, the Africa-Monkey argument was another indication of racism by Western scientists. Therefore, because of our history of colonialism and slavery, the first impulse of African leaders and opinion formers was to defensively repudiate such Western claims with a display of nationalistic garb ... In Nigeria in 1985, it was difficult to meet one person who did not view HIV/AIDS as a 'disease of the white man', and the African connection theory as more evidence of the Western association of Africa with everything negative. Well-meaning people who dared to preach abstinence or condom use as a way to curb the spread of HIV were routinely laughed at as victims of malicious Western propaganda. (Adeyemi, 2001)

Though there is little research on the prevalence of these attitudes, reports from a variety of countries indicate widespread use among African citizens of subversive acronyms to describe AIDS such as 'American Invention to Discourage Sex' and 'Syndrome Imaginaire pour Decourager l'Amour (Imaginary Syndrome to Discourage Sex)' (e.g., Mwadi, 1995; Schoepf, 1991). Surveys from the United States and South Africa suggest that HIV/AIDS conspiracy beliefs, though held by a minority, are nonetheless quite prevalent, ranging from 10 to 60% in different sub-populations of Africans and African-Americans (Grebe & Nattrass, 2012; Nattrass, 2013). Conspiratorial and dissident beliefs about HIV/AIDS may resonate with African populations and with populist leaders who use these messages as a semiotic strategy to project power and generate community (Wedeen, 1999).

This pan-African discourse has been tempered somewhat in light of increasing donor attention to HIV/AIDS and political pressure from highly visible social movements and transnational activist networks (Mbali, 2013), but policy legacies remain observable in the speed and degree of countries' scale-up of recommended HIV/AIDS programming (Lieberman, 2007, 2009).

Public opinion and policy feedback

A government is considered 'responsive' if it 'adopts policies that are signalled as preferred by citizens' (Przeworski, Stokes, & Manin, 1999, p. 9). These signals may include public opinion polls; various forms of direct political action, including demonstrations; and, during elections, votes for particular platforms (Przeworski et al., 1999). A government that is responsive to citizens' concern about HIV/AIDS will develop a policy that responds to their constituents' policy preferences as emitted through public signals. In a country with a low HIV prevalence rate or in which HIV/AIDS is seen as a disease specific to certain marginalised groups, the saliency of HIV/AIDS as a priority social issue should be low and governments will be more likely to align with the priorities of donor organisations (Lieberman, 2009). However, in a country with a high HIV prevalence rate, concern over spiralling infection rates should be empirically sufficient to engage the collective imagination of the public such that they demand some form of a response from government.

However, research on policy-making also suggests that public opinion is a two-way street. Party platforms may not only reflect the public's expressed positions, but may also structure their interests around broad ideological principles, acting as 'transmission belts' of interests (Boix, 1998). Further, voters' uncertainty about policies influences politicians' electoral strategies and platforms (Stokes, 1999). Politicians may wager that voters' preferences can be swayed and actively constructed through a process of 'policy feedback' – a reciprocal relationship whereby the public's preferences affect policy, and subsequent policy then affects preferences, and so on (Hetling, McDermott, & Mapps, 2008). Leaders may venture that HIV/AIDS denialism or a questioning of Western biomedical hegemony will register with the public at large and that they will come to accept a pan-African response. This feedback process may be further affected by political competition, when parties adopt competing pan-African and Geneva Consensus rhetoric or strategically realign their rhetoric to attract donor funds. Furthermore, because donors are more likely to engage with countries that are receptive to Geneva Consensus policies (so-called *donor darlings*), policy legacies may be compounded over time (Lieberman, 2009).

Individual, structural and ideological explanations for HIV/AIDS policy-making

Previous efforts to explain government policy responses to HIV/AIDS have tended to either place a primary emphasis on individual leadership and personalities in explaining different countries' policy approaches, or have emphasised structural and institutional explanations, marginalising the role of individuals or targeted advocacy. Researchers who have focused on individual personalities of leaders have suggested that the political 'commitment' of leaders, often measured in terms of public pronouncements of key political leaders, are the major driving factors behind the aggressiveness of policy responses (e.g., Fox, Gore, Goldberg, & Bärnighausen, 2011; Putzel, 2004). For instance, in sharp contrast with countries adopting a pan-African response, in Botswana, President Mogae quickly declared HIV/AIDS a national emergency and announced a plan to make treatment access universal, investing national resources and partnering with funders, thereby securing ART for 90% of those in need. Likewise, President Museveni in Uganda is well known for his early embrace of aggressive prevention policies through a 'zero grazing' campaign (Youde, 2007), and the Diouf administration in Senegal took an early lead in countering the epidemic by bringing together religious leaders across the country even with modest infection levels (Putzel, 2006). Governments have also evolved over time, initially questioning the severity of the epidemic or calling it un-African, but later embracing the epidemic. Several former heads of state, including former president Kuanda of Zambia and Chissano of Mozambique, have become Champions for an AIDS-Free Generation following tepid responses while in power. While not focusing on the issue during their presidencies, Nelson Mandela and Bill Clinton have become leading figures in the HIV/AIDS field after retiring from their executive posts. In Uganda, Museveni's seemingly effective early embrace of HIV/AIDS as a disease threatening the nation (and the military particularly) soon gave way to an emphasis on the promotion of abstinence-only education after the introduction of the PEPFAR (Epstein, 2007; Patterson, 2006; Youde, 2007). Individual accounts, such as these, tend to stress the agency of leaders as 'cultural entrepreneurs' in endorsing and legitimising either 'mainstream' or 'oppositional' HIV/AIDS beliefs (Nattrass, 2013).

Structural accounts, by contrast, downplay the role of specific leaders or influential individuals/organisations, and instead emphasise institutional factors that influence the responses that countries have. Dionne (2006), for instance, analyses the role of competitive elections in influencing HIV/AIDS resource allocations, hypothesising that the shorter time horizons of leaders who face frequent re-election will lead to a more muted response than executives who expect to be in power for longer. She finds evidence that countries with regular elections (i.e., shorter executive time horizons) have lower levels of government spending on health, but have more comprehensive HIV/AIDS policy. Gauri and Lieberman (2006) argue that ethnic and religious fractionalisation mutes policy responses to HIV/AIDS through a process of blame shifting – 'because social boundaries inevitably concern not only group differences, but also intergroup moral hierarchies in which groups occupy spaces of relative virtue or cleanliness, a dynamic of blame and shame about the pathogenesis of AIDS ensues' (p. 50). Patterson (2006) examines four structural factors that have influenced policy responses – centralisation of authority, patron-client relations, state capacity and government stability – and finds that different combinations of these factors interact to explain policy trajectories. Parkhurst and Lush (2004) attribute varying responses in Uganda and South Africa to differences in bureaucratic capacities, health care infrastructures and the role of external donors in addition to differences in political leadership. In general, structural accounts tend to downplay the importance of governments' rhetorical or stated positions on policy, whereas individual accounts place emphasis on these elements.

Following Youde (2007), this paper takes a middle ground approach. It acknowledges the pivotal role of influential individuals in the symbolic politics of HIV/AIDS, which can have a profound effect on the saliency of HIV/AIDS to citizens by serving as a signalling device communicating government stances on HIV/AIDS. At the same time, the paper places policy responses in the broader political context and set of incentives faced by leaders and political parties in countries. While not discounting the idiosyncratic roles of individual leaders, this paper aims to situate these policy responses in the larger policy context of post-colonial African states.

Previous research on public opinion on HIV/AIDS in Africa has not examined attitudes towards HIV/AIDS policy responses explicitly comparing attitudes in countries that are considered policy leaders and policy laggards. Prior structural accounts also do not stress the role played by ideology and partisan politics in shaping HIV/AIDS politics and policy, while individual accounts have not linked support for HIV/AIDS conspiracy to political beliefs and post-colonial ideology, instead viewing these beliefs as emanating from 'mis-information' or moral panics in times of uncertainty about a terrifying new disease (e.g., Nattrass, 2013; Treichler 1999, p. 15). The goal of this paper is to examine whether there exists ideological congruence (Huber & Powell, 1994) between a government's response to HIV/AIDS (Geneva Consensus or pan-African) and the public's HIV/AIDS policy preferences. The hypothesis is that there should be congruence between incumbent party supporters and the regime's HIV/AIDS response, even in countries considered to be laggards. If a disconnect is found to exist between government policy and citizen attitudes, particularly among party faithful, this suggests a democratic deficit (see Figure 1, conceptual model). I expect that ideological congruence will either deepen over time, or may lessen due to increased external attention to HIV/AIDS and declining infection rates.

Methods

To examine the role of partisanship on attitudes towards government responses to HIV/AIDS, this study employs Afrobarometer data for eleven medium and high prevalence East and Southern African countries. The paper examines only medium and high prevalence countries since these countries have a higher stake in responding to HIV/AIDS, and citizens of higher prevalence countries, in theory, should be more engaged by this issue. Using prior classifications of countries policy responses (Desmond, Lieberman, Alban, & Ekström, 2008; Lieberman, 2009; Nattrass, 2008), three questions on public perceptions of government responses to HIV/AIDS and information on respondents' party affiliation, this paper examines the HIV/AIDS related opinions of core supporters of the party in power versus opposition party supporters to assess partisan differences in support for different government approaches to confronting HIV/AIDS.

Categorising country responses

Countries were first coded as policy leaders or laggards in their HIV/AIDS responses using existing coding schemes. The complexities of categorising countries' responses to HIV/AIDS and the adequacy of existing measures have been discussed elsewhere (Fox et al., 2011; Goldberg, Fox, Gore, & Baernighausen, 2012). Among other issues, a country's level of donor support, state capacity and informal institutions influence its ability to scale-up access to antiretrovirals and achieve other HIV/AIDS related goals. Two previous studies have ranked countries according to the adequacy of their domestic HIV/AIDS responses, adjusting for international inputs and domestic resource levels/ capacity (Desmond et al., 2008; Nattrass, 2008). Desmond et al.'s country ranking scheme assigns three codes to classify countries as above-expectation, meeting expectation and below expectation, whereas Nattrass classifies countries only as consistently above or below expectation. This study combines both classifications and codes countries dichotomously as either leaders or laggards in terms of their progress on scaling up care and treatment services including ARVs, PMTCT and orphan care, adjusting for their domestic resource base.

Applying this coding, the following countries were considered leaders (Botswana, Kenya, Malawi, Namibia, Uganda, and Zambia) and laggards (Lesotho, Mozambique, South Africa, and Zimbabwe) (summarised in Table 1). Tanzania was indeterminate because it was not previously coded but was retained in the analysis. These are admittedly very rough categorisations and as these classifications were made between 2006 and 2008, they reflect more recent policy effort. As found in Nattrass (2008), these adjusted codings generally conform to commonly held country 'reputations'. However, these codings may not capture every aspect of a country's overall response and the degree to which it conforms to a Geneva Consensus or pan-African response. For instance, in spite of being praised for its early success at HIV/AIDS prevention, Uganda has maintained a commitment to homophobia that puts it at odds with global consensus over human rights and best practices in HIV/AIDS prevention (Gettleman, 2010). Table 1 also shows ARV coverage rates for 2006 and 2010 and per person HIV/AIDS spending. Earlier estimates are difficult to locate for most countries. Some countries have recently improved their ARV coverage rates during this time in step with increasing donation programmes and Global Fund activity (see Table 1). As summarised in Table 1, none of these countries experienced any significant change in party leadership over the period assessed in this analysis. Several countries had elections in 2004 or 2005, but only in Malawi did a new party come to power. In South Africa's 2004 election, Mbeki remained leader of the African National Congress (ANC), though Jacob Zuma replaced him as head of the ANC in 2007.

Data sources and definition

Dependent variable: public support for national HIV/AIDS responses

To examine the dynamics of support for government HIV/AIDS policies, this article relies on public opinion data collected during four consecutive rounds of the Afrobarometer survey. Afrobarometer is an independent, non-partisan research project that measures the social, political and economic atmosphere in Africa (http://www. afrobarometer.org/). Surveys employ a national probability sample to ensure a represent-ative cross-section of all citizens of voting age. Four rounds of the Afrobarometer have included questions pertaining to countries' HIV/AIDS responses. The first round, fielded between 1999 and 2001, only includes two HIV/AIDS questions in three countries in Southern and Eastern Africa (South Africa, Uganda and Tanzania). Rounds two and three were fielded between 2002–2003 and 2005–2006, respectively, and included three HIV/ AIDS related questions in 11 East and Southern African states (Botswana, Kenya, Lesotho, Malawi, Mozambique, Namibia, South Africa, Tanzania, Uganda, Zambia, and Zimbabwe). Round 4 fielded in 2008/2009 included the same countries but only two HIV/AIDS questions. Surveys and sample sizes are summarised in Table 2.

Three questions from the Afrobarometer were examined:

Table 1. Country HIV/AIDS response codings.

Country	Elections producing a change in leadership	Nattrass (2008) coding	Desmond et al. (2008) coding	ARV coverage rate	ARV coverage rate	Domestic AIDS spending per capita	HIV Prevalence	Final coding[a]
Year		2006	2006	2006	2010	2007	2005	
Botswana	2008	1	1	100	93	764.86	24.1	Leader
Kenya	2002,[b] 2007	1	2	44	61	NA	6.1	Leader
Uganda	–	1	2	41	47	215.34	6.7	Leader
Malawi	2004[c]	1	2	43	67	60.74	14.1	Leader
Namibia	2004[d]	1	1	71	90	652.50	19.6	Leader
Zambia	2002,[e] 2008	1	2	35	72	172.66	17.0	Leader
Tanzania	2005[f]	NA	NA	18	42	NA	6.5	Indeterminate
South Africa	2004,[g] 2009	0	0	32	55	109.06	18.8	Laggard
Lesotho	2007	0	1	31	57	90.50	23.2	Laggard
Mozambique	2005[h]	NA	0	14	40	38.83	16.1	Laggard
Zimbabwe	2009	0	0	15	59	99.63	20.1	Laggard

Note: ARV coverage rates and domestic spending are for illustrative purposes only and did not factor into the coding.
[a]Leaders are defined as countries either meeting or exceeding expectation in HIV/AIDS service scale-up based on the combined codings from Nattrass (2008) and Desmond et al. (2008), both of which use 2006 estimates of HIV/AIDS service availability from UNAIDS.
[b]Kenya's first free and fair general elections producing a change in power were held in Kenya in December 2002.
[c]New party formed by Mutharika in 2005.
[d]President Pohamba elected in 2004, but no change in party since independence.
[e]MMD in power since 1991 until the Patriotic Front won in 2011.
[f]CCM in power since 1985.
[g]ANC in power since the end of apartheid in 1994. Zuma replaced Mbeki as PM in 2008.
[h]FRELIMO in power since independence.

Table 2.   Country sample sizes and year collected.

| Country | Round 1[a] | | Round 2 | | Round 3 | | Round 4[b] | |
	Sample size	Year	Sample size	Year	Sample size	Year	Sample size	Year
Botswana	1200	1999	1200	2003	1200	2005	1200	2008
Kenya	–	–	2400	2003	1278	2005	1104	2008
Uganda	2271	2000	2400	2002	2400	2005	2431	2008
Malawi	1208	1999	1200	2003	1200	2005	1200	2008
Namibia	1183	1999	1199	2003	1200	2005	1200	2008
Zambia	1198	1999	1199	2003	1200	2005	1200	2009
Tanzania	2198	2001	1200	2003	1248	2005	1208	2008
South Africa	2200	2000	2400	2002	2400	2006	2400	2008
Lesotho	1177	2000	1200	2003	1200	2005	1200	2008
Mozambique	–	–	1400	2002	1198	2005	1200	2008
Zimbabwe	1200	1999	1104	2004	1048	2005	1200	2009

[a]Provides data for only 1 question on issue salience.
[b]Provides data only for 2 questions on issue salience and approval of government's handling of AIDS.

(1)   How well or badly would you say the current government is handling the following matters, or haven't you heard enough about them to say? Combating AIDS.

(2)   Which of these statements is closest to your view? Choose Statement A or Statement B. A: The government should devote many more resources to combating AIDS, even if this means that less money is spent on things like education. B: There are many other problems facing this country beside AIDS; even if people are dying in large numbers, the government needs to keep its focus on solving other problems.

(3)   What are the most important problems facing the country that the government should address? [open-ended] AIDS among top 3.

The first question captures general attitudes towards the incumbent government's HIV/AIDS response. We expect that incumbent party supporters will approve of the government's response even in countries considered policy laggards, as well as in policy leaders. The second question is included as a proxy for endorsing a pan-African stance on HIV/AIDS with the implication that there are more pressing problems facing the country even in countries with skyrocketing infection rates, minimising the significance of HIV/AIDS as a policy priority. We expect that incumbent party supporters will endorse the view that resources should be put towards other issues besides HIV/AIDS in policy laggards and that the opposition will support this view in countries that are HIV/AIDS policy issues. The third question captures a similar pan-African attitude regarding the level of priority accorded to different policy issues. We expect that incumbent party supporters in HIV/AIDS policy laggard countries will be less likely to view HIV/AIDS as a top three priority for the country and more likely in leaders.

Independent variable: party identification

Individuals were coded as incumbent or opposition supporters depending on the party they reported as being close to. As a large proportion of individuals do not affiliate with a particular political party, a third category of 'unaffiliated' was created for these individuals.

Controls

Gender, age, education, income, having lost a loved one to HIV/AIDS and presidential approval were entered in the multivariate analysis as controls. Previous research has found that few demographic variables are correlated with support for government HIV/AIDS policy responses (Youde, 2012). Nonetheless, respondent demographics were entered to adjust for these characteristics. Research has found a strong association between those who have lost loved ones to HIV/AIDS and those who cite HIV/AIDS or health as a top national priority (Dionne, 2012; Dionne, Gerland, & Watkins, 2013; Whiteside, Mattes, Willan, & Manning, 2004). Furthermore, research has shown that approval of a government's performance on HIV/AIDS is related to general support for the regime (Youde, 2012). While we would expect supporters of a party to generally approve of that party, there may be party supporters who disagree with their government's specific HIV/AIDS policy. Therefore, we control for presidential approval in the adjusted analysis.

Data analysis

Rather than pooling countries, weighted percentages and adjusted odds ratios were derived separately for each country for the three measures of public support for governments' HIV/AIDS policy, to examine country specific relationships and trends. Results are reported overall and stratified by support for the incumbent party, opposition party or unaffiliated. Separate results are generated for the years 2002/2003 and 2005/2006 to observe any change over time and given that several countries did change heads of state even if not party leadership during this time period. Chi-square tests of association were run to test significant differences in support for HIV/AIDS policies across supporters of incumbents versus opposition and unaffiliated individuals. Adjusted odds ratios were derived for each country in rounds two and three (the two rounds for which data were available for all variables) to assess the relationship between party affiliation and support for HIV/AIDS policies adjusted for other factors that affect support. We hypothesise similarity in results among governments identified as policy leaders and similarity among governments identified as policy laggards.

The specific hypotheses tested in this analysis are as follows (see Figure 1):

(1) Support for how government is handling HIV/AIDS should be lower overall in countries that are laggards compared with leaders, but higher among core party supporters compared with opposition supporters.

(2) In countries that are considered policy laggards, incumbent party supporters will be more likely to approve of the government's HIV/AIDS response, endorse that resources should be spent on other issues besides HIV/AIDS, and less likely to rate HIV/AIDS as a high priority compared with opposition supporters.

(3) In countries that are considered HIV/AIDS policy leaders, incumbent party supporters will be more likely to approve of the government's HIV/AIDS response, endorse that more resources should be spent on HIV/AIDS, and rate HIV/AIDS as high priority compared with opposition supporters.

	Approval of Gov handling of AIDS		Put resources towards other issues besides AIDS		AIDS top 3 problem facing country	
	Incumb	Oppos	Incumb	Oppos	Incumb	Oppos
Leaders	+	−	−	+	+	−
Laggards	+	−	+	−	−	+

Figure 1.   Theoretical model of expected responses of incumbent and opposition supporters in HIV/AIDS policy leaders and laggards.
Note: While in both policy leaders and laggards supporters of the incumbent should be more likely than opposition supporters to approve of how the government is handling HIV/AIDS, they should differ with regards to the level of policy priority given to HIV/AIDS. In policy leaders, opposition supporters should be more likely to report that resources should be put towards other issues and less likely to rate HIV/AIDS as a major problem facing the country. By contrast, in policy laggards, the opposition should be more likely to want to press the government to be more aggressive in its HIV/AIDS policies and more likely to see HIV/AIDS as a major problem.
'+': more likely than reference group to endorse a policy position; '−': less likely than reference to endorse a policy position.

Results

National attitudes and changing assessments over time

Table 3 displays overall trends in public attitudes towards government HIV/AIDS responses for each country across the four time periods. Overall, support for how government is handling HIV/AIDS is high and has generally been increasing over time. A majority in each country believe that the government is handling HIV/AIDS well or very well, with the sole exception of South Africa. In South Africa support was at a low of near 40% in 2000 at the apex of Mbeki's HIV/AIDS denialism. Support increased in 2002, to near 50% as the government began to soften in its pan-African rhetoric and reached a high of 55% after significant concessions on PMTCT and treatment access had been made in the 2006 round, though support fell again in 2008 with Jacob Zuma now leading the country. Surprisingly, other HIV/AIDS laggards nevertheless enjoy high levels of support for how they are handling HIV/AIDS. Although dipping to 40% in 2005, in Zimbabwe nearly 70% of the public said the government was handling HIV/ AIDS well or very well in 2003 and 65% in 2008.

In spite of the high general support for government HIV/AIDS responses offered by the public at large, the public in most countries is largely split over whether the government should spend more on HIV/AIDS or should instead focus on other issues (see Table 3). In Namibia, Zambia and Zimbabwe, more than 60% of the population believed that resources should be devoted to other problems besides HIV/AIDS in 2002/2003; however, these attitudes decreased by 2005/2006. In four of the six HIV/ AIDS policy leaders, support for spending resources on other issues besides HIV/AIDS increased between 2002/2003 and 2005/2006, a period of rapid scale-up of HIV/ AIDS services, but also in policy laggards Mozambique and Lesotho. In South Africa, Tanzania, Zimbabwe, Zambia and Namibia, support for putting resources elsewhere decreased between 2002 and 2006.

In all four rounds of the survey, less than 10% of respondents ranked HIV/AIDS among the top three most important issues facing the country in most countries (Table 3). The exceptions are the three most economically developed countries in the region, South Africa, Botswana and Namibia, where nearly a quarter of the population ranked HIV/ AIDS among the top three problems facing the country. There is little discernible difference between policy leaders and laggards. The fact that wealthier countries had a higher percentage of respondents listing HIV/AIDS as a major issue facing the country

Table 3. Attitudes towards HIV//AIDS policy, 1999–2009.

Country	Country response	Government handling AIDS well/very well				Spend resources on other issues besides AIDS		Spend more on AIDS		AIDS among top 3 most imp problem facing country			
Year		1999/ 2000	2002/ 2003	2005/ 2006	2008/ 2009	2002/ 2003	2005/ 2006	2002/ 2003	2005/ 2006	1999/ 2000	2002/ 2003	2005/ 2006	2008/ 2009
Botswana	Leader	NA	77.9	91.8	94.2	46.9	61.5	46.9	35.8	20.2	29.1	27.1	10.7
Kenya	Leader	NA	82.4	73.5	76.2	36	58.5	58.7	34.4	NA	9.5	4.5	1.9
Uganda	Leader	77.1	76.9	84.6	70.4	46.7	48.5	52.1	45.6	0.4	7.2	5.9	4.6
Malawi	Leader	NA	50.3	58.9	82.4	43.2	56.6	47.1	40.3	1.0	2.7	1.0	1.8
Namibia	Leader	NA	66.8	71.8	70.9	59.0	53.7	35.2	40.6	10.7	28	23.2	9.8
Zambia	Leader	NA	67.9	74.9	74.5	64.5	52.3	33	37.3	0	3.2	5.6	1.2
Tanzania	Indeterminate	73	79.9	80.5	84.3	43.2	30.3	47.2	59.4	0.4	13.8	3.3	3.7
South Africa	Laggard	40.5	48.8	55.2	41.6	42.7	38.0	40.4	45.6	8.0	26.1	23.9	21.1
Lesotho	Laggard	NA	64.9	60.1	76.8	36.3	47.0	56.6	45.3	0.1	4.8	5.0	4.2
Mozambique	Laggard	NA	53.0	65.8	70.2	28.0	33.6	56.1	55.0	NA	14.4	6.3	4.5
Zimbabwe	Laggard	NA	69.3	39.4	64.8	69.8	63.4	27.5	29.9	3.3	6.5	7.8	0.4

could reflect wealthier respondents' broader post-material[3] attitudes, whereas respondents in poorer countries place a higher priority on meeting basic needs. Across all countries with available data there was a dramatic increase in the percentage of people reporting HIV/AIDS as a top problem between 1999/2000 and 2002/2003, likely reflecting a growing awareness of and concern about the epidemic. During the period under investigation, concern reached a high point in most countries in 2002/2003 and appears to have been declining since that time.

Partisan differences in HIV/AIDS policy support (unadjusted percentages)

Tables 4 and 5 show support for the three HIV/AIDS policy questions stratified by party affiliation for 2002/2003 and 2005/2006. In 2002/2003, in most cases the opposition is moderately (though significantly) less likely to approve of the government response to HIV/AIDS, suggesting that general support for a party may translate into more generalised support for the party's policies, as others have suggested (Youde, 2009). Only in Botswana was support consistent across incumbent, opposition and unaffiliated and in South Africa, contrary to expectation, the opposition was actually more likely to approve of the government's HIV/AIDS response. This may reflect deep divisions within ANC supporters, which is comprised of a broad cross-section of voters. The same trends held in 2005/2006 – in all countries, including South Africa, incumbent party supporters were more likely than opposition and unaffiliated individuals to approve of the government's handling of HIV/AIDS, except in Botswana where the same trends held as in 2002/2003.

With regards to whether resources should be put towards other issues besides HIV/AIDS and how HIV/AIDS ranks compared with other country priorities, the trends were mixed. The expectation was that in countries that are policy leaders, the opposition would be more likely to believe that too many resources are being spent on HIV/AIDS and that the government should focus elsewhere, whereas opposition supporters in policy laggards should want the government to do more to address HIV/AIDS. In Kenya and Malawi, both policy leaders, the opposition was indeed more likely to believe that resources should be put elsewhere, but the same was true for South Africa and Mozambique, policy laggards, indicating that opposition supporters were more likely to support pan-African policy responses in contrast with expectation. In Namibia, with an above average response, supporters of the incumbent were more likely to endorse that resources should be put elsewhere, suggesting dissatisfaction with the government's aggressive Geneva Consensus response. By 2005/2006, Botswana's opposition was also more likely to think that resources should be put towards other issues, conforming to expectation. Only in Zambia was the opposition less likely than incumbent supporters to say that resources should be targeted elsewhere. In Uganda and Malawi, opposition supporters were more likely than incumbent supporters to view HIV/AIDS as a top three problem in 2002/2003. In South Africa, the opposition was less likely to say that HIV/AIDS was a top three problem facing the country, in keeping with their endorsement that resources should be put towards other problems.

Adjusted differences in levels of support between incumbent and opposition supporters

The adjusted odds ratios, summarised in Tables 6 and 7, largely supported the descriptive results and few clear stories emerged. Incumbent party supporters were generally more likely to approve of the government's response, and opposition less likely. In a few of

Table 4. 2002/2003 support for government HIV/AIDS responses by party affiliation.

	Country	Government handling AIDS well/very well (%)				Put resources towards other issues (%)				AIDS top 3 problem (%)			
		Incumbent supporter	Opposition supporter	Unaffiliated	p-Value	Incumbent supporter	Opposition supporter	Unaffiliated	p-Value	Incumbent supporter	Opposition supporter	Unaffiliated	p-Value
Leaders	Botswana	76.8	74.1	72.7	.511	48.5	45.4	45.9	.461	28.2	34.1	27.9	.214
	Kenya	**81.2**	**76.8**	**75.1**	**.001**	57.7	64.9	57.9	.071	10.5	10.4	7.7	.108
	Uganda	77.5	76.5	73.7	.213	45.7	49.0	46.7	.782	**5.8**	**11.5**	**7.1**	**.004**
	Malawi	**55.1**	**38.4**	**47.2**	**.000**	**37.9**	**63.8**	**37.2**	**.000**	1.9	4.7	2.4	.075
	Namibia	**65.7**	**57.6**	**72.5**	**.007**	**63.8**	**52.5**	**50.7**	**.000**	28.7	27.2	26.9	.812
	Zambia	64.9	65.7	66.9	.111	63.3	68.1	64.2	.573	2.6	4.8	3	.400
	Tanzania	**80.4**	**66.2**	**77.5**	**.002**	41.4	49.2	44.1	.114	12.9	18.2	13.9	.279
Laggards	South Africa	45.8	48.1	44.8	.439	**36.0**	**55.5**	**44.4**	**.000**	27.2	23.4	26	.360
	Lesotho	50.7	40.9	47.8	**.040**	35.9	37.0	36.5	.634	4	4.8	6.2	.284
	Mozambique	**49.5**	**18.5**	**49.4**	**.000**	**27.9**	**53.7**	**25.6**	**.000**	13.4	20.8	15.3	.261
	Zimbabwe	**70.3**	**59.1**	**63.4**	**.000**	65.5	72.7	71.5	.321	5.5	3.6	7.5	.199

Note: Bold represents significant at $p < .05$.

Table 5. 2005/2006 support for government HIV/AIDS responses by party affiliation.

	Country	Government handling AIDS well/very well (%)				Put resources towards other issues (%)				% AIDS top 3 problem			
		Incumbent supporter	Opposition supporter	Unaffiliated	p-Value	Incumbent supporter	Opposition supporter	Unaffiliated	p-Value	Incumbent supporter	Opposition supporter	Unaffiliated	p-value
Leaders	Botswana	93.6	90.3	90.3	.161	**56.4**	**62.3**	**70.9**	**.000**	27.6	24.6	29.5	.359
	Kenya	**77.2**	**72.6**	**70.4**	**.003**	59.3	57.9	57.8	.330	4.9	4.2	3.7	.677
	Uganda	**86.3**	**82.3**	**82.4**	**.011**	**50.6**	**55.0**	**43.7**	**.000**	4.8	6.9	4.1	.125
	Malawi	**67.7**	**55.6**	**57.6**	**.007**	**58.5**	**59.2**	**53.0**	**.037**	1.6	0.8	0.8	.553
	Namibia	**70.2**	**80.6**	**69.3**	**.000**	52.0	55.8	57.1	.239	24.2	22.3	20.6	.501
	Zambia	**78.7**	**72.8**	**74.7**	**.014**	43.8	40.3	32.9	.055	6	7.2	4.4	.176
	Tanzania	**83.7**	**75.0**	**75.2**	**.008**	30.1	32.9	30.6	.135	2.9	5.6	3.9	.336
Laggards	South Africa	**64.3**	**47.0**	**45.6**	**.000**	**35.9**	**38.8**	**40.6**	**.017**	**27.5**	**18.9**	**22.5**	**.004**
	Lesotho	61.9	55.1	57.1	.082	46.5	51.6	41.5	.161	4.9	6.3	4.1	.593
	Mozambique	**66.4**	**49.5**	**70.6**	**.000**	54.9	50.5	59.3	.604	7	4	4.2	.193
	Zimbabwe	**53.1**	**30.8**	**39.5**	**.000**	31.8	27.1	31.3	.112	7.1	7.4	8.3	.831

Note: Bold represents significant at $p < .05$.

the policy leader countries in 2002/2003, the expected pattern of the opposition endorsing the belief that resources should be put towards issues other than HIV/AIDS did emerge. In Kenya and Malawi, supporters of the incumbent were less likely to endorse this opinion and supporters of the opposition were more likely. However, this relationship was reversed in Namibia, and in two policy laggards, South Africa and Mozambique, where the opposition was more likely to believe that resources should be spent on other issues, and incumbent party supporters were not more likely to endorse the view that more resources should be directed elsewhere besides HIV/AIDS (Table 6).

Reverse patterns from expectation also emerged with respect to individuals viewing HIV/AIDS as a top three problem facing the country. In Uganda and Malawi, incumbent supporters were less likely to view HIV/AIDS as a top three problem while opposition supporters were more likely to view HIV/AIDS as a major problem facing the country (Table 6). The reverse was the case in policy laggard South Africa, where incumbent party supporters were more likely to view HIV/AIDS as a top problem and opposition less likely, though weakly so. By 2005/2006, however, incumbent supporters in South Africa were much more likely than opposition supporters to approve of the government's handling of HIV/AIDS. This shift likely reflects the government's relenting in its pan-African rhetoric and the development of a plan to roll-out antiretrovirals. As in previous studies, whereas demographics were not strongly associated with support for HIV/AIDS policies, general approval of the president was associated with higher approval of the countries' HIV/AIDS response, and knowing someone who has died of HIV/AIDS was associated with higher support for more resources going to HIV/AIDS across most countries (results not shown).

Discussion

Increasing support for government handling of HIV/AIDS with decreasing support for more resources and declining concern

Previous studies have not examined how public reaction to governmental HIV/AIDS responses has evolved over time in different countries. In general, seemingly in lockstep with treatment scale-up, support for government HIV/AIDS policies has mostly increased over time. Support for the government's response in Botswana reached 94% in 2008/2009. Support for South Africa's response has remained among the lowest (averaging around 45% approval) compared with other countries and has fallen again in 2008/2009 after increasing in 2005/2006 with the roll-out of treatment scale-up beginning in 2003. At the same time, even as approval for government responses has increased, as treatment access has grown, particularly between the 2002/2003 and 2005/2006 period, support for putting more resources towards HIV/AIDS has declined in many countries. The percentage listing HIV/AIDS as among the top three most important problems facing the country peaked in most countries in 2002/2003 and appears to be declining following a similar pattern to global trends in attention to HIV/AIDS.

Policy leaders/laggards generally reflected in overall support for government HIV/AIDS response

Overall, policy laggards enjoyed lower support than policy leaders. One exception is Malawi, which started off with a low of 50% of the country approving of the response, but has risen to 80% by the 2008/2009 round. This may reflect more recent scale-up efforts as donor funds have become increasingly available. Yet, surprisingly, some

Table 6. 2002/2003 adjusted odds ratios, support for government HIV/AIDS responses by party affiliation.

	Country	Government handling AIDS well/very well			Put resources towards other issues			AIDS top 3 problem facing country		
		Incumbent (opposition ref.)	Opposition (incumbent ref.)	Unaffiliated (incumbent ref.)	Incumbent (opposition ref.)	Opposition (incumbent ref.)	Unaffiliated (incumbent ref.)	Incumbent (opposition ref.)	Opposition (incumbent ref.)	Unaffiliated (incumbent ref.)
Leaders	Botswana	1.11	0.89	0.75	1.24	0.81	0.77*	0.76	1.31	0.92
	Kenya	1.24	0.80	0.77**	0.73**	1.37**	1.04	1.08	0.92	0.77
	Uganda	0.97	1.02	0.82*	1.02	0.97	0.97	0.54**	1.80***	1.17
	Malawi	1.46**	0.68*	0.88	0.50***	2.01***	0.89	0.44*	2.25*	1.08
	Namibia	1.33	0.74	1.37**	1.51**	0.66***	0.62***	1.04	0.95	0.96
	Zambia	1	1.00	1.06	0.80	1.24	1.05	0.70	1.43	0.93
	Tanzania	1.43	0.69	0.98	0.65***	1.53***	1.23	0.75	1.32	1.04
Laggards	South Africa	0.83	1.20	1.08	0.49***	2.03***	1.38***	1.28*	0.78*	1.00
	Lesotho	1.23	0.81	0.92	0.88	1.13	1.19	0.91	1.09	1.13
	Mozambique	3.28***	0.30***	1.00	0.49**	2.02***	0.68***	0.66	1.50	1.17
	Zimbabwe	1.81***	0.55	0.66	0.94	1.06	1.14	1.27	0.78	1.55

*$p < .1$, **$p < .05$, ***$p < .001$.

Table 7. 2005/2006 adjusted odds ratios, support for government HIV/AIDS responses by party affiliation.

	Country	Approve of government handling of HIV			Put resources towards other issues			AIDS top 3 problem facing country		
		Incumbent (opposition ref.)	Opposition (incumbent ref.)	Unaffiliated (incumbent ref.)	Incumbent (opposition ref.)	Opposition (incumbent ref.)	Unaffiliated (incumbent ref.)	Incumbent (opposition ref.)	Opposition (incumbent ref.)	Unaffiliated (incumbent ref.)
Leaders	Botswana	1.47	0.68	0.66	0.8	1.24	1.78***	1.20	0.83	1.02
	Kenya	1.06	0.93	0.79	1.26	0.79	0.88	1.18	0.84	0.82
	Uganda	1.26	0.79	0.84	0.94	1.06	0.71***	0.98	1.01	0.86
	Malawi	1.24	0.80	0.91	0.81	1.23	0.99	1.34	0.74	0.84
	Namibia	0.60***	1.67***	0.94	0.87	1.13	1.34*	1.10	0.91	0.75
	Zambia	1.49*	0.67*	0.81	0.95	1.04	1.51***	0.96	1.03	0.56
	Tanzania	1.49	0.67	0.63***	0.98	1.01	1.02	0.53	1.88	1.05
Laggards	South Africa	1.63***	0.61***	0.57***	0.96	1.03	1.19*	1.53**	0.65**	0.75***
	Lesotho	1.12	0.89	0.89	1.21	0.82	1.14	1.71	0.59	0.49*
	Mozambique	1.24	0.80	1.43**	0.71	1.4	0.9	2.10	0.47	0.52*
	Zimbabwe	1.64**	0.61**	0.71*	0.72	1.38	0.89	1.00	0.99	1.19

*$p < .1$, **$p < .05$, ***$p < .001$.

well-known policy laggards, including Zimbabwe, have received broad popular support of nearly 70% of the population, begging the question of why government responses remain domestically popular in spite of their global condemnation internationally. Likewise, in South Africa, 40–50% of the population has consistently approved of the government's response in spite of its many gaffes and set-backs. It is also possible in the case of Zimbabwe and South Africa that respondents interpret broadly the issue of how the 'government' is handling HIV/AIDS, with government not primarily signifying the executive branch, but the broader legislative and bureaucratic bodies. For instance, in spite of Mugabe's homophobic rhetoric (Phillips, 1997, 2004), the country's former Health Minister, David Parirenyatwa, was viewed by many in the HIV/AIDS community as one of the few progressive members of the ZANU-PF who spoke openly and frequently about the extent of the epidemic (Batsell, 2005, p. 71). Likewise, in South Africa, much of the government, including members of the Medical Research Council and other government bodies did their best to work around the President and the Health Minister with some openly condemning their oppositional HIV/AIDS stances (Mbali, 2013). Previous studies have suggested that support for HIV/AIDS policies may serve as a proxy for more generalised support of leadership (Youde, 2009), or represent very real policy preferences among 515 many poor Africans with competing needs as more pressing proximal concerns take precedence over HIV/AIDS (Dionne, 2012).

Some differences in partisan support for HIV/AIDS responses, in both leaders and laggards

The adjusted results found significant differences in partisan support for government HIV/AIDS responses in a number of countries, but not primarily in the expected direction. Generally, as expected, the unadjusted frequencies find lower support for government response from opposition in both policy leaders and laggards, which may very well be reflective of general support for the party. After adjusting for approval of the Presidents' job performance, the significance in support for government policies is eliminated in most countries. Significant results ($p < .05$) are summarised in Figures 2 and 3, comparing hypothesised results with results from the adjusted analysis. There were few differences between policy leaders or laggards in terms of which groups were more likely to view HIV/AIDS as a priority. Contrary to expectation, incumbent supporters in policy laggards were not uniformly more likely to say that country resources should be directed to other problems besides HIV/AIDS or less likely to list HIV/AIDS as a pressing problem. Instead, in South Africa and Mozambique, the opposition was more likely to endorse the view that resources should be spent elsewhere besides HIV/AIDS. It may be that in these countries, certain opposition parties endorse an even stronger pan-African sentiment with regards to HIV/AIDS than the incumbent party or that supporters of the incumbent party are torn over the government's approach to handling HIV/AIDS. For instance, in South Africa, the ANC enjoys wide support across a broad spectrum of the voting public. Although support was generally stronger in South Africa among ANC supporters in 2005/2006, support for the government response in 2002/2003 did not differ across party lines – approximately 45% of individuals whether ANC aligned, unaffiliated or aligned with an opposition party supported the government's handling of HIV/AIDS even prior to the government relenting in the worst of its HIV/AIDS denialism. Most of the contestation on the countries' HIV/AIDS policy actually has come from different factions within the ANC, internal divisions, which would not be reflected in this analysis. Furthermore, the analysis did not stratify by race, which may significantly divide public

	Approval of Gov handling of AIDS		Put resources towards other issues besides AIDS		AIDS top 3 problem facing country	
	Incumb	Oppos/Unaffil	Incumb	Oppos/Unaffil	Incumb	Oppos/Unaffil
Leaders	+	–	–	+	+	–
Botswana						
Kenya		–	–	+	–	+
Uganda						
Malawi	+		–	+		
Namibia		+	+	–		
Zambia						
Laggards	+	–	+	–	–	+
South Africa			–	+		
Lesotho						
Mozambique	+	–	–	+		
Zimbabwe	+	–				

Figure 2.   Summary of results and correspondence with hypothesised relationships, 2002/2003.

opinion in South Africa across party lines. HIV/AIDS policy leaders Kenya and Malawi, on the other hand, followed the hypothesised pattern, at least in 2002/2003 prior to scale-up – opposition supporters were more likely to indicate that resources should be spent elsewhere besides HIV/AIDS. In Zimbabwe, incumbent party supporters consistently approved of the government's HIV/AIDS response in 2002/2003 and 2005/2006, in spite of the global criticism regarding the inadequacy of the regime's response (Price-Smith, 2007), also conforming to expectation.

Namibia, a policy leader, also presents some counterintuitive trends. In Namibia, incumbent supporters were more likely to endorse that resources should be spent elsewhere besides on HIV/AIDS in 2003, suggesting that they disagree with the government's aggressive HIV/AIDS policy. Also, in 2003 and 2005 opposition supporters were more likely to approve of the government's HIV/AIDS policies than incumbent supporters. This may also reflect internal divisions within the party as in South Africa, as well as the fact that there is an opposition party that has an even more pro-Geneva Consensus platform than the incumbent SWAPO party, which has led the country since independence. The lead opposition group, the Congress of Democrats (CoD), has pushed for even stronger provisions for care and treatment related to HIV/AIDS. The CoD lobbied in favour of the government's plan to roll-out ART, pushed for larger targets than those in the plan, and wanted to declare AIDS a national emergency, critiquing SWAPO for not going further (Lebeau & Dima, 2006).

Based on these results, refined propositions about the relationship between incumbent party support and HIV/AIDS responses are as follows: overall, for most countries, HIV/AIDS does not appear to be a highly partisan issue, with few differences between

	Approval of Gov handling of AIDS		Put resources towards other issues besides AIDS		AIDS top 3 problem facing country	
	Incumb	Oppos/Unaffil	Incumb	Oppos/Unaffil	Incumb	Oppos/Unaffil
Leaders	+	–	–	+	+	–
Botswana				+		
Kenya						
Uganda				–		
Malawi						
Namibia	–	+				
Zambia				+		
Laggards	+	–	+	–	–	+
South Africa			–	+		
Lesotho					+	–
Mozambique		+	–	+		
Zimbabwe	+	–				

Figure 3.   Summary of results and correspondence with hypothesised relationships, 2005/2006.

incumbent and opposition party supporters in their HIV/AIDS policy preferences or approval of government HIV/AIDS responses. In countries where HIV/AIDS is a partisan issue, it is not predictable which direction that support will go, that is, towards a Geneva Consensus or pan-African response. In some cases, political leaders may genuinely disagree with donors, and take an independent stance from the public. Where the public does demand a stronger state response, such as in South Africa, when facing pressures from core party constituents to adopt a more aggressive Geneva Consensus response, leaders may be forced to capitulate and ease pan-African responses. In other cases, like Namibia, leaders may genuinely agree with donors and ignore the preferences of party faithful who desire less attention to HIV/AIDS. Of course, in autocracies, leaders may be freer to ignore public demands, or alternatively, may be more adept at 'manufacturing consent', for instance, in Zimbabwe where incumbent party supporters as well as the public at large, approve of the government's HIV/AIDS response, however inadequate.

In the post-scale-up period, researchers have begun to question whether too many resources have been devoted to HIV/AIDS, and therefore, the degree to which donor funding is responsive to recipient needs (Esser & Keating-Bench, 2011; Shiffman, 2006) as well as citizen demands (Dionne et al., 2013). What the present analysis suggests is that, overall, African publics are divided over whether more or fewer resources should be put towards HIV/AIDS, and a large share of the population believes that resources should be devoted to other issues (a majority in 6 out of 11 countries by 2005/2006). Public opinion on AIDS as a priority issue has largely followed donor attention – the salience of HIV/AIDS increased with increasing global attention to the issue and has declined over time as HIV/AIDS has been criticised for receiving a disproportionate amount of attention. The levelling off of HIV/AIDS infection rates may have also contributed to a decrease in the sense of urgency to address the epidemic among the public. In some instances, it appears that there has been greater policy congruence between African citizens and donors, but a democratic deficit between African governments and African publics, notably in South Africa and Mozambique, where incumbent supporters exhorted their party to do more to address HIV/AIDS and overall approval of the governments' response was relatively low. In Namibia, incumbent party supporters thought their party was doing too much to address HIV/AIDS.

In these three countries, governments pursued policies that were at odds not only with the public at large, but also with core party supporters, suggesting a democratic deficit. While we might expect autocracies to produce democratic deficits, two of the three countries where we found some evidence of a democratic deficit are considered to be democracies – South Africa and Namibia (Diamond & Plattner, 1999). Another way of viewing the results, however, is that they suggest that at times governments have acted independently of both donor and public wishes. This interpretation would point towards explanations focused on individual leadership characteristics. Namibia's leadership embraced the Geneva Consensus approach in spite of opposition, just as South Africa pursued its pan-African response in the face of general disapproval among ANC supporters. Politicians refusal to pander to public opinion and preference for acting independently is at times viewed as a positive leadership characteristic (Jacobs & Shapiro, 2000).

Limitations

This study has several limitations. The questions used to proxy a pan-African response to the HIV/AIDS epidemic are not ideal and could be picking up other concerns, such as desire to put resources towards meeting basic needs among a majority of respondents who live in dire poverty. In addition, dividing countries into Geneva Consensus versus pan-African is not a straightforward process and is confounded by a number of factors. These include difficulties in separating markers of the domestic response from the response offered by international donors. In addition to country outcomes not reflecting a state's own effort, countries may strategically embrace rhetoric that they would be inclined to disagree with in order to attract donors, especially in very poor states. This effect is somewhat muted in the wealthier Southern African countries, and indeed these countries have adopted clearer independent responses. Finally, the development of political party identity in Africa is known to be quite weak with ethnic, tribal and patrimonial relationships underlying political support more so than a coherent ideology (Giliomee, 1999; Young, 1999). This is reflected in the large percentage of the public reporting themselves as unaffiliated in the analysis.

Conclusions

Across multiple Southern and East African countries, there is widespread endorsement for the idea that resources should be devoted elsewhere besides HIV/AIDS. This sentiment has increased in a number of countries over the period of HIV/AIDS scale-up, but was also quite prevalent prior to ART scale-up in both countries that took the lead and those that dragged their heals in their HIV/AIDS responses. There are, however, observable partisan differences in the attitude that resources should be spent on other issues besides HIV/AIDS, suggesting that political competition has factored into governments' HIV/AIDS responses, though the patterns that emerge are largely contrary to expectation. Namibia, a country that is now an HIV/AIDS policy leader, appears to have scaled up its response in spite of low support by core constituents for more resources being spent on HIV/AIDS. In policy laggards, South Africa and Mozambique, opposition party supporters, rather than incumbent supporters, were more likely to want resources to be spent on other issues besides HIV/AIDS, which is more in line with the government's tepid response. In most countries, including policy laggards, a majority approved of the government's response to HIV/AIDS and incumbent party faithful were more likely to approve of their government's response even accounting for overall support of the regime.

Donors should be cognizant of the domestic political dynamics at play in a country and should seek to better understand the political basis of pan-African HIV/AIDS rhetoric and responses. Rather than simply blaming and shaming HIV/AIDS policy laggards, which may only serve to deepen and reinforce pan-African responses, global health initiatives should seek to understand the domestic political cross-pressures faced by African political regimes. In some sense, the most intriguing finding from this analysis is the case of Namibia, where a government supportive of the Geneva Consensus faced cross-pressures from core supporters to devote fewer resources towards HIV/AIDS. That donors should consider bypassing recalcitrant governments if the public demands a more aggressive Geneva Consensus response is perhaps less objectionable (to some) than the notion that donors might go against the wishes of the public and provide more HIV/AIDS resources than demanded. Should donors respect the wishes of the public and provide fewer HIV/AIDS resources? From a practical perspective, the success of global health interventions ultimately depends on local receptivity (Dionne, 2012). As concern has risen that HIV/AIDS has crowded out other global health priorities (whether true or not) (Grepin, 2012), the saliency of HIV/AIDS has recently fallen as reflected in the public's changing prioritisation of the HIV/AIDS issue over time. Although not changing the overall conclusion that HIV/AIDS is a grave illness afflicting the continent, this disconnection among donor priorities, African leaders' policies, and public preferences raises questions about sources of legitimacy and respect for autonomy in global health as well as in domestic politics.

Notes

1. 'Geneva Consensus' refers to best practice, evidence-based responses to HIV as recommended by the World Health Organization (WHO) and the Joint United Nations Programme on HIV/ AIDS (UNAIDS), two international health institutions located in Geneva, Switzerland (see Gauri & Lieberman, 2006).
2. Here I use the term 'pan-African' to refer to oppositional HIV/AIDS responses adopted by African leaders that explicitly challenge the Western construction of HIV/AIDS with regard to treatment, prevention and behavioural approaches to addressing the epidemic and to explaining its spread. As described more below, this pan-African discourse on HIV/AIDS has taken a variety of forms. Other authors have discussed President Mbeki's use of pan-African rhetoric in crafting South Africa's response to HIV/AIDS and the influence of his notion an African Renaissance in influencing his personal beliefs on the subject (Butler, 2005; Nattrass, 2003).
3. See Inglehart (1997).

References

Adeyemi, Y. (2001). It's not too late to start saving lives in Nigeria. *Journalists Against AIDS (JAAIDS)*, *3*(2). Retrieved from http://thebody.com/content/policy/art13242.html

Batsell, J. (2005). *AIDS, politics, and NGOs in Zimbabwe*. In A. S. Patterson (Ed.), *The African state and the AIDS crisis* (pp. 59–78). Burlington, VT: Ashgate Publishing Company.

Boix, C. (1998). *Political parties, growth and equality*. Cambridge: Cambridge University Press.

Butler, A. (2005). South Africa's HIV/AIDS policy, 1994–2004: How can it be explained? *African Affairs*, *104*(417), 591–614. doi:10.1093/afraf/adi036

Cassidy, R., & Leach, M. (2009). Science, politics and the presidential AIDS 'cure'. *African Affairs*, *433*, 559–580. doi:10.1093/afraf/adp057

Desmond, C., Lieberman, E., Alban, A., & Ekström, A.-M. (2008). Relative response: Ranking country responses to HIV and AIDS. *Health and Human Rights*, *10*(2), 105–119. doi:10.2307/20460106

Diamond, L., & Plattner, M. F. (1999). *Democratization in Africa*. Baltimore, MD: Johns Hopkins University Press.

Dionne, K. Y. (2006). The role of executive time horizons in state responses to AIDS in Africa. *Comparative Political Studies*, *44*, 55–e77. doi:10.1177/0010414010381074

Dionne, K. Y. (2012). Local demand for a global intervention: Policy priorities in the time of AIDS. *World Development*, *40*, 2468–2477. doi:10.1016/j.worlddev.2012.05.016

Dionne, K. Y., Gerland, P., & Watkins, S. (2013). AIDS exceptionalism: Another constituency heard from. *AIDS and Behavior*, *17*, 825–831. doi:10.1007/s10461-011-0098-5

Epstein, H. (2007). *The invisible cure: Africa, the West, and the fight against AIDS*. New York, NY: Farrar, Strauss, Giroux.

Esser, D. E., & Keating-Bench, K. (2011). Does global health funding respond to recipients' needs? Comparing public and private donors' allocations in 2005–2007 Open Access Articles. Paper 2238. http://escholarship.umassmed.edu/oapubs/2238

Fox, A. M., Goldberg, A. B., Gore, R. J., & Bärnighausen, T. (2011). Conceptual and methodological challenges to measuring political commitment to respond to HIV. *Journal of the International AIDS Society*, *14*(Suppl 2), S5. doi:10.1186/1758-2652-14-S2-S5

Gauri, V., & Lieberman, E. (2006). Boundary institutions and HIV/AIDS policy in Brazil and South Africa. *Studies in Comparative International Development*, *41*, 47–73. doi:10.1007/BF02686236

Gettleman, J. (2010, January 3). Americans' role seen in Uganda anti-gay push. *New York Times*. Retrieved November 11, 2013, from http://www.nytimes.com/2010/01/04/world/africa/04uganda.html?_r=0

Grebe, E., & Nattrass, N. (2012). AIDS conspiracy beliefs and unsafe sex in Cape Town. *AIDS and Behavior, 16*, 761–773. doi:10.1007/s10461-011-9958-2

Grepin, K. A. (2012). HIV donor funding has both boosted and curbed the delivery of different non-HIV health services in sub-Saharan Africa. *Health Affairs, 31*, 1406–1414. doi:10.1377/hlthaff.2012.0279

Giliomee, H. (1999). South Africa's emerging dominant-party regime. In L. Diamond & M. F. Plattner (Eds.), *Democratization in Africa* (pp. 140–157). Baltimore, MD: John's Hopkins University Press.

Goldberg, A., Fox, A. M., Gore, R., & Baernighausen, T. (2012). Indicators of political commitment to respond to HIV. *Sexually Transmitted Infections, 88*, e1. doi:10.1136/sextrans-2011-050221

Hetling, A., McDermott, M. L., & Mapps, M. (2008). Symbolism versus policy learning: Public opinion of the 1996 U.S. welfare reforms. *American Politics Research, 36*, 335–357. doi:10.1177/1532673X07313736

Huber, J. D., & Powell, G. B. (1994). Congruence between citizens and policymakers in two visions of liberal democracy. *World Politics, 46*, 291–326. doi:10.2307/2950684

Inglehart, R. (1997). *Modernization and postmodernization: Cultural, economic and political change in 43 societies*. Princeton, NJ: Princeton University Press.

Jacobs, L., & Shapiro, R. Y. (2000). *Politicians don't pander: Political manipulation and the loss of democratic responsiveness*. Chicago and London: University of Chicago Press.

Lebeau, D., & Dima, E. (2006). Multiparty democracy and elections in Namibia. *EISA Research Report, 13*, 1–109. Retrieved from http://www.content.eisa.org.za/pdf/rr13.pdf

Lieberman, E. S. (2007). Ethnic politics, risk, and policy-making: A cross-national statistical analysis of government responses to HIV/AIDS. *Comparative Political Studies, 40*, 1407–1432. doi:10.1177/0010414007306862

Lieberman, E. S. (2009). *Boundaries of contagion: How ethnic politics have shaped government responses to AIDS*. Princeton, NJ: Princeton University Press.

Mbali, M. (2013). *South African AIDS activism and global health politics*. London: Palgrave McMillan.

Mwadi, A. (1995). The power to silence us. In E. Reid (Ed.), *HIV and AIDS: The global inter-connection*. New York, NY: Kumarian Press.

Nathanson, C. (2007). *Disease prevention as social change: The state, society and public health in the United States, France, Great Britain and Canada*. New York, NY: Russell Sage Foundation.

Nattrass, N. (2003). *The moral economy of AIDS in South Africa*. Cambridge: Cambridge University Press.

Nattrass, N. (2008). Are country reputations for good and bad leadership on AIDS deserved? An exploratory quantitative analysis. *Journal of Public Health, 30*, 398–406. doi:10.1093/pubmed/fdn075

Nattrass, N. (2013). Understanding the origins and prevalence of AIDS conspiracy beliefs in the United States and South Africa. *Sociology of Health and Illness, 31*(1), 113–129. Published online 25 April. doi:10.1111/j.1467-9566.2012.01480 page 1–17. Forthcoming in the printed edition, Vol. 31, no. 1: 113–129.

Parkhurst, J. O., & Lush, L. (2004). The political environment of HIV: Lessons from a comparison of Uganda and South Africa. *Social Science and Medicine, 59*, 1913–1924. doi:10.1016/j.socscimed.2004.02.026

Patterson, A. (2006). *The politics of AIDS in Africa*. Boulder, CO: Lynne Reinner.

Phillips, O. (1997). Zimbabwean law and the production of a white man's disease. *Social and Legal Studies, 6*, 471–491. doi:10.1177/096466399700600402

Phillips, O. C. (2004). (Dis)Continuities of custom in Zimbabwe and South Africa: The implications for gendered and sexual rights. *Health and Human Rights: An International Journal, 7*(2), 82–113.

Price-Smith, A. T. (2007). Vicious Circle – HIV/AIDS, state capacity, and national security: Lessons from Zimbabwe, 1990–2005. *Global Health Governance, 1*(1), 1–24.

Przeworski, A., Stokes, S., & Manin, M. (1999). *Democracy, accountability and representation*. New York, NY: Cambridge University Press.

Putzel, J. (2004). The politics of action on AIDS: A case study of Uganda. *Public Administration and Development, 24*(1), 19–30. doi:10.1002/pad.306

Putzel, J. (2006). A history of state action: The politics of AIDS in Uganda and Senegal. In P. Denis & C. Becker (Eds.), *The HIV/AIDS epidemic in sub-Saharan Africa in a historical perspective* (pp. 171–184). Retrieved from http://rds.refer.sn/IMG/pdf/AIDSHISTORYALL.pdf

Schneider, H. (2002). On the fault-line: The politics of AIDS policy in contemporary South Africa. *African Studies, 61*, 145–167. doi:10.1080/00020180220140118

Schoepf, B. G. (1991). Ethical, methodological and political issues of AIDS research in Central Africa. *Social Science and Medicine, 33*(7), 749–763. doi:10.1016/0277-9536(91)90374-L

Shiffman, J. (2006). HIV/AIDS and the rest of the global health agenda. *Bulletin of the World Health Organization, 84*(12), 923. doi:10.2471/BLT.06.036681

Stokes, S. (1999). What do policy switches tell us about democracy? In A. Przeworski, S. Stokes, & M. Manin (Eds.), *Democracy, accountability & representation* (pp. 98–131). London: Cambridge University Press.

Treichler, P. (1999). *How to have theory in an epidemic: Cultural chronicles of AIDS*. Durham and London: Duke University Press.

Washington, H. A. (2007, July 31). Why Africa fears Western medicine. *New York Times Op-Ed*.

Wedeen, L. (1999). *Ambiguities of domination: Politics, rhetoric, and symbols in contemporary Syria*. Chicago, IL: University of Chicago Press.

Whiteside, A., Mattes, R., Willan, S., & Manning, R. (2004). What people really believe about HIV/AIDS in Southern Africa. In N. K. Poku & A. Whiteside (Eds.), *The political economy of AIDS in Africa* (pp. 127–151). Aldershot: Ashgate.

Youde, J. (2007). Ideology's role in AIDS policies in Uganda and South Africa. *Global Health Governance, 1*, 1–16.

Youde, J. (2009). Government AIDS policies and public opinion in Africa. *Politikon: South African Journal of Political Studies, 36*, 219–235. doi:10.1080/02589340903240161

Youde, J. (2012). Public opinion and support for government AIDS policies in sub-Saharan Africa. *Social Science and Medicine, 74*(1), 52–57. doi:10.1016/j.socscimed.2011.10.008

Young, C. (1999). Africa: An interim balance sheet. In L. Diamond & M. F. Plattner (Eds.), *Democratization in Africa* (pp. 63–83). Baltimore, MD: Johns Hopkins University Press.

Index

Note: Page numbers in **bold** type refer to figures
Page numbers in *italic* type refer to tables
Page numbers followed by 'n' refer to notes